Working With
African American
Males

Working With African American Males

A Guide to Practice

Larry E. Davis
Editor

SAGE Publications
International Educational and Professional Publisher
Thousand Oaks   London   New Delhi

Copyright © 1999 by Sage Publications, Inc.

For information:

SAGE Publications, Inc.
2455 Teller Road
Thousand Oaks, California 91320
E-mail: order@sagepub.com

SAGE Publications Ltd.
6 Bonhill Street
London EC2A 4PU
United Kingdom

SAGE Publications India Pvt. Ltd.
M-32 Market
Greater Kailash I
New Delhi 110 048 India

Printed in the United States of America

Library of Congress Cataloging-in-Publication Data

Main entry under title:
    Working with African American Males: A guide to practice/
edited by Larry E. Davis
        p. cm.
    Includes bibliographical references and index.
    ISBN 0-7619-0471-9 (cloth: acid-free paper)
    ISBN 0-7619-0472-7 (pbk.: acid-free paper)
    1. Afro-American men—Health and hygiene. 2. Afro-American men—
Mental health. 3. Afro-American men—Family relationships. 4. Afro-
American men—Social conditions. I. Davis, Larry E.
    RA448.5 .N4W67   1999
    613.0423'08996073—ddc21   98-40277

This book is printed on acid-free paper.

99 00 01 02 03 04 05 7 6 5 4 3 2 1

Acquisition Editor:	Jim Nageotte
Editorial Assistant:	Heidi Van Middlesworth
Production Editor:	Wendy Westgate
Editorial Assistant:	Nevair Kabakian
Typesetter:	Lynn Miyata
Cover Designer:	Ravi Balasuriya
Indexer:	Molly Hall

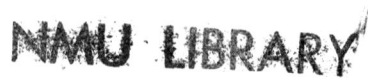

Contents

Acknowledgment

I owe a special thanks to the African and Afro-American Studies department for providing me with a nurturing environment in which to edit this book. My colleague and friend Professor Gerald Early, director of the program, and his staff, Adele Tuchler and Raye Riggins, were ever present with encouraging words when my efforts got bogged down with the "inevitable delays" of editing a volume such as this. I also want to acknowledge Rebecka Rutledge, a doctoral student, and Rayvon Fouche, a postdoctoral student, both of whom were associated with the African and Afro-American Studies department during the editing of this book. Thanks for your wonderful and sometimes very late-night discussions on gender and postmodernism.

Each of the many contributors to this volume deserves a kind word for making and remaking the many requested changes to their manuscripts. Their willingness to fine-tune their individual chapters has resulted in a much improved final product. Thanks are also due to both Professor Charles Garvin of the University of Michigan School of Social Work and to Jim Nageotte of Sage Publications for their thoughtful guidance and editorial assistance.

As those of you who have edited lengthy manuscripts or books are aware, without the support of committed research assistance, projects of this type would take forever to complete—so I say thanks to Karen Sutton and Raqiyyah Abdal-Aziz for their loyalty and for seeing this project through from beginning to end. And also to Rudolph Clay, I say thank you for being a librarian who is always there when you need him.

Finally, I owe a great deal of thanks to faculty and staff at the George Warren Brown School of Social Work. First, let me thank my dear friend the dean, Dr. Shanti Khinduka, for doing what he has always done—given me all that I needed to have a chance at success. Others have also been unwavering in their support: Nancy Vosler, David Cronin, and Michael Powell. Last, when during the course of editing this volume I became ill, my colleague Michael Sherraden stepped in to keep the momentum of the project going until I could return—thank you, your efforts were very much appreciated.

Introduction

African American males are arguably the most visible group of males in America. Unfortunately, however, only that which is negative about them tends to be remembered. Moreover, many in America have only recently acknowledged African American males as even being men, as it has become less popular and advantageous to be one. Commonly, African American men are seen as caricatures of super athletes and heartless villains and rarely as real men who are fathers, sons, husbands, and friends. Too infrequently does our society perceive African American males as being like most men: average individuals who struggle in their personal lives with social, physical, and economic problems. Even less frequently are they seen as individuals who are deservingly in need of help. But no African American male is exempt from an inexcusably high risk of being murdered, imprisoned, unemployed, uneducated, and experiencing on a daily basis both institutional and personal forms of racism. Despite some substantial achievements in the 1960s and 1970s, African American men enter the 21st century facing what may be their most difficult times since slavery. For them, there are few safe havens: The larger white community is both afraid of and hostile toward them, and the African American community is often a violent and dangerous place.

Most notably through the works of Na'im Akbar, Phillip Bowman, Lary Gary, Haki Mahatubuti, Robert Staples, Richard Majors, John McAdoo, Robert Taylor, and Jewelle Taylor Gibbs, we now have a wealth of information on the "at risk" status of African American males. Few Americans are unaware that African American males experience lots of jail time, little job time, troubled school time, sporadic family time, and truncated lifetimes. Hence, what is now needed are greater efforts to use what is known to eradicate the exigencies experienced by African American males. It is time to use the considerable wealth of collective wisdom at our disposal. As a researcher, I do not advocate that we cease to employ research as a tool in this effort, but I do believe that researchers must also recognize that we will never explain away "all the variance." We will never have all the answers or possess all the resources we would like. Still, we must attempt to do what we can with what we have, in the ways available to each of us. To a greater extent than we have in the past, we must attempt today to make useful that which is known.

It was in this vein that I asked the authors of this volume to write their chapters. They were asked to provide the reader with both their knowledge and wisdom about a given topic. They were asked to think beyond what they, and others, had previously written. The contributors to this volume have eagerly and with great success done this. The interventions proposed in this volume are, for the most part, direct; that is, they outline working with African American males individually, in families, or as part of a community or group. All, however, have recognized the need to pay attention to social, economic, and political factors that impinge on the lives and well-being of all African American males. The result is a practical, nonpolemic, "hands-on" book.

Although this book covers broad areas of concern, it was impossible to cover each and every aspect of African American male life that warrants attention. Certainly, different areas might also have been included, and even those addressed here might have been addressed differently. In addition to providing a diversity of topics, the book also focuses on diverse groups of African American males—for example, young boys, adolescents, gay men, and older men. Each of the groups selected could easily have had an entire volume devoted to it. Perhaps future efforts of this type may find it beneficial to focus more in-depth on either a single problem or a select subgroup of African American males. Surely these writers, with different intellectual priorities, will vary in their approaches, but we hope they will sustain this unique race- gender practice focus.

This volume is an interdisciplinary effort and benefits from the perspective of educators, anthropologists, sociologists, economists, psychologists, social workers, and psychiatrists. The result is a broader vision of solutions to problems confronting African American males than could be obtained from any single profession alone. It was my original aspiration that the diversity of academic disciplines included in this volume would contribute to its reaching a more diffuse audience than a book written by individuals from a single discipline. Ideas that might otherwise be confined to one group have the potential here to be read by "professional outsiders," who may then, in turn, employ what are for them new and alternative practice interventions. Yet, despite the professional diversity among these authors, they share considerable conceptual ground. Throughout the collection of chapters, a number of key themes prevail, such as the importance of African American culture, the church, the economic environment, and client reliance on informal helping networks. Common also among these chapters is the focus on the strengths and resiliency of African American males themselves.

This practice guide is divided into six sections, addressing six different areas of concern. Each section is preceded by a brief introduction, which provides a backdrop for the chapters that follow. Part I focuses on the delivery of services intended to enhance the mental health of various groups of African American males. Although these chapters have, in general, a common goal, the practice issues and dynamics addressed vary considerably, as do the populations for whom interventions are proposed. Moreover, the traditional one-on-one clinical practice scenarios of working with clients, are insightfully addressed from varying practice traditions.

Part II is devoted to health. The quality of health among African American males is among the lowest of any group in our society, In response to this situation, Part II provides guidelines for working with African American males who have experienced or are at risk of experiencing social and emotional difficulties as a consequence of specific health problems, for example, cancer and diabetes. This section also provides suggested interventions to prevent violence among young African American males and to reduce their engagement in risky behaviors such as drug and alcohol use. Hence, this section has a twofold purpose: first, to assist in the resolution of emotional problems that are a consequence of health difficulties, and second, to reduce or eliminate behaviors engaged in by African American males that are injurious to them. Each of the chapters in this section provides both causative theory and accompanying intervention strategies.

Part III addresses education. Although their overall high school graduation rate continues to improve, African American youth remain at risk of being educationally unprepared for tomorrow's workforce. Hence, the goal of this section is to provide guidelines for getting African American boys educationally "on track" and increasing the probability that they will stay there. Key among the strategies offered to enhance the education of African American youth are the suggestions that we better understand the dynamics of the educational process for these youth, keep better track of the most mobile students, enhance the way they perceive and respond to each other, and make the school itself a safer place to be.

Part IV addresses familial relations. As is true for most individuals, the quality of life for African American males is significantly affected by the quality of their interactions within their families. Hence, this section is devoted to the enhancement of familial relationships among African American males. First, it provides practitioners with strategies to work more effectively with African American men in family practice. However, in addition to the traditional concerns of family practitioners, this section also gives attention to working with those fathers who are, or have been, incarcerated. Moreover, this section informs practitioners on how to work with teen fathers to enhance and promote their roles as providers and protectors, Last, attention is devoted to treatment strategies designed to reduce domestic violence and enhance positive nonviolent interactions between African American males and their partners.

Part V is devoted to criminal justice. The number of young African American males who find themselves entangled in the criminal justice system is staggering. The resulting human, social, and economic cost to our society is also staggering. Indeed, this section addresses a concern that has immediate implications not only for African American youths but for all who are concerned with social order and safety. The chapters in this section address efforts to reduce crime and delinquency among African American youths. These chapters make programmatic suggestions that practitioners can employ to reduce delinquency, enhance prosocial behaviors, and improve the social environments of all African American youths.

Part VI is devoted to economic enhancement of African American males. This book comes at a time when African American males are increasingly challenged in their efforts to fulfill their roles as providers. Important strategies are provided to enhance their skills and readiness to interface with the workplace. Although it is true that many African American males are "doing well," significant numbers are being lost to an "invisible underclass." Hence, among its other contributions, this section provides the practitioner with insights as to how and why having assets—that is, investments in our society—would serve to enhance the overall social functioning of African American males.

Who should use this book, African Americans, whites, other nonwhites, women, high-, middle-, or low-income practitioners? The answer is, of course, all of the above. Again, the goal is to assist those who wish to improve or expand their skills with this population. Still, I would be less than candid if I did not say that implicit in many of these chapters is the underlying assumption that the reader needs to increase his or her practice familiarity with African American males. This need was a major motivation for the initiation of this project. No other group of men is as likely to be provided services by those who "differ" from themselves. Rarely can they expect to receive health, mental health, educational, or employment services from those of the same race, gender, or class. On the contrary, they are often helped by those who have had little exposure to them and even less practice experience with them. This book cannot, of course, improve the intervention efforts of those who do not value African American men, nor of those who do not truly wish to provide services to them. But for those whose major obstacle to the delivery of satisfactory services to African American males is the absence of specific information, skills, and insights, this volume will help their practice efforts substantially.

To my three sons
Amani, Naeem, and Keanu

May they grow up to be good men
and good at being men.

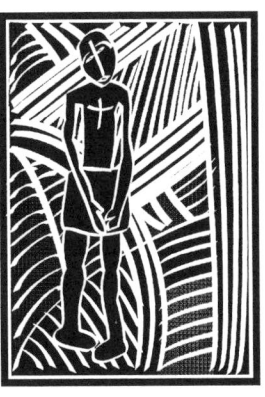

PART I

Mental
Health

The mental lives of African American men continue to be complicated, made difficult not only by everyday events but also by the strains of race and class. Especially difficult during these times is the normal social, emotional, and psychological development of young men. Contributing to their difficulties are societal changes that have taken place regarding the expectations of what is appropriate male behavior. Many African American males, in the effort to improve themselves, now wonder if they should talk more or listen more, be kinder or stronger, attempt to make more money or focus instead on their emotions? Make no mistake, seemingly contradictory expectations such as these have been suggested for virtually all men, without regard for their race.

So what makes African American men unique? Could their expectations be different from those of most men, or unrealistic? Actually, there are no data to suggest that either is the case. No, it is not that their aspirations differ significantly from those of other men, but rather it is their inability to realize their aspirations which most profoundly effects them and makes them different (Bowman, 1989; Gibbs, 1988; Staples, 1991). They are required to develop in ways that are deemed "normal," but they are frequently required to do so in environments that are hostile to their efforts (Chestang, 1976). Most of all, it is their perception of limited life opportunities that has most influenced their perception of what it takes to be a man. Young African American men engaging in "tough guy" behaviors intended to compensate for both real and perceived threats to their manhood are common fixtures in most urban areas. These behaviors, captured by such terms as *cool pose*

(Majors & Billson, 1989) and *hypermasculinity* (Wilson, 1991), often suggest superfluous risk taking and an undue readiness to engage in violence. Even among those African American males who have managed to satisfy traditional definitions of manhood, via economic and professional success, the stresses associated with this process often produce incapacitating rage, fear, and paranoia (Cose, 1993; Grier & Cobbs, 1968).

Unfortunately, many who deliver mental health services know little about African American men, and many others are inclined to perceive them as a culturally homogeneous group. But, like other groups of men, they constitute a diverse and varied population. Specifically, it has been suggested that older African American males represent a forgotten minority within a minority. Similarly, the mental health of African American male subgroups such as the elderly, gays, and preadolescents are sometimes completely overlooked. Clearly, mental health practitioners must expect to treat a more diverse group of African American males. They must also be prepared to treat these diverse groups with appropriate clinical frames of reference.

In part, because African American males are known to underuse mental health services (Broman, 1987; Neighbors, 1985), this section has three goals: first, to improve the cultural sensitivity of mental health services delivered to African American males; second, to enhance the clinical skills and thereby the willingness of practitioners to work with this group of men; and third, to encourage greater diversity among the types of African American males who are seen by mental health practitioners.

CHAPTER 1

Therapeutic Support Groups for African American Men

ANDERSON J. FRANKLIN

Like most men (Levant & Pollack, 1995; Meth & Passick, 1990), most African American men do not talk about personal issues or share vulnerabilities with each other (Ridley, 1984). Black men, however, will talk about how their skin color, physique, and physical and psychological presence determines their acceptance, both within the African American community and in society as a whole. Many African American men believe that succeeding is difficult, in spite of their competency and experience. Therefore, therapeutic support groups for African American men can serve as a special outlet for discussing these common feelings and thoughts about being black and male in today's world.

Black men might be motivated to join a support group as an opportunity to sort out the presumptions about how they are perceived and treated as men of African descent. Another way to enhance the appeal of the group is by showing the utility of countering the personal impact of perceived racist treatment on fulfillment of personal life goals. In addition, emphasizing the informality of the group process presents the interaction as approximating typical conversational exchanges among African American men.

Black men are wary of "genuine talk," which exposes uncharacteristic emotions, immobility, struggle with weaknesses, or lack of knowledge. There is almost no discussion of emotional issues among black men because they see such talk as a weakness that runs counter to the image of strength they seek to project.

MALE GENDER ISSUES

Unlike other men, African American men must deal with thoughts, emotions, and behaviors that are triggered by what their skin color and physique uniquely mean to others. Negative responses to these visible attributes are the source of many conflicts, forming barriers to success for black males and triggering intrapsychic consequences. Complicating these external circumstances are intrasocietal expectations about gender role fulfillment that collude in the creation of racial gender stereotypes. Masculinity is no longer a simple matter. It is now construed more as a *gender role strain paradigm* featuring contradictions and inconsistencies, considerable violation of gender roles, overconformity out of perceived failure, and imposition through socialization of stereotypes and norms, with the threat of severe consequences for deviating from expectations (Pleck, 1995).

For African American men, masculinity can also be conceived within the gender role strain paradigm, wherein racism serves as a unifying theme (Jones, 1997). In this way, gender role expectations are derived from adaptive responses to life circumstances shaped by the prejudice and discrimination experienced by African American men. This might be seen in, for example, the cool, unflappable posture of black youth described by Majors and Billson (1992).

Fulfillment of male roles is especially complex for African American men when the conceptions of masculinity among black men conflict with those of the larger society.

These issues are enormously powerful in the lives of black males; the emotional force and insidiousness of race-coded circumstances can easily overwhelm the goal of taking personal responsibility for one's life. This is where the therapy group serves its most important purpose. It can assist individual black men in understanding and managing a balance between external social factors, such as racism, and internal psychological factors, such as disillusionment and self-doubt.

MANAGING INVISIBILITY

The group can also help to manage the stress of being treated like an invisible man and not a person of worth (Franklin, 1993, 1997). When white people treat black men as if they are invisible during interpersonal encounters, this manifests historical attitudes and conceptions about African American men wherein the black male is ignored and unacknowledged. Many African

American men believe it is this attitude and form of treatment that compromises their opportunities and contributes to their marginal position in so many arenas of life (e.g., education, employment, positions of power). Black men often believe that when they succeed and their positive contribution is acknowledged, it is at the expense of their ethnicity—their race is either minimized or they are singled out as an exception. When their behavior is seen as negative, however, their race is highlighted to perpetuate a caricature.

Because skin color and maleness are so emotionally loaded for black males, a paradox has been created. When people ignore an individual's genuine personality, talents, and contributions, that person feels unacknowledged, in effect, "invisible." But, on the other hand, when black men appear to pose a threat or challenge, their physical and psychological presence is undeniable.

Therefore, the visibility of black men is experienced as a dilemma, inconsistent and depending on societal stereotypes, assumptions, and priorities of racism. Managing the stress from this interpersonal dilemma can lead to considerable confusion and disillusionment among black men.

PERSONAL ISSUES

A support group for black men can also allow time to sort out other personal issues, such as family relationships and friendships, and to reevaluate individual life goals—subjects that are rarely discussed by black men beyond a superficial level. Using each other as a genuine resource and support is difficult for many black men because of gender expectations to be a "man" and racial expectations to be a "brother." Making others believe that everything in your life is always OK or under control and that you are successfully managing pressure is a significant male value.

At substantial psychological cost, black men struggle to hold true to gender and racial expectations. Doing so creates a personal dilemma contributing to the manner in which responsibilities and commitments are fulfilled.

ESTABLISHING THE GROUP

Starting

There are many African American men and women who privately acknowledge the need for a support group for black men but do not know how to get men to participate. In my experience, group members came from several sources. Some patients in individual or couples treatment were candidates for this type of group experience. Referrals from other practitioners were also solicited. Spousal or partner referrals played a significant part because many black women, sensitive to the struggles of their men, saw the group as relevant for them. An important recruitment strategy was contacting black professional organizations and colleagues, informing them of the focus and purpose of the group. Likewise, making formal presentations to agencies and conferences broadened the network referrals. Using a male peer network of friends and acquaintances as advocates was also very useful.

Although the following describes the start of a therapeutic support group for African American men within a private practice, some of the considerations are relevant to forming groups for black men in public agency-based programs.

In spite of the numerous legitimate issues for black men to discuss in a group, resistance to participating is high because of the stigma of therapy among African American men. I decided that interest and participation from black men would best be achieved by forming the group around this perspective: Because society's treatment of and response to the black male's race and gender are a major factor in life success, it is important to be able to handle these complex issues successfully.

The group was designed to get black men to pierce superficiality and start genuinely talking and sharing with each other. An appeal was deliberately made to affirm the need for a new view of fraternal values. The purpose of this group was declared as an effort to empower black men to achieve their personal life goals and to remove personal barriers blocking that objective.

Screening Candidates

Candidates for the group were met in several individual consultation sessions to determine their suitability for membership. Each was encouraged to discuss the following issues: How have his experiences as a black man in society affected him? What does he see as specific issues for black men? Has his race and gender affected his ability to achieve, and, if so, could he offer personal life examples? Why does he want to join such a group, and what does he expect to gain from it? Prospective members were also asked whether they had any prior experience with individual or group therapy.

Substance Abuse

People at risk for or with chronic mental disorders were excluded. Substance abuse history and active use were carefully evaluated to determine whether the use was so severe as to be disqualifying for group membership, in which case a referral to a treatment program was made. Past users in recovery were eligible.

Confidentiality and Commitment

The final topics explored in the consultation sessions centered around the importance of confidentiality and commitment. Because trust is seen as a sensitive issue among black men, discussing the vital role that confidentiality plays in permitting uninhibited participation from each member was carefully reviewed, and assurances about confidentiality were made.

In a discussion of commitment, candidates had to understand that each member was making a commitment to attend group meetings regularly, viewed his commitment to the group as a barometer of his behavior in life, and would hold others accountable.

Establishing Ground Rules and Educating About the Group Process

Ground rules become important in establishing a group experience for black men, because trust, power, and control are fundamental gender and racial issues in the lives of black men. Agreements were developed about sharing information and whether any disclosures about the group process could be made, even to loved ones and significant others. This also addressed the often verbalized community wisdom that "we don't air our dirty linen in public." When a new member joined the group, the men collectively reaffirmed the need for confidentiality and were given a chance to discuss their understanding, perceptions, expectations, and misgivings about how their personal life experiences would be protected by group members.

Commitment was also discussed, with the initial meetings focused on members' intentions to honor the pledge to attend regularly and on time. These early meetings were also dedicated to talking about the group process and gaining a collective understanding about the group purpose, goals, and personal interpretations of them.

The men were asked to share particular apprehensions about making disclosures, and the difference between sharing facts and personal vulnerabilities was delineated. It was carefully explained that the group had to have time to coalesce and form a bond before serious issues could be confronted. This therapist-led discussion was important to maintain reasonable levels of expectation about group process and outcomes. Also discussed was integrity and how it determined what each individual would get out of the process.

It was important to have a full discussion of these areas because most members had never been involved in a group. This education process also lessened the mystique about therapy as "mind reading," or a disarming process that exposes and makes you vulnerable. For black men, not only is this a great gender taboo, but it also puts at risk their survival skills within a racist society.

Group Leader and Orientation

The group leader was an African American man whose style was informal, recognizing the effectiveness of informality with black men, particularly in facilitating early stages of member participation and group cohesion (Davis, 1984; A. Sutton, 1996). In addition to guiding the group process, the therapist used an integrative psychotherapeutic approach.

An integrative approach to psychotherapy draws on different modalities considered most effective for presenting issues in treatment (Stricker & Gold, 1993). For example, cognitive behavioral techniques were employed when the group focused on restructuring interpersonal skills about trust, communication, and anger and stress management. There were times, however, when group sessions followed a more psychodynamic approach, particularly when exploring such issues as sources of anger, self-esteem, immobility in careers, and relationship commitment. Therefore, a particular learned skill of the therapist was relying on clinical judgment, often consistent with conventions of treatment modalities, for both active and passive interventions.

Being an African American man made it easier for the therapist to join with the group, and it enhanced the group process. Particularly useful was his knowledge and use of black slang and idiomatic expressions; he was also mindful of how intentions can be masked in what is commonly known among African Americans as "getting over" behavior (Hecht, Collier, & Ribeau, 1993).

However, the possible advantage provided by matching race and gender does not preclude group leaders of different personal or racial attributes from working with black men in groups. Genuineness, commitment, and personal comfort along with professional skill are essential group leader attributes that also contribute to working effectively with black men.

Composition of the Group

Some gender and racial issues were represented in the group, composed of five middle-class African American men, all employed in white collar/

professional positions, all but one college educated, and ranging in age from 25 to 45. Two were married, two were never married, and one was divorced and single. This group had been meeting for more than a year. Although middle class by current income status, like many in their position, they were the first generation to be college educated, coming from families and childhoods of limited financial means. They contended with an extended family struggling to survive. A prominent theme in the lives of these men and many other African Americans who have recently achieved middle-class income status is adjusting to and managing the expectations of family and friends, given their presumed success.

Length of the Group

Leading therapeutic support groups for African American men has been a major part of the author's career. Therefore, the length of these groups varies, in part depending on how longevity is evaluated. Members may join an ongoing group, with selective admission of new members to maintain a critical core of six. Consequently, members have participated from 6 months to 3 years. In several instances, a core of four members have remained for 3 years. On rare occasions, past group members have returned to join a different group.

In addition, new members are assisted in their first session, when current members revisit the introductory group phase. The group pauses in its discussion of current issues while each member again shares his initial purpose in joining the group, personal commitment to the group, and his understanding and valuation of group rules. After current members share their views, the group leader invites the new member to share his reasons for joining, his commitment to the group, his understanding of the rules, and any further information about himself he chooses to reveal.

ISSUES FOR BLACK MEN

The kinds of issues black men bring into a group process vary in their context but are consistent in subject and psychodynamic themes. Some of the primary areas of concern are the absence or inaccessibility of fathers, relationships with women, fulfillment of commitments, and achievement of personal goals.

Father absence or inaccessibility becomes a significant topic as the men struggle with how their fathers interacted with them and and how that influenced their childhood and adult development. Some fathers who had been physically present in the home were emotionally inaccessible and offered little active guidance on how to manage emotions. The men feel that the way their fathers modeled how to be a man and handle responsibilities is not a pattern they can follow now as adults. There is much discussion about preparedness for manhood in a society that treats black males within a legacy of stereotypes, malevolence, and discrimination.

These discussions create particular pitfalls for therapists, and black therapists especially, because African American men are inclined to overly politicize and externalize blame for their personal circumstances, then look to each other, and the black therapist, for validation of their opinions. Although the therapist must be aware of the legitimacy of such views, the group process in helping African American men must continue to explore personal responsibility for individual circumstances.

Anger toward fathers is abated by their own hardships as black men and their ability to fulfill male role expectations for their partners, spouses, and/or children. Acknowledging their own realities tempers their discontent with their own fathers' absence or inaccessibility. The discussion became more consistent with Bowman's (1992) research conclusions that structural inequalities existing for black men in employment opportunities create a unique strain on their role as providers.

Job instability has nurtured distrust of black men as providers in black male and female relationships. This situation is at the heart of many black men's beliefs about themselves as men who are committed to secure and protect their family in spite of the barriers of racism. Moreover, when role expectations are unfulfilled, the integrity of the male-female relationship unravels; in some cases, the female partner becomes the more effective head of household. This often creates a racial and gender identity crisis for the black man. It is a crisis created by conceptions about how trust, power, and control are to be manifested and negotiated between partners, as well as what constitutes respect and the experience of dignity.

One of the efforts of the therapist is to help the men connect their concerns about employment with their complaints about how they are viewed by black women. The loss of mutuality and respect in a relationship can breed conflict. Not being the providers they want to be, not fulfilling the expectations of their partners and society as a whole, quickly becomes disillusioning to black men and their partners. In their efforts to overcome the barriers presented by racism, and the belief that it determines their circumstances, black men can lose sight of how personal responsibility plays an intricate part in life outcomes.

LEADING PHASES OF THE GROUP

The group process has an initial, middle, and mature phase. In the initial phase, there are great expectations along with apprehensions. The expectations for a group are consistent with the belief that these sessions offer a unique opportunity for black men to discuss intimately their feelings about everyday hassles of being black men. Furthermore, the men accept this challenge with confidence derived from their belief that the therapist is a black male professional who can identify with their life circumstances and bring his expertise and training to the process.

In one special group intervention, the therapist had to build on these expectations. The therapist's selective sharing of self helped alleviate initial apprehension among the men. This was accomplished while framing and discussing the reason for the group. The therapist talked about his own awareness of how black males are treated, sharing his own understanding and giving personal anecdotes. This was then combined with his professional knowledge and experiences.

In these early sessions, the men were also invited to share their views of how black men are treated and how they believed these views were relevant to the special focus of the group. In these initial sessions, the group leader's intent was to keep discussion on the common, less personally vulnerable issues. This objective keeps the process closer to more familiar conversational topics among black men, thus helping to reduce apprehension caused by misguided beliefs about groups and therapy. The process also allows the men to feel each other out, using their usual interpersonal style of communication. It also allows the therapist to witness these personal styles and learn something further about the men. Keeping the discussion going by sharing anecdotes and subsequently surface feelings about competency as a black man builds the prerequisite comfort level among the men, along with group cohesion.

In the middle phase, the focus on everyday life as a black man is still very salient as a catalyst for the group process. The group leader encourages the men to verbalize their frustrations more and to speak about how they feel during encounters they experience and how they would solve the unique circumstances of their life.

In the mature phase of the group process, most major pretenses, along with the communication games between the men, have subsided, making possible more personal disclosures about vulnerabilities. Trust has developed to the point where greater confidence and reliance on the advice and personal support of each other is apparent. A major contributor to achieving this level of group intimacy is the men's commitment to come regularly to sessions over an extended period of time.

The mature phase allows for more of the traditional form of group therapy interventions. This is in part because the men are at a point where they can begin confronting vulnerabilities and personal responsibility for their behavior. Likewise, the group begins to achieve a level of consistent interpersonal integrity; what the men share reinforces self-understanding and provides the catharsis from their input consistent with group outcomes (Yalom, 1995). Managing the unique gender and racial stress is better understood, with better perspective about the individual's control over larger societal issues in contrast to personal responsibility in spite of them.

CONCLUSION

Therapeutic support groups for African American men can provide them with an opportunity to change conventional ways of relating to each other. Thus, the need to encourage a different kind of fraternal support built on better ways of using each other and the community to change their life circumstances becomes ever more urgent.

By framing the support groups as a forum for discussing life as black men, as well as appealing to the need to restructure the way African American men communicate with each other, their typical resistance to therapy-like situations can be reduced. Careful attention, however, must be given to the selection of group members to increase the chances of success in keeping participants and making the group work.

This particular objective is also important for establishing that such groups can exist and be seen as beneficial. It is crucial to communicate this potential among the larger audience of African American men. For example, after some time in the group, members report as much disbelief as curiosity among friends and acquaintances about their participation in a men's group. It is not uncommon for their male friends to confide that they would like to be in such a group while at the same time admitting they wouldn't know how to approach such an opportunity if available.

CHAPTER 2

Group Work With Sexually Abused African American Boys

SHIRLEY SALMON-DAVIS
LARRY E. DAVIS

A frican American boys who have been sexually abused have been under-studied, underreported, and underresponded to (Finkelhor, 1986; Pierce & Pierce, 1985; Russell, 1983; Wyatt, 1985). This comes as no surprise to many, as male sexual abuse generally has received scant attention. Fortunately, this is less true today than in the past (Bolton, Morris, & MacEachron, 1989; M. Hunter, 1990; Mendel, 1995; Peters, Wyatt, & Finkelhor, 1986; Urquiza & Capra, 1990; Violato & Genius, 1993). Boys who are victims of sexual abuse have been found to experience a large range of difficulties: guilt, depression, low self-esteem, sleep disturbances, social withdrawal, behavioral problems, and emotional disturbances (Rogers & Terry, 1984; Sebold, 1987). All instances of child sexual abuse, whether perpetrated against African Americans or other racial groups, are harmful and negatively affect these youths. The intent of this chapter is to provide the reader with guidelines to work effectively in groups with sexually abused 9- to 13-year-old African American boys.

What is sexual abuse? We define child sexual abuse, whether by consent or force, as genital exposure, fondling, masturbation, cunnilingus, fellatio, and vaginal or anal intercourse between a child and a person of any age. It is unknown exactly how many African American boys are sexually abused in any given year. However, given that African Americans are about 12% of the population, and there were some 500,000 sexual abuse cases reported in 1992 (McCurdy & Daro, 1993), we estimate that about 12% of the sexual

15

abuse cases occurred among African Americans and, as was true for whites, that a third of these occurred among males. Should we bother to even make a racial distinction? That is, are there sexual abuse differences between African American and non-African American boys? Unfortunately, there is little research or literature on this phenomenon.

A study by Pierce and Pierce (1984) helps us to address this question. Their study, which offers significant insights, suggests that African American children who have been sexually abused appear to differ from white victims in a number of important ways: (a) They may be younger; (b) they may be more reluctant to acknowledge their victimization, despite the fact that their abuse may be reported sooner; (c) their abuse may be more likely to be reported by a physician than a social worker; (d) they are more likely to remain at home after their abuse; (e) their families are likely to be younger and poorer; (f) perpetrators are less likely to live in the household of the victim, and these households are less likely to include the natural father; (g) their perpetrators may be less likely to engage in oral sex, and as is true for whites, their perpetrators are most likely to be male; (h) their mothers tend to be less likely to reject information that the abuse occurred and less willing to tolerate the abuser; (i) families are less likely to be referred to treatment if the father lives in the household; and (j) there is a greater probability that the perpetrator will be arrested. Although these noted differences are probably not exhaustive of those features unique to sexually abused African American youths, they give practitioners factors to consider during their group treatment efforts.

WHY USE GROUPS?

Group work has been used with considerable frequency in the treatment of girls (Faller, 1988; Gil & Johnson, 1993; Mandell & Damon, 1989; Sturkie, 1983). However, group work is also an efficacious method of treatment for sexually abused boys (Berliner & Ernst, 1984; Kitchur & Bell, 1989; Porter, 1986; Porter, Block, & Sgroi, 1982). Groups allow boys the opportunity to share their experiences with others like themselves. This is a critical dynamic, as children who have been sexually abused commonly withdraw and isolate themselves. Hence, the group has the potential to reduce isolation and social stigma and improve a youth's social skills. African Americans boys, for whom the peer group is often a strong source of support, may welcome the chance for group affiliation. Here, they may draw on peer support in the recovery and healing process.

TREATMENT ISSUES

The major clinical issues for sexually abused African American boys can be captured under three major categories: feelings about self, feelings about others, and feelings in relationship to others.

Feelings About the Self. Youth who have been sexually abused commonly have feelings of guilt, shame, dirtiness, and powerlessness. They may view themselves as "damaged goods." The sense of powerlessness may be acutely strong, as feelings of impotence are a frequent consequence of any form of victimization. At the same time, it is particularly important for African American male youth to perceive themselves as being able to "take care of themselves." Being tough, cool, and in control is often crucial to their perceptions about becoming a man and maintaining a sense of masculinity (Connor, 1995). Often, African American boys have an exaggerated sense of maleness in the form of "bravado, hyper-masculinity and cool" (Majors, Tyler, Peden, & Hall, 1994; Wilson, 1991). Consequently, the sense of powerlessness or loss of personal control that accompanies sexual abuse has potentially significant and damaging implications for these youths. In this sense, a sexual abuse experience and its accompanying feelings of power-lessness may be more damaging to the self-perception of masculinity among African American youth than among white youth.

Some children who have been abused by a male fear they will become gay. They sometimes believe that they must *be* gay for a male to have abused them. Those sexually abused by males may fear that others finding out will tease them, calling them gay or "faggot." These children may know of other children who have been abused by a male; witnessing such name calling about others has reinforced their fears. And given that the African American community has a reputation for responding negatively to homosexuality in general, their fears of being labeled gay or homosexual are understandable (Boykin, 1996; Newman & Mussonigrro, 1993).

Many children feel guilty or disloyal for having "told on their abuser." Clearly, those children who disclose their abuse take a great risk. It is possible that they will not be believed, and even if they are, they may be blamed for their own abuse. Still other youths may experience feelings of confusion. They may ask "why me?" They blame themselves not only for causing the abuse but also for not doing something to stop it. They may report having both good and bad feelings from the abuse. Some children experienced pleasurable physical feelings from their body's natural responses at the same time that they emotionally and mentally wanted the abuse to stop. And for some boys, the physical contact during the abuse may be the only major source of "positive" social attention they received from others. Finally, some boys may fear that they will become sexual abusers themselves.

Feelings About Others. Boys who have been sexually abused experience negative feelings not only about themselves but also about those with whom they have interacted. This may include feelings of loss, for what was once a good relationship with the abuser. Even more traumatic, in some instances, the child may not be believed and find rejection from virtually everyone. However, it should be remembered that in comparison with white mothers, African American mothers may be less rejecting of information that the abuse occurred (Pierce & Pierce, 1984). And finally, there is also a possibility that the child may experience further loss by being removed from his home for protective intervention.

Common among sexually abused African American boys are feelings of abandonment and neglect. Also common are feelings of anger and rage toward his family, which may be perceived as not protecting him, not stopping the abuse, or not believing his earlier disclosures about the abuse. At the same time that he is feeling anger toward those who have abused him and possibly toward those who failed to prevent it, he may fear retaliation from the abuser and/or his family for disclosing the abuse. There may also be a great deal of fear about the legal and court process. Recounting the details of the abuse can be frightening. Moreover, most fear the possibility of facing the abuser in the future.

Feelings in Relationship to Others. African American boys who have been sexually abused typically experience feelings of fear and embarrassment about the social stigma of having been abused. This may be manifested in the fear of being rejected by their families and others for being "different" or strange.

These boys may also experience feelings of vulnerability and lack of protection by a caretaker who did not see the risk and potential of abuse. In particular, the absence of an African American male authority figure with whom to work out his trauma, a youth may feel that the damage to his sense of masculinity has gone unrecognized. Given the high percentage of female-headed families in the African American community, not having a reliable confidant is a reality for many African American boys (a male group leader is especially critical in these instances). In this sense, an African American boy's perceptions of a female caretaker's failure to acknowledge this issue may contribute further to his feelings of rage and depression. These feelings may be especially strong among those children who gave indications that they were being abused, such as nightmares, bed-wetting, and verbal hints. Therefore, it is common for boys who have been abused to experience anger at parents or caretakers for not being approachable enough to encourage his disclosures. Often, youth are aware that their parents' or caretakers' negligence contributed to their problems. These boys may believe that their caretakers' personal problems or issues, such as substance abuse, interfered with their ability to care for, protect, and respond to them appropriately.

The sexual abuse experience may have understandably lessened a boy's willingness to trust adults in the future. He may feel apprehensive about becoming a member of a group to discuss his experience. Indeed, he may question whether either the leaders of the group or the group members can be trusted. Finally, he may have little faith in group therapy itself, questioning whether it will really help him or only serve to humiliate him further.

GOALS FOR TREATMENT

Establishing clear and realistic goals for sexual abuse victims is one of the most important tasks for the group leader. The failure to establish a good picture of what is to be accomplished will likely result in inadequate outcomes. In general, the establishment of goals for each youth must be directed toward enhancing his ability to move and grow beyond the traumas he has experienced. Although the treatment goals for each boy will differ according to his particular situation and history, the following are some of the most important and basic treatment goals.

Goals for Boys Who Were Abused

1. *Stop the abuse.* Although typically the abuse has stopped before entry into group work, it is important to determine that it has in fact stopped. As part of this effort, it is also important to teach the child self-protection.

2. *Reduce feelings of trauma and shame.* Virtually all youths who have been sexually abused experience trauma, shame, guilt, and dirtiness. Hence, professional workers must make reducing these feelings a primary task.

3. *Learn about the effects of sexual abuse.* Workers should attempt to obtain specific information on the consequences that sexual abuse has had for each youth. For example, a boy's ability to trust has probably been impaired by this experience. He may also be unclear or confused about

personal boundaries and gender roles. (Male and female co-leaders may prove beneficial in helping to resolve this latter issue.)

4. *Learn appropriate social skills.* Boys may have inappropriate or deficient social skills. Learning, for example, how they come across to other people and how to behave and communicate appropriately will serve to lessen their social isolation.

5. *Learn about the cycle of abuse.* Because many youth who are abused later abuse others, this goal is both treatment and prevention. These youth must break this cycle and free themselves from potential pathology.

Goals for Boys Who Abuse

Unfortunately, children who have been sexually abused will often abuse others. Therefore, it will often be difficult for the practitioner to determine if a population is true to its classification, that is, whether it consists solely of youth who are abused or also includes boys who are abusers. Commonly, it is only after two or three sessions that a particular boy in a sexual abuse group can be identified as having also abused other children. Hence, it is crucial to approach practice with groups of abused youths with the awareness that one could be, and frequently is, working with both abused and abusers simultaneously. Therefore, even if the group is for "the abused," the leaders should be prepared to work with abusers also. For these youths, we have identified three primary goals.

1. *Learn how to stop their abusive behavior.* All sexually abusive behavior must stop. Education about feelings, thoughts, and behavior is important in this process. Children are taught to avoid high-risk behaviors and specifically to have no unsupervised contact with other children. Each child is helped to develop a repertoire of activities he can engage in when faced with unwanted thoughts. Part of this process is to teach boys to recognize the antecedents (triggers) of their sexually abusive behaviors.

2. *Accept responsibility for their abusive behavior.* Each offender must take full responsiblity for his abusive behavior. This means fully owning his behavior without minimizing or externalizing or projecting blame onto others (Salter, 1988).

3. *Learn to express empathy and make amends with victims.* A prior sexual abuser should make amends with those whom he has abused. These youths should also learn social skills and relationship building, which may include information on pre-dating and dating behaviors.

GETTING THE GROUP STARTED

Structure. Beginning a group for sexually abused African American boys is a moment often fraught with anxiety for the boys, and perhaps even for the leader. It is important to have a structured format that helps contain the boys anxiety level. The group leaders may elect to organize meetings around various themes, for example, feelings about self, feelings about others, guilt, shame, anger, and so on. However, a too highly structured format may create a barrier that keeps children from expressing crucial issues and topics for treatment; many children who have been sexually abused re-enact through play or action their horrific experience. A group that allows children enough space to play and act out their experiences while ensuring the safety of other children thus seems best (Berlinger & Ernst, 1984). Furthermore, groups containing only members identified as having been abused should be closed, with no new members added after the second session. This allows members to develop a more rapid degree of trust and safety.

The Place and Time. The group should be conducted in a safe, comfortable, and nonthreatening environment. Ideally, the environment should include a positive African American presence. If an agency in question does not meet these criteria, the worker may want to seek permission to meet in church or some other African American community facility where a group of African American boys meeting on a weekly basis would not be conspicuous or out of place. We recommend meeting periods of 60 to 90 minutes.

Group Size and Frequency. The group size should be six to nine members. We recommend 10 to 12 session cycles, with about 4 weeks' break between cycles. The fact that we have employed the term *cycle* suggests that it may be necessary to continue to see some or all of the group members again. It is possible that their goals and those of the leader may have only been partially met during a particular cycle. In addition, while members need to be informed that there is an official end to their treatment, they should also understand that it is possible to begin anew if they or significant others deem it necessary. The recommended 4-week break between cycles has advantages for children as well as the group leaders; both members and leaders are able to take a break from therapy and are able to make assessments and evaluate the progress and effectiveness of their efforts. The leaders may also use this time to bolster their environmental intervention efforts.

Phases of Group Development

A period of 10 to 12 sessions is long enough to allow the group to become cohesive and to work through the normal stages of group development as outlined by Garland, Jones, and Kolodny (1965): pre-affiliation, power and control, intimacy, differentiation, and termination. It is important that those leading groups have some understanding of these phases so that they might anticipate and respond more appropriately to the behaviors of their boys.

During the initial *pre-affiliation phase,* group members are likely to exhibit approach-avoidance behaviors. Even though many of these boys will be happy to receive the attention of a "helper," they are also likely to feel some embarrassment and hence reticence about being in a group for sexually abused boys. The leader can help this process by engaging in activities that reduce the members' initial anxiety, such as providing a snack (a good idea at all meetings) or engaging members in a conversation about their favorite pastimes and heroes.

Once they have overcome their initial feeling of wanting to leave, members move on to a *power and control phase.* Here, we often see blatant struggles for power and status between African American boys. Members are likely to engage in name calling, cursing, and shoving matches. Some of this name calling may take on sexual and even racial overtones. The leader should not conclude that he has lost control of the group or that the group is deteriorating but, rather, understand this as a normal process (Hack, Osachuk, & Deluca, 1994). These youth are merely attempting to control others by hurting them in ways that they themselves have been hurt and controlled. Setting limits on the extent of this behavior (Schacht, Kerlinshy, & Carlson, 1990), the leader might use these occasions to discuss what and why some racial and sexual language has in the past been hurtful to them and why they now employ it against others.

However, once having established some rudimentary pecking order among themselves, the boys are likely to move on to an *intimacy phase.* This phase is characterized by group cohesion. Here members are likely to share the more intimate details of their sexual abuse. For example, they may disclose their age when they were abused, their relationship to the abuser, and how long the abuse continued. They more readily discuss the identities of their perpetrators and the nature of their sexual acts. It is also here that group members may reveal that they themselves have sexually abused others. The worker should exploit the spirit of this phase by encouraging members to support and trust one another. The group leaders should also use this period to build normative support among the group members against the future sexual abuse of others.

Members will soon move beyond mere cohesion and begin to see and accept each other as distinct individuals who are similar yet different from themselves—the *differentiation phase*. It is through the process of recognizing the different experiences of others and the acceptance of these differences that members also acquire greater acceptance of themselves. The group leaders can facilitate this process by clarifying and pointing out the differences among the group members, for example, differences in their perpetrators.

Once achieving some of their goals, the members may begin to move apart—*the separation phase*. In addition, boys may begin to seek out alternative sources of social and emotional support, for example, Boy Scouts or team sports. While encouraging this process, the leaders will witness some members who feel themselves ill prepared to leave the group. These members may return to an earlier phase of acting out, for example, inappropriate sexual language and behavior. These members are foremost exhibiting feelings of insecurity. They should be informed of their existing gains and of the future availability of the leader and alternative sources of help.

LEADERSHIP

Working with African American boys who have been sexually abused is always heart-wrenching work. The leaders need to have worked through their feelings and attitudes about sexual abuse. Also, it is wise to have inspected oneself for potential biases against African American males, a feeling that both non-African Americans and African Americans often harbor. Sexually abused males may have traditionally received insufficient attention in part because it was thought that males could not be abused if heterosexual. Given the sexual stereotypes associated with African American males, it is probably less conceivable to some that they could be sexually abused. Obviously, this type of thinking is erroneous, and practitioners who work with African American youths must resist falling victim to it.

We recommend that these groups have co-leaders. Moreover, we suggest that these groups be led by male and female co-leaders (Adams-Tucker & Adams, 1984; Lubell & Soon, 1982; Shilkoff, 1983). The presence of male and female co-leaders will afford the group members an opportunity to witness appropriate sex-role behaviors and cooperation. It is especially important that at least one of the co-leaders be an African American male. The African American co-leader should provide clinical intervention as well as model gender roles, appropriate masculine behavior, and cooperation between the sexes.

CURATIVE INTERVENTION PROCESSES

All interventions employed by the group leaders should have as their fore-most intent the promotion of physical and emotional safety for all group members. Critical to this process is trust. Indeed, the first crucial task for the group leader is to establish trust with members. Yet, youth, who have been sexually abused are among those least likely to trust adults (Einbender, 1991; Mandell & Damon, 1989; Porter et al., 1982). Also, when relating to representatives of the establishment, African Americans frequently possess a sense of "healthy cultural paranoia" (Grier & Cobbs, 1968). Because of their frequent negative encounters with those representing the system, African Americans are justifiably cautious in dealing with any professional.

Of course, if the group leader is non-African American, the task of establishing trust is further exacerbated (Davis, 1985). However, there is evidence that the race of the practitioner may be less important, in some instances, than his or her level of experience (Cimbolic, 1972). It would seem that the leaders must simply demonstrate patience, be persistent, and behave in ways that demonstrate to group members that they can be trusted. Unfortunately, there is no shortcut to establishing trust when working with groups of sexually abused African American boys.

Beyond the establishment of trust, we believe that there are six group processes that most clearly benefit sexually abused African American boys. Irving Yalom (1995) refers to these processes as curative factors. We advocate that the leader actively and purposefully intervene in ways to promote their occurrence within the group.

1. *Universality.* Boys will benefit from the awareness that they are not alone. The awareness that other African American boys have also experienced sexual abuse serves to lessen their feeling of deviance, isolation, and shame. The leader may promote this process by asking members to share their experiences with the other members.

2. *Instilling hope.* Seeing other boys in the group get better, resolve issues that they share, is beneficial. Often, those who have already completed a cycle may relay to new members the benefits of their group experience. Hence, the leader may want to ask a previous group member to return to a group for a given session to serve as a role model.

3. *Group cohesiveness.* Luckily, African American boys, like other boys, tend to be gregarious, so it comes naturally for most of them to want to be part of a group. The aspect of belonging and feeling close to other members who understand and accept them reduces their sense of social isolation and

fear. Any activity that promotes a positive group identity might foster this process, for example, working on a project together.

4. *Interpersonal learning.* Most boys need to improve their social skills in getting along with people. Because one of the effects of sexual abuse is often social isolation, their social skills may have become impaired. Hence, they may need to learn how to socialize appropriately with peers. The leader may teach these youth how to share, for example, by devising a method for them to equitably share their snacks or group responsibilities.

5. *Catharsis.* Members benefit from being able to say what is bothering them, instead of holding it inside. It is important that these boys be able to express thoughts and feelings of shame and outrage. The group may be the only safe place that these youth have ever had to release these feelings. However, because African American youth frequently need to maintain an image of being in control and "cool" (Majors et al., 1994), they may be reluctant to express their feelings of pain and shame. The leader may need to repeatedly foster the idea that it is not "uncool" or unmanly to express feelings.

BEYOND THE GROUP

Given the economic status of African American children, at least half of the children seen by group workers will probably be from poor families. Subsequently, leaders of these groups must pay special attention to the possible social or economic constraints on these boys. For example, there is a real possibility that a boy will be unable to move away from a known perpetrator, or that a mother may have to continue to rely on child care that is suspect and unreliable. This does not mean that efforts to prevent future offenses will be futile but, rather, that greater effort and the possible employment of more sources for monitoring the youth may need be employed, for example, family services, courts, and fictive kinship networks.

Moreover, despite sometimes having the pejorative reputation for being "a wild and crazy place," the African American community is really quite conservative. This is probably what accounts for the fact that African American perpetrators are even more likely to be prosecuted than their white counterparts (Pierce & Pierce, 1984). And although it is true that the larger community or "'hood" is often a hostile place for African American males, it also has many underused resources. For example, fraternal groups such as 100 Black Men, Alphas and Kappas, and Rites of Passage commonly engage in outreach efforts directed at African American youth. The church, in

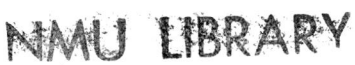

particular, has always served as a valuable resource for families and individuals in need within the African American community. Group leaders should attempt to make contact with organizations such as these in their efforts to restore sexually abused African American boys. For example, they may attempt to determine the potential benefit of enlisting a family minister or pastor. Pastoral support may take the form of providing information and insights into a particular youth. A member of the clergy may also serve to encourage the family to support the group leaders' therapeutic efforts (Boyd-Franklin, 1989).

The group leaders may also find it useful to engage in a pregroup home interview (Kitchur & Bell, 1989). Such an interview will allow the workers to assess the social context of these boys. Specifically, a pregroup home visit will allow the leaders to assess the family's interest in the boy attending the group, foster rapport with his parents or caregivers, and give the workers a better feel for the boy's safety and physical environment.

Finally, it is impossible to outline in this chapter all possible extragroup contingencies, but group leaders may want to keep in mind what we call the *FARC* approach. First, be *flexible* in their work with these youths and their caregivers as many will have less control over their environments—for example, bus schedules, unreliable child care. Second, be *active*: An existential, laissez-faire, laid-back approach may suggest, to those whose lives are frequently in crisis and in need of immediate action, that the leaders are too far removed. Third, always indicate *respect* when interacting with these boys and their caregivers. Although this is a good rule to follow with any population, African Americans are often flagrantly disrespected by representatives from the system and are keenly sensitive to discourtesy. Last, the leaders should attempt to be as *concrete* as possible in both their language and methods. The goals of our "talking therapy" are sometimes too vague. African Americans appreciate clear and explicit suggestions regarding the interventions being employed and the outcomes to be expected.

CONCLUSION

The intent of this chapter has been to provide readers with guidelines to work effectively with African American boys who have been sexually abused. Sexual abuse is one of the most damaging, painful, and ugly experiences possible in the lives of children. Those who lead groups of sexually abused African American boys have, so to speak, their work cut out for them. It will be demanding and exhausting work, and group leaders must employ all the resources at their disposal in the treatment of these youth. Leaders of these groups must have both patience and compassion in working with a population of young boys who have been grossly wronged.

Yet, despite the traumatic nature of sexual abuse among these boys, it should be remembered that a tremendous strength of African American youth is an ability to overcome what would seem insurmountable events. Indeed, much of the success of African American males can be attributed to "individual and family resilience, the ability to 'bounce back' after defeat or near defeat, and the mobilization of limited resources while simultaneously protecting the ego against a constant array of social and economic assaults" (Daly, Jennings, Beckett, & Leashore, 1995, p. 42). Group leaders must stay cognizant of these facts and come to their groups expecting the continued improvement and success of all their members.

CHAPTER 3

Psychiatric Treatment of Older African American Males

F. M. BAKER

This chapter will begin with a description of the demographic characteristics of older African American males, review the historical events occurring during the development of the black American elder, and discuss the importance of a biopsychosocial perspective in the assessment of the older African American male. Then, it will consider specific diagnostic concerns and the assessment of cognitive function, affective symptoms, and psychopathology in the evaluation of the older African American male requesting mental health services and discuss strategies for engaging him in therapy. It will conclude with a discussion of specific treatment options.

DEMOGRAPHIC CHARACTERISTICS OF THE OLDER AFRICAN AMERICAN MALE

As a group, African Americans make up 12% of the total U.S. population. About 11% of black Americans are age 65 and older (National Center for Health Statistics, 1991). A total of 21% of older Americans will be minority group members in 2050 (Angel & Hogan, 1991), and African American elders will account for 24% of the minority elders at that time (Angel & Hogan, 1991).

The older African American population is diverse. Although 33% have incomes below the poverty level, 67% have incomes above $30,000 per year (Gottlieb, 1996). Education varies: 4% completed college, 18% completed high school, and 18% have had no formal education. Older African American males experienced limited educational opportunities and restricted options for employment, due to legalized segregation in their youth. Many worked in unskilled jobs in the construction industry, which placed them at risk for injuries and exposure to environmental toxins. A smaller number had careers as businessmen, teachers, preachers, lawyers, and physicians (Baker & Lightfoot, 1993).

Access to health care was restricted in the developmental years of the older African American male due to segregation and restricted income. Diets high in salt and saturated fat resulted in obesity, diabetes, hypertension, heart disease, stroke, and cancer (Jerome, 1988). The black American elder has an average of five active medical problems (Harper, 1992; Jerome, 1988). Hypertension, obesity, osteoarthritis, glaucoma, goiter, and gout are the most frequent medical problems observed in older African Americans (Harper, 1992; Jerome, 1988; National Center for Heath Statistics, 1991). Cancer is also a concern. Malignancies of the prostate, lung, and esophagus among older African American males are of particular concern because of the significantly lower 5-year cancer survival rates for African American males in comparison to white American males (Baquet, 1988). These multiple medical problems increase the risk of depression, an episode of delirium, and/or drug-induced psychotic episodes (Baker, Lavizzo-Mourey, & Jones, 1993).

HISTORICAL EVENTS OCCURRING DURING THE LIFE SPAN OF THE OLDER AFRICAN AMERICAN MALE

People called African Americans today are the great-, great-, great-, great-grandchildren of people who were born, predominantly in West Africa, captured in local wars and sold into slavery, and whose descendants survived and attained freedom in the United States. As young children, black American elders of the 1990s may have heard of the black cowboys of the West (Miller, 1991) and the buffalo soldiers, black men who served in the cavalry and in the U.S. Army in segregated units in the 1890s (Powell, 1995). In their adolescent years, stories about the period of the Harlem Renaissance and its black artists and jazz musicians may have stimulated them to emulate the creativity of these artists (Baker & Lightfoot, 1993). In the 1930s, black American elders, then in their teens, may have joined their families as part of the black migration to the midwest, west, and northern United States because of the Great Depression (Baker & Lightfoot, 1993). The assault on returning African American World War I soldiers by white Americans in several U.S. cities, called the "Red Summer," may have been passed on as oral history with the medals of the relative who served in World War I. Today's black American elders may have been among the Tuskegee airmen who participated in the "Noble Experiment" to train black American men as fighter pilots for World War II—at that time a controversial program. The heroes of the older African American male of the 1990s include Charles Drew, M.D.; General Benjamin O. Davis, Sr; General Benjamin O. Davis, Jr.; Jackie Robinson; Ralph Bunche; and U.S. Supreme Court Justice Thurgood Marshall. The leadership of the Rev. Martin Luther King, Jr. in the Montgomery bus boycott and the subsequent civil rights movement may have directly expanded opportunities for older African American males when they were in their twenties (1940s) and thirties (1950s). The Black Revolution of the 1960s contrasted the nonviolent, negotiating approach of Dr. King and the confrontational approach of the Black Panther movement, which advocated "power to the people" now. The separatist approach advocated by Malcolm X, as the spokesperson for the Black Muslim movement (Haley, 1992), recalled for black American elders, now in middle age, the need for a homeland emphasized by Marcus Garvey when they were in their teens (Griffith & Baker, 1993).

Emerging role models for African American elders in their middle age years included Dr. King, General Colin Powell, Magic Johnson—fighting a chronic disease (AIDS)—and in the entertainment field, Bill Cosby and Denzel Washington. Successful African American male role models may have had to overcome adversity in their lives, including substance abuse (Haley, 1992; Mfusi, 1996).

Black American elders were in old age when the Million Man March was held on October 16, 1995, in Washington, D.C., bringing males of African origin from across the nation to emphasize the importance of family and brotherhood within the African American community. Black American elders may have recalled the 1940 threat of A. Phillip Randolph, President of the Union of Sleeping Car Porters, to organize such a march for better benefits for union members.

IMPORTANCE OF THE BIOPSYCHOSOCIAL PERSPECTIVE IN THE ASSESSMENT OF THE OLDER AFRICAN AMERICAN MALE

The biopsychosocial perspective of Engle (1977, 1980) has particular relevance for the older African American male. Because the older African American male has an average of five medical problems (biologic sphere), he is at risk of early death (before age 67) and has the lowest survival rate of any U.S. age-sex-racial grouping (Angel & Hogen, 1991). Because the role of stress (psychologic sphere) in the generation of hypertension and peptic ulcer disease has been established, the chronic stress of surviving in a society that featured legalized segregation in his childhood and young adult years increased his risk for the development of medical illness (biologic sphere) (Baker, Lavizzo-Mourey, et al., 1993).

In late life, the psychological stressors faced by the surviving older African American male are varied. They include the loss of family and friends due to death. If retirement income is restricted to social security benefits, the elder may only be able to afford housing in a high-crime, drug-infested urban area or resource-poor rural area. Applications for recertification for eligibility for Medicaid funds and social security benefits may result in frustrations and interpersonal conflicts as the elder struggles to understand forms and procedures established for people with a high school education, which he may lack.

The social sphere of the black American elder includes family, friends, and his church (Taylor & Chatters, 1986a, 1986b). Although many African American males were denied the opportunity to obtain positions of power and authority within the larger American society, even with a college education, many older African American males were active in their churches throughout their lives. If it exists, the extended family and the social network evolving from church provide important resources for the black American elder throughout his life span.

Elderly African American males in their 80s and beyond continue to hold important roles as the elders in their families and their churches, contributing to their sense of productivity and self-worth in their retirement years (Taylor & Chatters, 1986a, 1986b)—which then contributes to the lower rates of suicide among black American elders (Baker, 1994b; Griffith & Bell, 1989), particularly those residing in the South. About 59% of older black Americans reside in the southeastern United States (Harper, 1992).

EVALUATION OF THE OLDER AFRICAN AMERICAN MALE

Too often, the evaluating clinician fails to establish key demographic data beyond age, sex, race, and marital status. Knowledge of the education completed, work history, and significant social supports are crucial to understanding the resources and coping capacities that the older African American male brings to the initial psychiatric interview. A few authors have emphasized the importance of reviewing the personal history of an older patient in the context of the historical events that have occurred during the person's life span, termed a life review (Baker, 1982, 1987; Colarusso & Nemiroff, 1987).

Diagnostic Considerations

Misdiagnosis of psychiatric symptoms has been an ongoing concern for older African American males with psychiatric problems (Adebimpe, 1981b; Griffith & Baker, 1993; Wilkinson & Spurlock, 1986). In the 1950s, African American males who presented with psychotic symptoms were more likely to be diagnosed as having schizophrenia. A differential diagnosis of Major Depressive Disorder (Adebimpe, 1981a, 1981b), bipolar disease (Bell & Mehta, 1979; Jones, Gray, & Parson, 1981), schizoaffective disorder (Baker, 1995), or substance-induced mood disorders (Bell et al., 1985) was infrequently considered. In the 1990s, it is essential to explore whether the black American elder has had any history of substance abuse, has ever had a history of head trauma with loss of consciousness, or has had any exposure to toxic industrial chemicals. Each of these factors could cause the psychiatric symptoms observed.

If the older African American male has a prior psychiatric history, it is important to review the specific symptoms reported and the context of their development because of the pattern of misdiagnosis among African American patients (Bell & Mehta, 1979; Bell et al., 1985; Coleman & Baker, 1994; Jones et al., 1981). Only a few studies have rigorously rediagnosed older African American patients using the *Structured Clinical Interview for the Diagnostic and Statistical Manual* (SCID). In one such study of 13 patients with known psychiatric disorders (Baker, 1995), the diagnoses were changed in 31% (*N* = 4) of cases from schizophrenia disorders to affective disorders based upon the SCID interview. In 54% of these patients (*N* = 7), new *DSM-III-R* (American Psychiatric Association [APA], 1987) diagnoses were identified, mainly anxiety disorders and phobias.

Assessment of Cognitive Function

The assessment of cognitive function is an important component of the mental status examination (MSE). The Mini-Mental State Examination (MMSE) has been found to be an effective screening instrument for cognitive impairment among African Americans with at least an eighth-grade education (Baker, Robinson, & Stewart, 1993; Folstein, Folstein, & McHugh, 1975).

For people with less than an eighth-grade education, the Short Portable Mental Status Questionnaire (SPMSQ) is an important alternative; it also includes an adjustment for education (Fillenbaum et al., 1990; Pfeiffer, 1975). It is an important tool that can be helpful for patients with limited formal education, particularly older African American males. Norms for the SPMSQ were developed in a population that included elderly, rural residing African American males and females.

Assessment of Affective Symptoms

An additional component of the evaluation should be an assessment for the presence of affective symptoms. It is important to remember that older African American males are stoic and may not report feelings, which they identify as signs of weakness. If experiencing a major depressive disorder, the black American elder may report "difficulty concentrating," "aching all over," "being angry all the time," and "being evil" (irritable and verbally hostile toward family and friends). Additional complaints may include having difficulty sleeping and a change in appetite or weight. This atypical presentation of depression with somatic complaints and denial of symptoms is seen frequently among African American males and should be explored. The violent confrontations and episodes of violence for some males may be precipitated by an underlying depression (Griffith & Bell, 1989). The clinician must remember that all the symptoms in the *DSM-IV* (APA, 1994) criteria may not be reported by the African American elder and may even be denied when asked during the interview.

The Center for Epidemiologic Studies of Depression (CES-D) Scale (Radloff, 1977) has been found to be a more effective screen than the Geriatric Depression Scale for the presence of depressive symptoms in older African American males and females (Baker, Vellie, Friedman, & Wiley, 1995). Because of the report of somatic symptoms among older African American males, it is important to select a screening instrument that includes these questions.

It is crucial to ask about the presence of passive suicidal thoughts by asking "Have you ever wanted to go to sleep and not wake up?" Active suicidal ideation should be directly addressed: " Have you ever had thoughts about wanting to harm yourself. . . to end your own life?" The presence of a suicidal plan should be clarified: "How would you attempt to end your life?" If the plan is well detailed, the potential for implementation is increased and action should be taken to prevent the older African American male patient from acting on his suicidal ideation. Immediate referral to an emergency room or a crisis treatment setting is indicated if the African American elder will not contract for safety and has no social support network.

Assessment of Psychopathology
(General Symptoms of Mental Disorders)

The Short Psychiatric Evaluation Schedule (SPES) was developed by Pfeiffer (1979) for use as a screening instrument for psychopathology in the elderly. Its Yes/No response format enables it to be administered in less than 10 minutes, even to severely impaired patients. It can provide useful information about the types of symptoms reported by the black American elder.

Rationale for the Use of Screening Instruments

Using standardized instruments will enable the clinician to establish a baseline and then to follow the change in scores during the course of treatment. As insurance companies and managed care groups request documentation of the efficacy of treatment, the demonstration of a decline in a score in psychopathology (SPES) and affective symptoms (CES-D) and an improvement in MMSE scores (or SPMSQ scores) will facilitate a communication about the benefits of treatment for the specific patient.

ENGAGEMENT OF THE OLDER
AFRICAN AMERICAN MALE IN TREATMENT

The establishment of the patient-therapist relationship should begin in the evaluation process. Because of the diversity within the African American community, it is important to establish the educational background and work history of your patient. The personal resources and experiences of a retired African American physician will be different from those of an African American male who was a construction worker. The therapist interaction with each of these males must be sensitive to the different life courses of these males and must use language that will facilitate communication with them (Baker, 1994a; Spurlock, 1982; Wilkinson & Spurlock, 1986).

If the black American elder has experienced exclusion or frank hostility in prior attempts to obtain medical care, the health care setting may have negative associations for him. Hypervigilance and defensive behavior may characterize his initial interactions in anticipation of another rejection or misinterpretation or selective listening to his concerns and complaints. Or the older African American male patient may be very comfortable in the psychiatric setting based on a successful prior treatment or prior psycho-analysis. Understanding the role of the psychiatric patient will enable this black American elder to effectively present his reasons for returning to treatment.

Whatever the economic level, educational background, and past treatment history of the black American elder patient, the acknowledgment by the therapist of obvious difficult times in the patient's life course and the therapist's recognition of the capacity of the older African American male to survive these stressors should facilitate the patient's understanding that the therapist is carefully listening and capable of empathy with his life experiences.

Clarifying the people in the social network and among the close confidants of the black American elder will facilitate the establishment of the psychosocial context that brings the patient into treatment; it also may be an important resource for him. Interviewing an accompanying family member, friend, or significant other can provide an important corroboration of the data obtained from the patient as well as providing specific information about the changes in the patient observed by someone who is most familiar with him. If your patient has had any prior negative experience(s) with health care settings, the presence of a trusted confidant can help him feel more at ease in the mental health care setting (Baker, 1994a; Jones, Gray, & Jospitre, 1982).

TREATMENT OF THE AFRICAN AMERICAN MALE

Early in the treatment process, the therapist must establish the patient's definition of mental illness. Does the patient identify his psychiatric symptoms as symptoms of mental illness? Are the symptoms believed to result from the working of roots, from a hex, or from a voodoo curse? Does the patient fail to perceive that his thoughts or behavior are unusual? Part of the initiation of treatment may be the clarification of the symptoms that he is experiencing as a mental illness with a specific diagnosis and a description of the range of treatments available for that mental illness (Baker, 1994a; Baker & Lightfoot, 1993).

Having established the diagnoses with the aid of screening instruments, interviews with pertinent significant others, and a review of prior records (if they exist), it is important to carefully describe the specific treatment to be provided and its expected outcomes. The indications for the proposed treatment and the reasons that you are recommending it should be presented in detail in language comprehensible to the older African American male patient. If feasible, the older African American male should be encouraged to be an active participant in the choice of treatment options.

Because of the probability that the older African American male will be taking multiple medications for medical and mental illnesses, it is important to be alert for the possibility of drug interactions. Reviewing the symptoms of such interactions with the black American elder is an important part of the treatment process. Using lower doses of psychoactive medications and increasing the dose slowly are important strategies. Such an approach will identify the minimal effective dose of medication required, minimize the potential for side effects from the medication, and decrease the potential for drug interactions.

The specific ethnic and racial background of the therapist may or may not be pertinent to the treatment (Jones et al., 1982). A prior negative experience with a therapist of a different racial and/or ethnic group, who related to the patient based on the therapist's preconceived stereotype of African American males, will make the establishment of a therapeutic alliance more difficult until the transfer issues are identified and resolved. A negative transference may occur, also, with an African American male therapist who is viewed by the patient as a domineering or demeaning father or uncle who made his early developmental years difficult. The African American therapist who comes from a different socioeconomic group may experience difficulty relating to an African American male who is homeless or a chronic alcoholic and whose life experience is very different from that of the therapist. Although this would be true, also, for a northern European or Asian American therapist of middle or higher socioeconomic class, the older African American patient and African American therapist both may expect that their common experience as black Americans will initially facilitate open communication. If this does not occur, both the patient and the therapist may experience a sense of loss, or in some instances betrayal (Baker, 1994a).

Therapists who are significantly younger than the black American elder may have no understanding of the impact of specific societal events on that person's life course. The use of group therapy, composed of patients from the same birth cohort, is an effective treatment option. Such group therapy will provide consensual validation of the common experiences that group members lived through and a recognition of the strengths needed to survive difficult times (Baker, 1985). Additional benefits of group psychotherapy with older patients include facilitating an awareness of the expression of affects associated with key life events of group members. The group provides a setting for working through unresolved feelings toward specific people in the lives of group members as specific transferences emerge.

CONCLUSION

The engagement of the older African American male patient in effective treatment readily occurs when the therapist is sensitive to the unique history of the individual patient in the biopsychosocial context of his development within the larger American society. Listening to the patient to understand the experiences and coping capacities that have resulted in his current psychiatric symptoms will enable the patient to participate in developing a treatment plan that can be effectively implemented because of the commitment of the African American elder to it.

CHAPTER 4

Counseling African American Men

COURTLAND C. LEE

This chapter offers direction for counseling with African American men. Crucial issues and strategies for counseling African American men are presented. Although much has been written about counseling men in recent years, very little of this literature has focused on specific issues of counseling with African American men. The literature suggests that while there are issues common to counseling all men (Moore & Leafgren, 1990; Scher, Stevens, Good, & Eichenfield, 1987), the unique psychological and social pressures on African American men make mental health intervention with this client group particularly challenging (Gary, 1985; Gary & Berry, 1985; Jones & Gay, 1982, 1983; Lee, 1990; Lee & Bailey, 1997; Washington, 1987). To provide a framework for counseling African American men, a number of important issues need to be considered. These include racism, problems of aggression and control, cultural alienation, self-esteem, dependency, help-seeking attitudes and behaviors, and racial identity status (Gary, 1985; Gary & Berry, 1985; Jones & Gay, 1982, 1983).

RACISM AS A PRECIPITATING FACTOR OF MENTAL HEALTH CHALLENGES FOR AFRICAN AMERICAN MEN

When discussing important issues in counseling with African American men, it is important to stress that, as a client group, members differ significantly in terms of their socioeconomic status, educational attainment, lifestyle, and value orientation. However, all African American men share the common reality of racism (Gary, 1985; Gary & Berry, 1985; Jones & Gay, 1983). Although reactions to this oppressive dynamic may differ, its persistence significantly affects the quality of life for African American men and should be considered as a significant factor in both problem etiology and counseling intervention (Gary, 1985; Gary & Berry, 1985; Jones & Gay, 1983). The stresses of daily life are compounded for African American men by both overt and covert racism. As mentioned previously, racism operates, in many instances, to limit African American men from a full measure of life-sustaining employment and the ability to support a family (Jones & Gay, 1983; Staples, 1978). In addition, racism has spawned a number of negative stereotypes about African American manhood (Cazenave, 1981; Gibbs, 1988; Jones & Gray, 1983; Majors & Bilson, 1992; Oliver, 1984; Staples, 1978). These stereotypes include the notions of being socially castrated, insecure in their male identity, and lacking a positive self-concept.

The historical persistence of racism has significantly affected the mental health of adult African American males. The general inability to totally fulfill masculine roles has made anger, frustration, diminished self-esteem, and depression pervasive mental health issues for African American men (Gary, 1985; Gary & Leashore, 1982; Hilliard, 1985; Jones & Gray, 1983; Lee, 1990; Lee & Bailey, 1997; Washington, 1987).

Significantly, African American men have developed a number of ways of coping with and adapting to the dynamics of racism and its inherent challenges, many of which may manifest themselves as presenting issues in counseling. Several of these are discussed in the following paragraphs.

Problems of Aggression and Control. The problems that African American men experience with aggression and control often present themselves in one of three ways. First, African American men may exhibit too much control over their anger, frustration, or other strong emotions, resulting in repression or suppression of such affect. Second, they may exhibit too little control over such emotions. In this case, they often demonstrate limited or immature coping skills. Finally, African American men may engage in inappropriate channeling processes in which they direct strong emotions inward. Such channeling can often lead to stress-related illness such as hypertension (Myers, Anderson, & Strickland, 1989) or maladaptive behaviors including substance abuse (Redd, 1989).

Cultural Alienation/Disconnection. Often perceiving themselves to be marginalized or powerless in American society, many African American men cope with their anger, frustration, or sense of hopelessness by disconnecting from meaningful personal relationships or roles valued by society. Such disconnection often leads to cultural alienation. With a limited sense of interconnectedness and a perceived sense of rejection by many sectors of society, the attitudes, behaviors, and values of many African American men often reflect significant disengagement from the world of work, family, and community. This cultural alienation often leads to an identity built on an "outlaw" or "outsider" image among many African American men.

Self-Esteem Issues. The general inability to totally fulfill masculine roles often contributes to diminished self-esteem among African American men. An internalized negative self-image generally results when African American men perceive that they are socially or economically handicapped by negative stereotypes or exclusion from a full measure of employment opportunities. Such perceptions may lead to concerted and often misdirected efforts to assert manhood and attain a sense of self-esteem. In many instances, such efforts result in maladaptive or antisocial behaviors.

Dependency Issues. The dimensions of coping and adaptation among African American men can often be related to issues of dependency. African American men often relieve environmental or interpersonal stress by developing unhealthy or unproductive dependencies. For example, the release of anger, frustration, or other negative affect may be associated with a dependency on drugs or alcohol. Similarly, the release of such affect may be linked to dependency on a process. This might be seen among men whose problem-solving or coping behavior consists of a relatively constant process of maladaptive or violent behavior.

Help-Seeking Attitudes and Behaviors Among African American Men. In considering these issues, it is important to examine the help-seeking attitudes and behaviors among African American men. Consistent with the literature on counseling men in general, African American men, as a rule, do not seek counseling. In many cases, African American men consider the need to seek traditional counseling as an admission of weakness or as "unmanly." Although this is a phenomenon that can be observed among men from a number of racial or ethnic groups, it takes on a different dimension for African American men. For many of them, doing anything that seems unmanly can threaten a masculine self-concept already diminished by society's views and stereotypes of African American manhood. As a rule, therefore, African American men are generally socialized to not open up to strangers.

African American men often find counseling, however, within community kinship networks (Taylor & Chatters, 1989). For example, many men will seek out family members or close and trusted friends for help with problem solving or decision making. They may also seek the guidance of a minister or other religious leader associated with the black church. In addition, African American men have traditionally found counseling services in community centers of male social activity such as barbershops, taverns, or fraternal/social organizations. These are places where men engage in informal conversation and significant male bonding. Such centers allow men to informally, and often indirectly, discuss personal issues with trusted confidants in a nonthreatening atmosphere.

In many instances, African American men are referred for counseling by some societal agent, be it judge, social worker, or probation officer, after they have committed some offense against the social order. Counseling, therefore, becomes a forced choice, and the implicit goal is rehabilitation or punishment. It is not unusual, therefore, to find many African American men approaching the counseling process with apathy, suspicion, or hostility. The resistant attitude about counseling may be a defense mechanism among many African American males (Majors & Nikelly, 1983; Vontress, 1995). African American men generally view counseling as an activity that is conducted by agents of a system that has rendered them virtually powerless. The counseling process, therefore, may come to be perceived as another infringement on African American manhood (Lee, 1990; Lee & Bailey, 1997).

Racial Identity Status. Issues such as those discussed contribute greatly to the racial identity status of African American men. Racial identity development has spawned significant scholarly interest in counseling. Counselors and psychologists have conceptualized and investigated the process by which individuals develop an identity as a racial being (Atkinson, Morten, & Sue, 1993; Cross, 1995; Helms, 1990, 1995).

The development of racial identity has traditionally been conceptualized as an evolutionary linear stage process (Atkinson et al., 1993; Cross, 1971, 1995) or, more recently, as a dynamic personality status process in which racial information is simultaneously interpreted and internalized at various levels (Helms, 1995). It is important to point out that most models of racial identity development in the United States have been developed in a context where people of European origin have been in a position of social and cultural dominance with respect to other groups. The perceptions of this cultural privilege held by people from ethnic minority groups have profoundly influenced attitudes they hold of themselves and European Americans as racial beings (Atkinson et al., 1993; Helms, 1990, 1995).

Racial identity development, therefore, occurs in a milieu characterized by complex social interaction among individuals from ethnic minority groups and the European American majority in the United States. Helms (1995) describes how African Americans evolve through a series of information-processing statuses as they develop a racial identity. These statuses reflect a person's view of self, a view of others in the same racial minority group, a view of other minority groups, and a view of those individuals from the majority racial group.

Responsive counseling with African American men must be predicated on an understanding of racial identity development. It is important for a counselor to have some idea about how an African American male client is processing information about racial matters and his sense of himself as a racial being.

A FRAMEWORK FOR COUNSELING WITH AFRICAN AMERICAN MEN

Although the issues discussed above may present barriers to effective counseling with African American men, they also provide the basis of a framework for effective intervention with this client group. A number of key factors make up this framework:

◆ *Developing rapport.* Given the possible degree of alienation or distrust of the counseling process, it is important to find ways to make an initial personal connection with African American male clients. Counselors may need to adopt an interpersonal orientation when counseling with African American men. Such an orientation places the primary focus on the verbal and nonverbal interpersonal interactions between counselor and client as opposed to counseling goals or tasks (Gibbs, 1980).

◆ *Pacing the engagement of the actual counseling process.* It is important to pace the counseling relationship and be mindful of engaging in therapeutic work too rapidly with many African American men. The process is often more effective if it evolves naturally from a personal relationship, based on openness and trust, that emerges between the counselor and the client.

◆ *Counselor self-disclosure.* It is important that a counselor be prepared to self-disclose, often at a deep and personal level, to an African American male client. A counselor's willingness to forthrightly answer direct, and often intimate, questions about his or her life increases credibility and promotes rapport with many African American men in counseling. A counselor should only self-disclose, however, to the level of his or her comfort about revealing personal information to a client.

◆ *Introspection process.* Given cultural alienation or disconnection among many African American men, a counselor may need to foster a climate that encourages client introspection. The veneer of aloofness, strength, and control characteristic of alienation among African American men may preclude the sharing of intimate feelings, which is generally a major aspect of the counseling process. Counselor credibility and openness can promote a climate that will facilitate an introspection process with many African American male clients.

◆ *Spirituality.* Counseling with African American men can often be enhanced if a counselor can engage clients in an exploration of how they approach living and dying (i.e., spirituality). Helping clients to explore their sense of spirituality or personal meaning in life can provide a focus for processing issues of alienation, anger, or frustration. Such an existential/philosophical exploration can only be facilitated if rapport and trust have been established.

◆ *Racism-sensitive counseling.* Counseling with African American men must be predicated on a sensitivity to the dynamic of racism. Although there is a great deal of variation in the effects of racism on the psychosocial development of African American men, its influence on the quality of their lives cannot be overstated. A culturally responsive counselor, therefore, should factor this variable into problem etiology and resolution as appropriate. It is important to avoid discounting clients' perceptions of how this dynamic affects their lives.

◆ *Psychoeducational counseling.* Counseling should be viewed as an educative process for many African American men. The primary focus of the process may need to be developing new skills or behaviors to deal more effectively with social and economic challenges.

CRUCIAL STAGES IN A COUNSELING PROCESS
WITH AFRICAN AMERICAN MALES

The counseling framework can be seen in the following crucial stages of a counseling process with African American men. The stages are similar in their structure and content to a framework advanced by Gibbs (1980) for conceptualizing the initial response of African Americans to the use of mental health consultation. Gibbs suggests the importance of considering an interpersonal orientation in mental health interventions with African Americans. This clinical orientation focuses on process rather than content in interpersonal interactions. Adopting such an orientation requires interpersonal competence, which is the ability to evoke positive attitudes and to obtain favorable responses to one's actions. Culturally responsive counseling with African American men, therefore, is predicated on promoting an interpersonal orientation. The following five stages imply interpersonal competence on the part of a counselor.

Stage 1: Initial Contact/Appraisal Stage

On entering counseling, many African American men will be aloof, reserved, passive-aggressive, or openly hostile. Conversely, they may be superficially pleasant and appear to acquiesce to the counselor's wishes. Underlying such behavior may be hostility toward or a lack of trust in the counselor and the therapeutic process. At this stage, therefore, personal authenticity on the part of the counselor is critical. It is critically important that an African American male client see the counselor from the outset as genuine or "being for real."

Stage 2: Investigative Stage

Equalitarian processing will characterize this stage. In specific terms, this may consist of attempts on the part of an African American male client to minimize any social, economic, professional, or educational distinctions he perceives between himself and the counselor. A client may seek to relate to the counselor on a level that minimizes degrees, licenses, and other forms of professional identification. An African American male client may "check out" the counselor by investigating possible areas of personal commonality that exist between them. It is important, therefore, that a counselor become comfortable with stepping outside of his or her professional role to interact with an African American male client at such a level of personal commonality.

Stage 3: Involvement Stage

It is at this stage that an African American male client often decides whether he can identify with the counselor as a person. This decision is generally predicated on open and honest self-disclosure on the part of the counselor. At this stage of the counseling process, a client will often engage in an identification process that is characterized by asking the counselor personal questions. The counselor's ability to get personal and engage in self-disclosure with an African American male client can often promote a sense of trust and facilitate movement into a working counseling relationship.

Stage 4: Commitment Stage

At this stage, an African American male client generally makes a decision about whether or not he can trust and work with a counselor. This decision is usually based on his evaluation of the counselor as an open and honest individual that he can relate to on a personal level.

Stage 5: Engagement Stage

At this stage, the client makes a decision that the counselor is "for real" and can be trusted. This is the working stage in which the counselor and client engage in the process of counseling.

The following case study highlights some of the possible issues and challenges associated with counseling African American men:

Lawrence is a 55-year-old African American male. He is currently a mid-level manager with a major electronics firm. He is married with three children. His wife is a middle school counselor in an urban public school system. Lawrence and his family live in a middle-class suburb of a major city. His oldest child is a student at a prestigious university, and his other two children attend a math/science magnet secondary school.

Lawrence grew up in a working-class neighborhood in a large city. His father worked two manual labor jobs to support Lawrence, his mother, younger brother, and sister. Today, Lawrence's sister is a nurse; she is married and lives with her family in a distant city. His brother became involved in drugs during adolescence and is now serving time in a nearby prison for manslaughter.

When he graduated from high school, Lawrence enlisted in the Marine Corps and served a tour of duty in Vietnam, where he was wounded and received the Purple Heart. On his discharge from the Marines, Lawrence got married and started his family. He also enrolled in college part-time. After 6 years of working full-time in a factory and attending college part-time, Lawrence received a B.S. degree in electrical engineering. He was then hired as a management trainee by the electronics firm. He was the only African American hired as a management trainee.

Recently, Lawrence's performance at work has been slipping. He appears at work looking tired and, according to his boss, often seems detached from his coworkers. Suspecting problems at home, Lawrence's boss suggests that he talk with the firm's employee assistance counselor.

Lawrence is extremely reluctant to talk with the counselor. He initially attends the counseling sessions because he feels that has been ordered to do so. Lawrence gradually reveals to the counselor, however, that he has recently been under a great deal of stress. His father passed away several years ago, and now he finds that he must take care of his mother, who is beginning to have health problems. This, in addition to paying college tuition for his oldest child and addressing the needs of his two younger children, has begun to strain his relationship with his family. Lawrence says he and his wife are constantly arguing over finances and other family matters. He also never seems to have time for his children and seems to be constantly yelling at them.

However, he is most upset because he has watched younger white males with less experience advance beyond him in the management of the firm. In many instances, Lawrence was responsible for the initial training of these men. When he has discussed his progress in the company with his supervisor, he has been told that these younger employees attended better training programs and their knowledge of the electronics field is more current. This, despite the fact that his performance evaluations have always been outstanding. He claims he has watched white men in the company form networking groups that have generally excluded him. He knows that the key to advancement in the firm lies in being a part of one of these groups. Lawrence reluctantly confides to the counselor that he has begun drinking to deal with his stress, fears, anger, and frustration.

Case Interpretation

Lawrence is an African American man dealing with a significant amount of stress in his life. His anger, frustration, fears, and perceptions of racism have actually moved him beyond stress to a state of distress. Ironically, he did what the system expects and sought the so-called American Dream. He got an education, honorably served his country in a time of crisis, found gainful employment, worked hard, raised a family, and joined the ranks of the middle class. His achievements refute many of the statistics and stereotypes associated with black men in contemporary American society.

Despite his accomplishments, however, Lawrence perceives that he has not been able to fully participate in or cash in on the American Dream. Although his financial and family challenges are characteristic of many middle-class American men, the dynamics associated with his ethnicity play a major role in Lawrence's perceptions. Despite his qualifications and job performance, he has been unable to feel fully integrated into his work setting. More important, he has not been afforded the opportunity to advance in a manner commensurate with his job performance.

Lawrence considers his failure to move up the corporate ladder a reflection of how he, as an African American, is viewed and treated in the workplace. It is obvious that he has reached the infamous "glass ceiling," which confronts many ethnic minorities and women in the workplace. It is a barrier that is characterized by racial or gender insensitivity and exclusion in the workplace. This unseen but pervasive barrier generally stifles both talent and career goals. It can also have a damaging effect on many aspects of an individual's life. For African Americans, this barrier to career advancement has fostered significant amounts of anger among members of the middle class (Cose, 1993; Thomas, 1993). This is certainly the case with Lawrence.

Significantly, Lawrence's anger, frustration, and the associated stress have begun to affect the quality of his home and family life. His perceived inability to fulfill his multiple masculine roles of provider and head of his family have severely affected his well-being.

Presenting Issues

As is often the case with African American men in counseling, the major presenting issue in Lawrence's case is anger. He is angry at a system that has thwarted his ability to reach his full potential. Lawrence appears to have channeled this anger and the other strong emotions associated with it inward, which has no doubt precipitated his drinking. As his level of stress rises, he attempts to cope by disconnecting from his environment, both at home and in the workplace.

It is obvious that being constantly passed over for career advancement has severely affected Lawrence's self-esteem. As family pressures increase, his ability to fulfill increasing responsibilities as a provider is in direct proportion to his inability to advance professionally. Lawrence's career stagnation is particularly hard on him because, in his perception, the only thing blocking his advancement is the color of his skin.

Counseling Intervention

Initial Contact. At the outset, it was important to gain Lawrence's trust and allay his fears about talking about personal issues to a stranger. The counselor wanted Lawrence to see him as a person first, mental health professional second. The counselor adopted an interpersonal approach that was focused more on the relationship between the two of them than on any specific counseling goals. The counselor engaged Lawrence in conversation about a variety of nonthreatening issues (e.g., sports, events in the community, the firm's ranking in the electronics field, etc.).

Appraisal. As Lawrence and the counselor continued to talk over the first few sessions, it was obvious that they had much in common. The counselor was forthcoming with information about his own family origins, educational background, and military experience. It turned out that Lawrence and the counselor shared similar political views, religious views, and opinions about the local sports teams. Several times, Lawrence asked direct questions about the counselor's home and family life. The counselor, although not altogether comfortable in revealing such information, was generally open and honest with Lawrence. Although Lawrence had not yet revealed anything of any substance related to his anger and frustrations, he and the counselor established a solid personal relationship. This was evidenced by the fact that Lawrence began to refer to the counselor as "my man."

Lawrence and the counselor shared much in common. If this had not been the case, however, it would have been important for the counselor to be open with Lawrence in a personal way. Finding ways to equalize the status between Lawrence and the counselor would have been an important aspect in establishing a counseling relationship.

Involvement. Lawrence began to reveal his anger at the firm's promotion policies. As he spoke, his anger became increasingly evident. It was important at this point for the counselor to let Lawrence tell his story and vent his anger. As his story unfolded, Lawrence would periodically turn to the counselor and ask "You understand what I'm saying?" or "You see where I'm coming from?" This was Lawrence's way of checking to see if the counselor was really hearing what was being said. It was important for the counselor to answer these questions in a forthright and often personal way. In other words, Lawrence needed to hear from the counselor, "Hey man, I've been there."

Commitment. After several sessions, it was obvious to Lawrence that the counselor was someone he could definitely talk to and possibly work with. Lawrence proclaimed that the counselor was "alright!" With this stamp of approval, he proclaimed that he was ready to work with the counselor on finding concrete solutions to the challenges facing him. In Lawrence's words, it was "time to take care of some business."

Engagement. At this point because of the personal nature of the professional relationship that had been established between himself and Lawrence, the counselor encouraged Lawrence to explore meaning in his life. He asked Lawrence to consider how he saw himself as a human being, a man, and as an African American. He asked what meaning being an African American man had for him. The counselor encouraged Lawrence to consider what gave his life meaning as an African American man. Lawrence talked about the importance of family, God, and work to his life. Lawrence claimed that all of these things were important to him because things were so bad for black men in general.

As the meaning and purpose of his life became more focused for Lawrence, the counselor helped him to see the interrelatedness of his challenges: He now bears the financial responsibility for not only his children but his ailing mother as well. Career advancement would no doubt make this responsibility easier to bear. However, the glass ceiling appears to be preventing him from moving up the corporate ladder to greater economic reward. All of this contributes to his sense of anger and frustration, which affects his relationships both at home and work. It also has him questioning his worth as a man. At this point, Lawrence was ready to engage in a plan of action.

His first step was to admit that he was drinking too much and that this excessive behavior would not effectively relieve his stress. The counselor helped him to engage in a concrete problem-solving process. The primary goal was to find ways to channel his strong emotions more effectively. Lawrence and the counselor explored a variety of options.

Lawrence decided that one way to deal with the drinking and relieve stress was to get some exercise. He had played some basketball in high school and had put a net in his driveway for his children's recreation many years ago. In the past, he had enjoyed, "shooting hoops with his kids." The counselor suggested that he might find time to shoot baskets again with his two younger children. This would not only provide him with exercise but would help him reconnect with his children as well.

While his wife and children went to church on a regular basis, Lawrence did not. He and the counselor also discussed the possibility that spiritual direction within the African American religious tradition might be important in dealing with his challenges. The counselor strongly supported Lawrence's decision to attend church again with his family on a regular basis. The counselor and Lawrence considered ways that this could become important family time. Part of family time would include talking about and planning for family challenges with his wife.

A particularly difficult family issue and one that, heretofore, had not been discussed was Lawrence's relationship with his incarcerated brother. Lawrence visited his brother several times a year but had minimal contact with him. When talking about his brother, Lawrence got extremely emotional. He experiences tremendous guilt with respect to his brother. He discussed his regret at not having spent more time with his brother when they were both younger. Lawrence feels that if he had spent more time as a role model or mentor for his brother, perhaps the brother would not have gotten into trouble.

Lawrence made a commitment that part of his family time would be spent visiting his brother on a regular basis. Lawrence would use his visits with his brother as a time to reestablish his relationship with him and possibly help him plan for his life after incarceration.

With respect to his work situation, Lawrence discussed with the counselor the possibility of confronting his supervisor about his perceptions concerning racism in the firm's promotion practices. Lawrence rehearsed with the counselor what he might say to the supervisor about his concerns. His goal was to be able to state his perceptions about the promotion practices in a calm, logical, but forceful manner.

The counselor at this point also decided to engage in some advocacy efforts on Lawrence's behalf. He helped Lawrence network with several local civil rights associations that could serve as a resource in his efforts to affect the firm's promotion policies. He promised to help Lawrence locate and work with a lawyer in preparing a discrimination suit against the firm if that became necessary. The counselor also coordinated some training sessions on diversity issues in the workplace for the firm's management team.

Follow-Up

As a result of his efforts and the threat of external legal and political action, Lawrence was eventually promoted to an upper-level management position. His family-focused efforts also improved the quality of his home life. He had found important new ways to channel his anger. His drinking behavior moderated significantly. After terminating the formal relationship with the counselor, he would periodically drop by the counselor's office whenever he was feeling "stressed out" and needed to talk.

Reviewing this case, a culturally responsive counselor would need to address the challenges associated with issues such as those that confronted Lawrence with intervention at the interpersonal and systemic levels. The first level of intervention involves the direct service to the client. There is much that a culturally responsive counselor can do to help empower a client like Lawrence to effectively challenge his stress, fears, anger, and frustrations. Such service delivery must be predicated, however, on an understanding and appreciation of the culture-specific issues that may hinder or facilitate responsive counseling with African American men.

In addition to direct client intervention with a client like Lawrence, a culturally responsive counselor may need to intervene in the work setting to effect institutional change. In this case, the counselor readily assumed the role of advocate for Lawrence. As an advocate, the counselor intervened within the firm on behalf of Lawrence, and indirectly other minority employees, in a way that was designed to eradicate both overt and covert racism.

THE ISSUE OF COUNSELOR-CLIENT DISSIMILARITY

It is obvious in the preceding case that both the counselor and client were African American and male. This no doubt greatly facilitated the counseling process. In many instances, however, the clinical scenario will involve an African American male client and a counselor who is dissimilar in terms of gender and/or ethnic background.

Any counselor who engages in a therapeutic relationship with an African American male, therefore, must first examine his or her own attitudes, behaviors, and values. White counselors, for example, must consider the possibility that they have been afforded unearned privilege based solely on their race (McIntosh, 1989). It is important that they reflect on their life experiences as a way to understand the possible impact of this privilege on their counseling philosophy and technique. The focal questions for self-analysis are: Has being white afforded me advantages and opportunities in society? If so, what are these? Will an African American male client's perception of my privilege help or hinder my counseling effectiveness?

African American female counselors may need to examine their attitudes related to significant personal life experiences with African American males (e.g., fathers, brothers, sons, significant others, etc.). It is particularly important for African American women to evaluate possible "baggage" they bring to the counseling relationship based on past close personal interactions with African American men. They must constantly consider possible transference/ countertransference issues in clinical interactions with African American male clients that might originate from experiences in their personal lives. Such issues could seriously interfere with therapeutic effectiveness.

No counselor, regardless of his or her ethnic background, should attempt to counsel African American men unless he or she is perceived as being empathic and sensitive to cultural diversity. The challenge for any counselor working with an African American man is to develop a thorough knowledge of the historical dimensions of the African American male experience, an appreciation of the psychosocial effects of racism and oppression on African American male development, and an awareness of the rich subtleties of the African American cultural experience.

CONCLUSION

Within the panorama of the changing face of manhood in America, the realities of African American males often stand out in a striking and often troublesome manner. The challenges confronting Lawrence do not represent the experience of all African American men. However, this case does highlight the issues facing scores of African American men in contemporary society. The future status of African American men depends, in some measure, on the ability of counselors to help empower this client group for maximum psychosocial development and meaningful, productive lives. This will require not only an understanding of the social and cultural context that frames African American male realities but also a willingness to expand the boundaries of counseling practice.

CHAPTER 5

Responding to the Needs of the Gay Male Client

JAMES HERBERT WILLIAMS

A lthough there have been numerous studies on homosexuality among men, most have focused on European American males. In spite of this increasing emphasis on gay issues, comparatively little attention has been given to African American gay men. In the case of these men, no studies can claim a representative sample on which to base scientific assumptions. Much of the literature is based on qualitative research methods (e.g., case studies, convenience samples). This lack of strong empirical data presents a challenge in understanding the issues and needs of African American gay men. The purpose of this chapter is to examine information on African American gay men to facilitate the effectiveness of practitioners (e.g., social workers, psychologists, counselors) in meeting their service needs. The specific aims of this chapter with respect to African American gay men are as follows: (a) to provide a further understanding of African American gay identity development, (b) to determine the insights that can be gained from existing research focused on assisting human service professionals in working with these men, (c) to ascertain the extent of human service professionals' usage of environmental and interpersonal social supports (e.g., family members, community, peers), (d) to identify the methodological issues and gaps in understanding that emerge when examining existing research on these men, and (e) to identify and discuss models of effective interventions that will address their practice needs.

Traditionally, social science researchers have attempted to specifically differentiate between the sexual actions, tendencies, and psychological identities of individuals. Researchers have explored the distinctions between behavior, orientation, and identity. A normative set of definitions has been developed and used by social scientists. Homosexual behavior is viewed as the performance of the actual sexual acts committed by an individual with a member of the same biological sex (Savin-Williams, 1990). Sexual identity, by comparison, connotes a consistent, enduring self-recognition of the meanings that sexual orientation and sexual behavior have for an individual (Savin-Williams, 1990). In this chapter, the term *homosexual* is conceptualized to include both self-identity and specific sexual behaviors. The contemporary uses of the concepts *homosexual* and *gay* convey different meanings in the context of African American men who have sex with other men (Icard, Longres, & Williams, 1996). The explorations used in this chapter include both studies of African American men who identify themselves as having same-sex desires (Bell & Weinberg, 1978; Kinsey, Pomeroy, & Martin, 1948) and those who engage in repeated same-sex behavior but do not reveal their same-sex desires (Icard, Schilling, El-Bassel, & Young, 1992; Loiacano, 1989). Conventionally, the term *gay* is used to refer to the former and *homosexual* is used to refer to the latter (Boykin, 1996; Greenberg, 1988; Icard et al., 1996). The review of reported studies indicates that methodology using both quantitative and qualitative designs have been used to investigate various social issues of African American gay men.

In our society, there is a ubiquitous assumption of heterosexuality. We generally assume that a child born to heterosexual parents will develop into a heterosexual adult. The development of a gay male identity has been defined as a process wherein an individual progresses from an assumed state of heterosexuality to an open affirmed state of homosexuality (Loiacano, 1989, 1993). Scholars have developed various models that conceptualize the stages and processes through which an individual progresses in developing a gay identity (Cass, 1979; Icard, 1996; Minton & McDonald, 1984; Troiden, 1979). Many of these models postulate similar stages throughout this progression. These stages are described in the following order: (a) exiting heterosexual identity—the recognition that one's sexual orientation is not heterosexual; (b) the development of a personal and social homosexual identity status—developing a sense of stability regarding thoughts, feelings, and desires; (c) developing a gay intimacy status—the development of dyadic relationships; and (d) the eventual acceptance and integration of one's gay identity—the entering of and connection with a gay community (D'Augelli, 1994; Icard, 1996; Minton & McDonald, 1984; Troiden, 1979). Various researchers have explored issues of gender differences as related to these stages and have found that the development tasks are different across genders (Faderman, 1984; Groves & Ventura, 1983).

Few authors have investigated the challenges specifically encountered by African American gay men in their gay identity development (Boykin, 1996; DeMarco, 1983; Icard, 1986). Studies by Icard, (1986, 1996) and Boykin (1996) have discussed how the phenomenon of racism may affect the gay identity development of African American gays. They have also explored the multiple layers of prejudices experienced by African American gay men— from the European American heterosexual community, from the European American gay community, and from African American heterosexuals— which further aggravate the internal stresses of being a sexual minority. It is hypothesized that because of the multiplicity of identities, African American homosexuals seem less likely than European American homosexuals to be openly gay or consider themselves out of the "closet." For European American homosexuals, sexual orientation is all that distinguishes them from the dominant group (Boykin, 1996). Thus, one would think that, for European American homosexuals, sexual orientation would take on greater importance than it does for African American homosexuals, who routinely exist with an additional component of alienation from the dominant group (Boykin, 1996). There has been very limited research and literature exploring the relationship between racial oppression of African American gay men and gay identity development. Icard (1986) made the following observation on gay identity formation of the African American gay male:

> The interpersonal relationships that gays experience are critical to the development of a positive sexual identity, particularly during what has been described as the coming-out period. Interpersonal relationships with others who also are gay have been recognized as facilitating congruence intra-psychically as well as interpersonally. For many Black gays, however, gay interpersonal relationships do not provide the kinds of positive consequences that have been defined as so important to the closure of the individual's sexual identity. (p. 90)

Culturally, African American gay men are descendants of African Americans living in a society dominated by heterosexual European Americans, and thus they are treated as marginalized people within a further marginalized sector of our society. To be African American, male, and gay in the United States is to challenge the basic assumptions of society by simply existing (Monteiro & Fuqua, 1993/1994). The theories of African American development concerning social and racial identity formation contain structures of specific stages, behaviors, or social outcomes similar to European Americans (Cross, 1991; Cross, Parham, & Helms, 1991; White, 1984). These theories postulate that African American social and racial identity development is built on the more spiritual, physical, and sociocontextual elements of a person's life (Akbar, 1991a; Nobles, 1991). The cultural duality of African Americans as a subgroup and the bicultural experience of African American gay men in a culture dominated by European heterosexuals can be a tremendous source of stress and pressure in the development of ethnic and sexual identities.

Human service workers are being increasingly challenged in responding to the social and emotional needs of African American gay men. It is essential that practitioners develop a strong practice knowledge to work with this population. To be an effective practitioner among African American gay men, intervention services must be germane to the culture of this client population. We cannot assume that inferences developed from research on European American gay men can be applied when working with African American gay men.

LITERATURE

Kinsey et al. (1948) provided the initial scientific investigation on human sexuality, using a diverse sample of both European American and African American males. His research was significant in discerning that sexual behavior occurs on a continuum ranging from exclusively heterosexual to exclusively homosexual. Although Kinsey's work was groundbreaking in the field of human sexuality, it was not without its limitations when explicating male homosexual behavior. Most of the men classified as homosexual in Kinsey's sample were men currently serving a prison sentence, and this bias provides questionable information about homosexual behavior in the general population (Harry, 1990). Building on Kinsey's research, Bell and Weinberg (1978) used a sample consisting of exclusively homosexual men from San Francisco and Chicago to systematically compare sexual orientation identities and race differences. The constraints of these two initial studies limited their ability to provide more pertinent information about the family and community environment of the African American gay.male. Research by Bell and Weinberg involving African American gay men developed insightful information through comparisons with heterosexuals by broadly examining the diversity within the homosexual community. Johnson (1982) conducted the first study on minority gays that did not use European American gay males as a comparison group. Notably, his work brought attention to the issues of racial and sexual identification of African American gay males. One shortcoming of this study was the geographic representation of the sample, which was composed entirely of African American gay men from San Francisco. The distinctness of San Francisco's liberal social climate would also be a limiting factor in drawing conclusions from Johnson's findings to generalize about African American gay men in other parts of the country. In addition, the participation rate of African American gay men in Johnson's study was less than half of those who were contacted. This response rate raises subsequent concerns about the generalizability and accuracy of findings. Notwithstanding these limitations, Johnson's study is considered a landmark piece of research on African American gay males and is frequently cited. Johnson's observation regarding the importance of social support from the European American gay community and the African American community in developing the self-concept of African American gay men has supported further qualitative research on the development of a homosexual identity among this population group (Loiacano, 1989).

Other researchers have focused more closely on the social and environmental factors (e.g., depression, AIDS knowledge and beliefs, high-risk sexual behavior, violence, drug and alcohol use, grief and loss) of African American gay males (Cochran & Mays, 1994; J. Hunter, 1990; Icard & Traunstein, 1987; Mays et al., 1992; Newman & Muzzonigro, 1993; Peterson et al., 1992, 1995; Rotheram-Borus et al., 1992; Rotheram-Borus & Koopman, 1991). J. Hunter's (1990) study of violence against gay youth offers two important contributions to research on African American gay men. It is one of the few studies denoting the need for direct consideration of the social needs of African American gay youth. Furthermore, this investigation is of particular interest for helping practitioners in that the data was from case records. This study unveiled the significant factor that violent assaults by family members are common among African American gay youths. J. Hunter (1990) also found that these youths reported high levels of assaults from their peers, and many reported that they had, on more than one occasion, considered suicide. Similarly, Newman and Muzzonigro (1993) showed that African American gay adolescents, in families with traditional values (e.g., valued religion, marriage, having children), were subjected to disapproval from their family members and reported feeling different from other boys. Notwithstanding that these findings are based on a very small sample, the study provides a forum for exploring the relationship between ethnic heritage, family values, and sexual assault among gay youth of color.

The 1991 National Survey of Men, which includes a comparative analysis of European Americans, African Americans, and other men of color, provided more controversial results than other prevalence studies. The National Survey of Men is acclaimed for challenging conclusions from previous surveys showing that gays and lesbians accounted for about 10% of the general population. Using a probability sample, this survey found that a low percentage of the men identified themselves as gay (Billy, Tanfer, Grady, & Klepinger, 1993; Tanfer, 1993). Moreover, this survey placed a greater emphasis on the actual sexual behavior of the men and not how they identified themselves. The respondents of this study were specifically asked to self-identify as gay. Researchers have discovered that, within the gay community and especially within communities of color, it is difficult for men who have sex with other men to admit their homosexual orientation (Icard, 1986, 1996; Icard et al., 1996; Johnson, 1982; Loiacano, 1989, 1993). In his study using a sample of college students, Belcastro (1985) found that 9% of African American males who identified as heterosexual also indicated they had received oral sex from another man, and 5% had performed oral sex on another man. Apparently, many men who are engaging in man-to-man sexual activities do not identify themselves as gay or homosexual. Results of the National Survey of Men suggest that researchers and practitioners must continue to explore ways of understanding homosexuality among African American gay men and how sexual orientation is interpreted in the African American community. Today, it is common for communities of color to have a perception of homosexuality as a European American phenomenon (Icard et al., 1996; Katz, 1976).

A significant proportion of research and scholarly writing on the sexual orientation of African American men in the past 10 to 15 years has been related to the epidemic of HIV/AIDS (Ernst, Francis, Nevels, Collipp, & Lewis, 1991; Morin, 1993; Peterson et al., 1992, 1995; Peterson & Marin, 1988; Ryan, Longres, & Roffman, 1996; Siegel, Bauman, Christ, & Krown, 1988; Wright, 1993). Although, AIDS is probably the most devastating catastrophe that all homosexual men must face, the high incidence of AIDS among African Americans has provided cause for directing this attention toward African American gay men. In their study of gay and bisexual men in San Francisco, Samuel and Winkelstein, (1987) found no differences in risk factors of HIV infection between African Americans and European Americans. Studies have revealed that it is important for practitioners to consider social class and economic factors as well as the person's culture for a better understanding of homosexuality and sexual behavior in African American men (Peterson et al., 1992). The results of the Samuel and Winkelstein study showed that males who practiced unprotected anal intercourse were more likely to be poor, to have been paid for sex, or to have used injection drugs.

In summary, a review of previous research indicates the following gaps were identified: (a) Most of the empirical studies were conducted on small samples, limiting their generalizability; (b) many of the studies used qualitative methods (e.g., case studies, ethnographic interviewing); (c) most knowledge was obtained through studies comparing African American gay men and European American gay men; (d) most of the information obtained about African American gay men was developed from samples taken in large urban areas (e.g., New York, Chicago, San Francisco); and (d) the research on African American gay men has focused primarily on social problems (e.g., HIV/AIDS, drug use, alcohol use). These gaps raise questions concerning the usefulness of many of these studies for developing competent practice for professionals in providing effective interventions with African American gay men. It is important that knowledge be further developed that is general to all social classes, ages, and geographical regions, employing larger samples of African American gay men.

HOMOSEXUALITY AND THE AFRICAN AMERICAN COMMUNITY

One of the primary issues that African American gay men face is their relationship with their families and communities (Beam, 1986; D'Augelli, 1994). Joseph Beam (1986), in his essay "Brother to Brother: Words From the Heart," defined the environment as larger and more complex and encompassing than one's living room:

> When I speak of home, I mean not only the familial constellation from which I grew, but the entire Black community: the Black press, the Black church, Black academicians, the Black literati, and the Black left. Where is my reflection? I am most often rendered invisible, perceived as a threat to the family, or I am tolerated if I am silent and inconspicuous. I cannot go home as who I am and that hurts me deeply. (p. 231)

Boykin (1996) notes that homophobia is omnipresent in the African American community. He indicates that this is not only evident in the rhetoric of African American religious institutions, in writing, and in the scholarly works of African American intellectuals, but it is also apparent in African American music and entertainment:

Unfortunately, homophobia in black America is not confined to the writings and speeches of black intellectuals. In the black community at large, homophobia and heterosexism reach all demographic groups, men and women, heterosexuals and homosexuals, the young and the old, the famous and the unknown. The views may differ from one group to another, but in all of them, homophobia and heterosexism are frequently seen not as prejudices but as survival skills for the black race or the black individual. (p. 167)

Many African American intellectuals associate homosexuality with the decline of the African American community. Homosexuality in the African American community is postulated to be an outgrowth of European American racism or a breakdown of the African American family (Asante, 1980; Hare & Hare, 1984; Staples, 1982). Hare and Hare (1984) view homosexuality in the African American community as a by-product of African American family disintegration. They further posit that homosexuality does not promote African American family stability, and it is a phenomenon of the European society and culture (Hare & Hare, 1984).

Following the 1969 Stonewall riots in New York City, when gay men resisted a police raid, the European American gay community began to organize for activism. By the 1980s, gay liberation was well developed, but many African American gay men felt the movement was not seriously concerned with their existence except as sexual objects (Beam, 1986). African American gay and bisexual men find acceptance and social support difficult to attain in their communities. They are not only confronted by prejudices against homosexual conduct within the African American community (Beam, 1986; Ernst, Francis, Nevels, & Lemeh, 1991; Icard, 1996; Icard et al., 1992; Stewart, 1991), but they are also exposed to racist attitudes and beliefs in the predominantly European American gay community (Boykin, 1996; DeMarco, 1983; Icard, 1996; Loiacano, 1989; Stewart, 1991). Knowledge about the attitudes of African Americans toward homosexuality is thus important for understanding an important part of the cultural milieu of African American gay and bisexual men. Popular conjecture and data from nonrandom samples have suggested that African American homosexuals are not as openly rejected by family and community as European American homosexuals. Although the perception of support is hypothesized, the moral stigma associated with being a homosexual in the African American community may still be great (Bell & Weinberg, 1978; Bonilla & Porter, 1990; Greaves, 1987; Staples, 1982). It has also been commonly accepted that homosexuality finds less tolerance in the African American community at large. This low level of social tolerance among fellow African Americans is thought to be the basis for the disproportionately high number of closeted gay men in the African American community.

Results of research exploring the differences in attitudes between African Americans and European Americans toward homosexuality have been mixed (Bonilla & Porter, 1990; Ernst, Francis, Nevels, & Lemeh, 1991; Herek & Capitanio, 1995). In their study, Herek and Capitanio (1995) found that negative attitudes toward homosexuality were widespread in their sample, which included 391 African American heterosexuals, but were less prevalent among European Americans. Attitudes of African American heterosexual men were more negative toward homosexual men than were those of female heterosexual African Americans toward homosexual women. It is interesting that African Americans do not usually think of African American men in connection with the word *gay*. These findings support the hypothesis relating to the difficulties experienced by African American homosexual men in developing a sexual identity. In the Herek and Capitanio study, African Americans and European Americans had similar attitudes concerning attributions of choice in sexual orientation. For European Americans, the acquisition of beliefs that homosexuality is not a choice may be related to personal interaction with a gay man. For African Americans, however, attributions about the degree of choice associated with homosexuality—and sexual orientation—appear not to be contingent on having personal contact. It is hypothesized that African American beliefs and attitudes may be shaped by a cultural construction of sexuality (Herek & Capitanio, 1995). This cultural construction may support previous findings showing a higher prevalence of bisexuality among African American men and stronger frequency of male-to-male sexual behavior by African American men who self-identify as heterosexual (Mays, 1989; Peterson, 1992; Ryan et al., 1996). The Herek and Capitanio (1995) study proposes the possibility that African American social constructions of heterosexuality and homosexuality may differ from those prevalent in the European American communities.

In another study comparing African American and European American tolerance for homosexuality, Ernst, Francis, Nevels, and Lemeh (1991) found that there is a greater condemnatory orientation toward homosexuality in the African American community. They found that the differences across races appear to be gender-specific. The significant differences between the races were attributed to the large differences between African American females and European American females (Ernst, Francis, Nevels, & Lemeh, 1991). It is hypothesized that the reasons for these disparities may be related to African American women's perception of a decreasing marriage pool of available African American males. Religious attitudes and religiosity are other factors underpinning the negative attitudes against homosexuality in the African American community (Boykin, 1996; Butts, 1988; Hayes & Oziel, 1976; Icard, 1996; Larsen, Cate, & Reed, 1983; Larsen, Reed, & Hoffman, 1980; Mays et al., 1992; Peterson et al., 1992; Taylor, 1988; Tinney, 1986). The moral condemnation of homosexuality is especially salient in African American churches. The AME (African Methodist Episcopal) Church is on record as being opposed to homosexuality (Greaves, 1987; Staples, 1982). It is generally agreed that the church has an influential place in African American culture and has an impact on almost every aspect of African American life (Taylor, Thornton, & Chatters, 1987). By many measures, African Americans are considered to be the most religious group of people in the world (Brashears & Roberts, 1996). Other cultural groups (e.g., Latinos, European Americans) are considered more tolerant on the moral dimension of attitudes toward homosexuality than African Americans, and this is probably due to the strong religious condemnation of homosexuality by the African American church and the centrality of the church in the African American culture (Bonilla & Porter, 1990; Boykin, 1996; Staples, 1982). Due to close familial bonds and kinship networks in the African American community, rejection by the family due to homophobia or a diagnosis of AIDS may more profoundly isolate African American gay men than European American gay men (Logan & Joyce, 1996). In addition, most African American gay men hide their sexual orientation within their community, which precipitates internal struggles over self-devaluation and alienation and generate anxiety about possible disclosure and rejection (Dowd, 1995).

MAJOR ISSUES FOR PRACTICE

Research has shown a definite bias in the perceived belief of mental health professionals regarding the psychological makeup of African Americans. Many mental health professionals believe African Americans to be less sophisticated than European Americans (Solomon, 1992). It is egregious that much of the social science knowledge about African American homosexual men has been amassed from small sample sizes, case studies, and personal stories. These research studies provide practitioners with only a marginal perception of the day-to-day lives of African American homosexual men. The lack of strong empirical data reduces the effectiveness of the work of practitioners who are seeking the most compelling techniques to deal with the social and interpersonal problems of African American homosexual men.

To adequately serve this population, it is imperative that culturally relevant practice models be developed. Most studies conducted with homosexual men have been focused on social problems (e.g., HIV/AIDS, substance abuse, alcoholism), and only a few of these have been conducted on African American homosexual men. Furthermore, issues of homosexuality are inherently absent from material on practice with minorities and on men within specific minority groups. (Ewalt, Freeman, Kirk, & Poole, 1996; Green, 1995; Lum, 1996).

Notwithstanding this lack of research support and studies on African American homosexual men, some recurring themes emerge from the existing literature that can be instrumental for informing practice. Some of the major themes that needs to be addressed in the practice setting should include (a) identity issues—understanding the perception of self by the African American homosexual male—within his racial groups, sexual orientation groups, and community; (b) the complexities of the relationships—family and friends—for the African American homosexual male; and (c) the responses of the African American community to the homosexuality of African American males. These themes should guide practice models with this population.

The fundamental purpose of human service practice can be perceived as the enhancement of adaptations between individuals, families, groups, communities, and their environment (Meyer, 1993). It would appear that human service practitioners would be the leaders in developing effective models for working with the gay male population, and particularly with gay men of color. Furthermore, given some of the contemporary discourses on homosexuality (e.g., homosexual identities, homosexual couples, same-sex marriages), it would be expected that research and intervention literature on the subject would more frequently appear in publication.

Practice with African American homosexual men should begin with the actual or potential problems the client is experiencing related to their client systems. It is important that practitioners identify those client problems for which services may be needed. This is initially done by analyzing the biopsychosocial factors related to the client's problems and building on the clients personal and environmental strengths. A proactive approach to intervention would aim at obtaining more basic knowledge that could be used across a range of services and, more important, in primary prevention and early intervention.

Social identity refers to reference group orientation, that is, those groups to which an African American man will attach himself and of which he will feel a part. Community integration is the objective component of identity because it describes the groups, organizations, and interpersonal networks that define the everyday experiences of individuals. Because communities compete for the allegiance of members, individuals often feel drawn to more than one community. African American homosexual men will feel the pull between allegiance to the African American community and to their involvement in the gay community.

Some researchers conjecture that there are various ways that African American homosexual men handle the issue of their connection and/or identification with a community (Boykin, 1996; Icard et al., 1996; Tinney, 1986). They may give total allegiance to one community—they may decide that they are gay and associate predominately in the European American gay community—or they may retain their commitment to their community of ethnic origin and maintain a closeted existence (Boykin, 1996; Icard et al., 1996; Tinney, 1986). It is important to note that the relationship between the African American homosexual man and the community may not be dichotomous but more of a multifaceted continuum. For example, African American gay men in interracial relationships may discover that it is difficult to be a part of either community. Gay interracial couples often face the scorn and derision of both racial groups. European Americans and African Americans criticize gays who cross racial lines. Icard (1996) describes the re-emergence of the African American gay community as a means of social support for African American gay men. Many gay-oriented service providers, such as *Gay Men of African Descent, The National Black Lesbian and Gay Leadership Forum,* and *Blacks Assisting Blacks Against AIDS,* have also emerged over the past 10 years in the large urban African American gay communities, predominately in response to the AIDS epidemic (Icard, 1996).

Often, African American gay men attempt to develop a dual identity, and this duality may range from a self-perception of themselves as predominantly gay or predominantly African American, thus creating the discourse regarding identity among gay men of African descent—African American gay or a gay African American (Beam, 1986; Simmons, 1991a, 1991b). This assumed cultural duality of the African American gay male is very analogous to the identity continuum of highly successful African American individuals, whose professional and social life has in many ways disconnected them from their communities of origin. Many African American homosexual men, however, appear to have the ability to accommodate both identities and ascertain the importance of both.

The degree of identity has direct implications for the types of services an African American gay man will use. For example, African American men who have sex with other men but do not identify themselves as gay or bisexual are less likely to use services focused toward the gay community (Ryan et al., 1996). The documentation of issues of social and cultural identity and the level of integration into the various communities is of fundamental importance to the practitioner. It is important for practitioners to understand all the variations of how an African American homosexual male self-identifies; this will help define the types of services African American homosexual men will use when in need of services. Many services designed for European American homosexual men are more likely to attract only those African American homosexual men who recognize and have a sense of comfortableness with their sexual orientation. Services designed for African American homosexual men are more frequently used by homosexual men who primarily see themselves as strongly connected to the African American community (Icard, 1996). As indicated earlier, it can also be assumed that African American men who have sex with other men and who do not self-identify as gay will feel awkward using either kind of service.

Models of interventions should be effective in distinguishing between the basic human needs and higher-order needs of African American gay men, such as belonging to a group and self-actualization. Regarding their social and economic status, African American gay men are very much within the same range as those of the majority of African Americans. A disproportionately large percentage of African American gay men are found among the undereducated, underemployed, unemployed, and homeless.

In 1978, Bell and Weinberg reported that African American homosexual men were generally more educated, more likely to be in skilled occupations, and more likely to be in occupational positions of public trust than African American heterosexual men. They also did not find significant differences between European American homosexual men and African American homosexual men on these indices (e.g., education, employment) of basic human needs. As previously discussed, the Bell and Weinberg (1978) study cannot be considered representative of the general African American population because their findings were developed from a nonrandom sample.

For intervention models to be effective in servicing African American homosexual men, it is critical that they have the ability to assess primary and secondary needs. If African American homosexual men are less able than European American homosexual men to meet their basic human needs, service providers will have to take this into account. Health and social service programs focusing on African American homosexual men will need to include service components that provide an array of services. These services must be multifaceted to assure that basic needs (e.g., food, housing, safety, employment training) and secondary needs (e.g., social supports, relationships, family) are met (Manns, 1981).

In working with African American gay men, it is important to assess the varying dimensions of their social support network (e.g., significant others, friends, family, professional networks). The practitioner should be cognizant that the perception of family and social supports among African American gay men may be somewhat different than perceptions within the heterosexual community. The existence of gay men on the margins of society at times forces them to develop alternative family structures. In their study of African American gay and bisexual men, Peterson et al. (1995) found that African American gay and bisexual men were least likely to seek help from family members and less likely to perceive family members as helpful with their concerns about high-risk sexual behavior. These results are in direct contrast with help-seeking data on European American gay men (Hays, Catania, McKusick, & Coates, 1990). These differences may be related to the difficulty of families in accepting the gay lifestyle of the African American gay male. Gay African American males may limit involvement with their families to avoid disclosure of their homosexuality (Peterson et al., 1995).

Notwithstanding these possible differences, family circumstances and dynamics are important areas of assessment for African American homosexual men (Icard, 1996). Many researchers consider the African American family as a primary resource for meeting the psychosocial needs of African American gay men (Icard, 1996). It is important not to overlook the importance of families in the lives of these individuals. For many African American gay men, the family of origin may provide a supportive network of personal relationships, and for others, the family relationship may be hostile and contemptuous. To the degree that the African American family holds traditional norms and values—high importance of religion, strong emphasis on marriage and children—the relationship of the African American gay man to his family may be more or less strained (Icard, 1996).

CONCLUSION

This chapter has examined information on African American gay men in an effort to provide practitioners with information to strengthen their skills in meeting the service needs of this underserved population. If research is intended to inform practice, it is apparent from the literature that only limited knowledge has been developed about African American gay men. African

American homosexual men have received limited focus and only moderate scholarly attention. This paucity of available information reduces the effectiveness of practitioners in working with this group of men. These insufficiencies clearly indicate the need for more empirical research on African American gay men beyond the current disease-focused research (e.g., AIDS, depression, alcohol). The building of knowledge regarding these psychosocial aspects will strengthen the practitioner's ability to be effective in resolving problems areas presented by these men. Furthermore, this lack of strong empirical data on African American gay men can limit their being understood by practitioners.

Practitioners should not assume that all African American gay men share similar experiences or that their experiences are always distinct from those of European American gay men. Although many African American gay men remain connected with the African American heterosexual community, some are more strongly affiliated with the developing African American gay community. Many African American gay men are gay-identified and participate in the larger gay community, including the use of social services and activities designed for that community. The literature on the connection with family and community among African American gay men has been mixed. Service use by these men may depend on level and types of identity with a social support network, community, and family. Notwithstanding the lack of information about this population, practitioners should always use cultural models that are sensitive to both racial culture and sexual orientation.

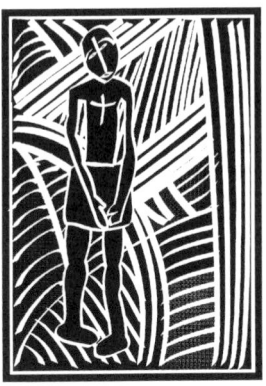

PART II

Health

A frican American males are among the least healthy of Americans. Not only are they more likely to be sick than other men, they are also likely to die sooner. For example, whereas the life expectancy for white males is approximately 73 years, it is only 65 years for African American males (U.S. Bureau of the Census, 1996). Unfortunately, African American males are at risk for a multitude of health difficulties—for example, accidents, substance abuse, homicide, cancer, AIDS, and hypertension. There is a saying that being black is hazardous to your health. Factors such as where they live, what they eat, and what they do for a living, as well as general access to quality health care, all serve to make this saying truer than it need be.

The goal of this section is to focus on the social and psychological aspects of health care with African American males. However, our attention is limited, as African American males face many more health hazards than we could possibly have addressed adequately in this brief section. The authors here have selected only three areas: risky behaviors (drug use and violence), cancer, and diabetes.

The first, cancer, is an all too familiar and well-known killer of African American males. It is safe to say that virtually every African American male fears the possibility of contracting prostate cancer. Hence, the concerns addressed are of potential concern to all African American males. Similarly, diabetes, which is often associated with trauma for low-income groups, is also a well-established killer in the African American community. As others have pointed out, diabetes is especially debilitating for African Americans (Chatters, 1991). Indeed, there are a variety of potential ailments associated with this disease: stroke, heart, kidney, and vascular disease, amputation, and blindness (Chatters, 1991, p. 203). Each of these health risks comes with its own social and psychological ramifications for both clients and practitioners.

A survey of African American health leaders indicated that they ranked reducing the risky behaviors of drug and substance abuse as most important in addressing the health needs of African Americans (Schneider, Greenberg, & Choi, 1993). The reader should keep in mind that this volume also contains a section on gangs, risky behaviors, and delinquency, so some of what might be said about substance abuse is addressed there, as well. However, not enough can be said about homicide. Indeed, homicide is the leading cause of death for African American males (U.S. Department of Health & Human Services, 1990). Familiar to most readers is the fact that the rate of homicide for African American males is seven to eight times that of whites. Hence, efforts that have as their focus the reduction and elimination of violence among African American males is of critical importance. Undoubtedly, the poor environmental and economic outlook for substantial numbers of young African American males contributes to violence as being part of their daily lives (Hammond & Yung, 1993). Therefore, any effort to enhance the health status of African American males must consider the overall life opportunities available to these men.

The interventions in this section suggest that practitioners need to be aware of the unique status of African American males. Specifically, practitioners need to know how the environment may serve to work for or against their efforts. The authors in this section also suggest that practitioners need to rely extensively on social support systems such as family, church, kin, and any social service agencies that can and should be brought into place during efforts to address actual or potential health hazards.

CHAPTER 6

Prostate Cancer in African American Men: Thoughts on Psychosocial Interventions

ROBERT PIERCE

Prostate cancer is the most commonly diagnosed disease among men. Studies show that one in five American men will develop prostate cancer in his lifetime (American Cancer Society, 1997; Jaroff, 1996), but early diagnosis and treatment increase the probability of surviving the disease (Freeman, 1990; Gambert, 1992). Studies also show that only a small percentage of men actively pursue medical intervention for this disease, and African American men in particular are less likely to seek intervention (Freeman, 1990). Some say the silence is because determining the exact cause of cancer is "like looking for a needle in a haystack" (Braus, 1996, p. 41). Others suggest that most men are extremely reluctant to talk or complain about their physical and emotional problems, much less share their fears and uncertainties about a disease that might render them impotent (Lewis, 1994). Henry's (name has been changed to protect his confidentiality) case was an exception. The catalyst that enabled this 64-year-old middle-class African American man to overcome his reluctance to talk about his fears and vulnerabilities with another man was his diagnosis of prostate cancer over 4 years ago and his struggle to cope with the physical and emotional pain that results from having the disease.

Most of us would agree that friendships, particularly during a crisis, are among the most important relationships we can ever have. Yet, men have difficulty forming close relationships with other men. Nardi (1992), for example, notes that because men risk rejection and feel vulnerable when expressing their emotions and feelings openly, men learn early to deny their need for close male-male friendships and, at some level, regard this need as unmanly or a sign of weakness (Seidler, 1992).

Henry's situation was different because he understood the benefits that could be derived from reaching out to a male friend for emotional support during a crisis period, a behavior many African American men, particularly middle-class black men, seem unwilling to do (C. Franklin, 1992). When African American men ascribe to the larger society's definition of masculinity, "many traits thought to be essential for the development of close friendships are lost" (p. 209). Consequently, ignoring this strong social taboo meant that Henry was willing to risk his masculine image of independence and self-sufficiency for the opportunity to receive emotional support from another man.

Henry's experience with the disease ultimately forced him to learn more about its etiology and psychosocial consequences. To some extent, Henry's knowledge and perception of prostate cancer are not that different from views held by other men. However, a significant number of African American men, particularly lower socioeconomic males, are only vaguely aware of prostate cancer and its warning signs (Berman & Wandersman, 1990). For example, Price, Colvin, and Smith (1993) examined the perceptions of 290 African American males, ages 38 to 78, about prostate cancer and found a tremendous gap in the subjects' knowledge of the disease. The authors note that many of their subjects could not recognize any warning signs of prostate cancer, and about 60% did not know they were more vulnerable than White men to contracting the disease. With findings like these, it is not surprising that so many African American men at diagnosis "have a lower proportion of local stage disease and a higher proportion of distant stage prostate cancer compared with white males" (Targonski, Guinan, & Phillips, 1991). Unfortunately, a late diagnosis indicates that the cancer has probably metastasized (spread to other parts of the body) and progressed to a higher level, making the disease more difficult to control and therefore more life-threatening. In this regard, Henry's reasons for sharing his story seem important. In Henry's words,

> Sharing my experience actually evokes some relief, beyond that, someone may benefit from reading this and that is worth the pain of telling my story. I hope that my talking about experiences will motivate men, particularly black men 40 and over, to be more proactive about the status of their health and thereby reduce their vulnerability to this deadly disease. Without question, becoming more assertive about one's health could spell the difference between successfully surviving prostate cancer and a more morbid outcome.

This chapter is arranged in four sections. The first section presents a brief overview of prostate cancer, the second section is Henry's story, the third section addresses treatment issues that emerge from Henry's story, and the fourth section outlines a number of recommendations for further research and practice.

THE PROBLEM

Cancer, regardless of the site, is a dreadful disease that affects every aspect of a person's life. According to Berman and Wandersman (1990), "the fear of cancer in the general population is probably more widespread and threatening than other nosophobias" (p. 85). In part, the perceived uncontrollability of cancer, plus the sense of fatalism usually associated with contracting the disease, account for much of the negative attitudes about the disease, they argue. The statistics support public fears: It is estimated that about 1,382,400 new cases of invasive cancer were diagnosed in 1997, and about 560,000 people died from the disease, about 1,500 per day (Parker, Tong, Bolden, & Wingo, 1997).

Prostate cancer, the leading cancer site among men (affecting about one in five) in the United States, accounted for 43% (334,500) of new cases and about 14% (41,800) of cancer deaths in 1997 (Parker et al., 1997). International data on age-adjusted death rates from prostate cancer reflect a similar degree of urgency surrounding this disease. For example, in the United States, between 1990 and 1993, the age-adjusted death rate was 17.5 per 100,000, which ranked 13th among 48 countries. More alarming is that recent data for the United States indicate the incidence of prostate cancer seems to be rising more rapidly among African American men than men from any other racial or ethnic group in the world (Clayton & Byrd, 1993). In fact, when compared to white men, the incidence rate for the disease is 66% higher for African American men (American Cancer Society, 1997), who also are twice as likely as white men to die from the disease; 43.9 per 100,000 vs. 21.1 per 100,000, respectively (Clayton & Byrd, 1993; Freeman, 1990). Even when comparing the total number of cancer deaths with deaths due to prostate cancer across five ethnic/racial groups (African American, Asian/Pacific Islanders, Native Americans, Whites, and Hispanics), racial disparities exist. For example, American Cancer Society (1997) data show that of the total number of cancer deaths of all types among African Americans (59,873) in 1993, 9.4% were due to prostate cancer. During the same period, of all cancer deaths among Asian and Pacific Islanders (6,636), 4.1% died of prostate cancer; among Native Americans (1,491 all cancer deaths), 6.0%; among Whites (461,891 all cancer deaths), 6.2%; and among Hispanics (15,743 all cancer deaths), 6.0%.

Studies by Gambert (1992), Littrup, Lee, and Mettlin (1992) show that early diagnosis and treatment of cancer correlate highly with a greater probability of surviving. Only a small number of African American men, particularly men from less fortunate circumstances, are diagnosed at an early stage when the prognosis for surviving the disease is more favorable. Because many African American men are only vaguely aware of cancer or its warning signs (Berman & Wandersman, 1990), it is not surprising that, at diagnosis, they are less likely to have local stage disease and more likely to have distant stage prostate cancer, compared with white males (Targonski et al., 1991). The intense fear people have about the disease to some degree explains the view that what you don't know won't hurt you (Berman & Wandersman, 1990). But a more advanced stage of the disease at diagnosis increases the likelihood that the disease has metastasized and is therefore more difficult to control. Of the 34,865 men who died of prostate cancer in 1993, about 8% were men 55 to 74 years of age, and 22% were men 75 years of age and older. Obviously, age and economic status are strong determinants of who survives prostate cancer. Braus (1996) notes that "state death records show that a disproportionate share of deaths due to prostate cancer occur among rural," older, politically powerless black men "who are less likely to visit a doctor in time to receive effective treatment" (p. 39).

Advances in cancer prevention, early detection, and improved treatment techniques have made it possible for more and more men to survive prostate cancer. Yet, a closer inspection of the data reveals that our so-called War on Cancer is not having the same positive impact on African American men that it has with other men. As long as African American men remain unaware of specific warning signs of prostate cancer: frequent urination; difficulty starting or holding urine; painful or burning urination and ejaculation; blood in the urine or semen; frequent pain in the hips, lower back, and upper thighs; and swollen lymph glands—and delay accessing effective treatment for the disease, the number of deaths will continue to rise.

HENRY'S EXPERIENCE

The Diagnosis and Decisions

In April 1992, a few weeks after completing my annual physical exam, I received the surprising news that I had prostate cancer. My blood workup revealed an elevated prostate-specific antigen (PSA), and the results of the digital rectal exam (DGR), ultrasound, and biopsy came back positive indicating the presence of cancer. Additional tests confirmed the diagnosis. No words could ever describe the mix of emotions I experienced. I was angry because this terrible disease could ruin my future and possibly take my life. I was frightened because I knew so little about prostate cancer, and at that point, there was little I could do to change the course of things. Besides, I thought only older men had to worry about contracting the disease. I also dreaded the idea of having to share the news with my family. Knowing that cancer, even cancer patients, frightens many people, there was no way I could predict their response to the news, and I did not want to hurt or be hurt by my own family. I was also very embarrassed about the diagnosis, mainly because the disease is known to cause impotence, and I had negative thoughts about having to deal with any aspect of my sexual dysfunction. I also realized that whatever the outcome, I would probably face it alone. Long ago, my spouse and I had given up on trying to share intimate fears and uncertainties. So, I figured, facing cancer would be no different. So, like many men, I was really naive about prostate cancer and its treatment. But why me?

The meetings with my internists and urologist, plus going through the required diagnostic tests, were isolating, totally overwhelming, and extremely frightening. Waiting for the next test was nerve racking because I sat for long periods of time. Afraid to talk, but wondering if my condition was any worse than the person sitting next to me. Numerous times I could feel myself giving in to fatalism and hopelessness, which often accompany a diagnosis of cancer. I tried to stay focused on my family and work, but it was extremely difficult to do. It was like being in a perpetual daze and nothing seemed to matter anymore. Eventually, I realized that I needed someone with whom I could share my frustrations and fears, someone who could be objective, nonjudgmental and sensitive to the fears of men. So I reached out to a long-time buddy whom I knew rather well, and who seemed really genuine and honest about people and their circumstances. Initally, our discussions and interactions were quite superficial and awkward. I really hated being this vulnerable in front of another man, particularly when discussing sexual issues. But as time progressed, our friendship became an invaluable factor in my ability to cope with the knowledge that I had cancer. So, regardless of the hour, what he was doing, or the focus of our discussion, my friend always took the time to listen.

I finally shared the news with my wife and our respective extended families. In their own way, they expressed their concern and encouragement and wished me well. In particular, my mom who "prayed on it" said that "God" would bring me through this. I'm not sure what my wife felt.

Surgery and Rehabilitation

Of the various treatment options (surgery [radical prostatectomy], external beam radiation, watchful waiting, cryosurgery [freezing the prostate gland], and hormonal therapy), I chose surgery. Although all treatments seemed terribly invasive, surgery appeared to offer the best long-term results. The surgery took place on June 10, about 2 months after the diagnosis. I was in surgery about 5 hours, and I can still feel the excruciating pain in my stomach. Except for the stomach pain and the struggle to cope with a catheter, my week in the hospital went well. My buddy either called or stopped by to monitor my progress and give encouragement, and for this and all the help he provided, I will always be grateful.

Once home, my convalescence was not smooth at all. I developed an abscess in my stomach that sent me back to the hospital. The abscess was the size of a grapefruit and caused all sorts of difficulties with my bladder. Because I had difficulty controlling my urine, I learned about incontinence, which, at times, caused problems and considerable embarrassment. I miscalculated once and wet on myself—a really devastating experience. I also developed a severe bladder infection that required learning how to catheterize myself.

Another difficulty I faced was accepting my new sexual self. My family composition has changed since my diagnosis almost 5 years ago. So starting over again in an intimate relationship is frightening. Given the impact of the surgery on my sexuality, I often questioned my self-worth and capacity to engage in an intimate relationship. Once I tried talking to my brothers about the problem, but as it usually is with men, it was easier for the guys to chat about their sexual exploits rather than sexual difficulties. My long-time buddy seemed to be the only male who would listen, not judge my capabilities, but give advice. I know that recovering from prostate surgery takes time (6 months to several years), but I must accept the fact that in all likelihood, my sexuality will never be the same as prior to my surgery. Being somewhat traditional, I had to be convinced that sexual pleasure and gratification goes beyond one's ability to achieve an erection. Trying to incorporate the essence of my friend's advice into my thinking is one of the most difficult challenges I have faced.

INTERVENTIONS

While every man's experience with prostate cancer is different, most men feel overwhelmed and confused by the disease and all it implies (Blum, 1990). Several themes in Henry's story reflect some of this dismay and confusion, and, if addressed, interventions with African American men might improve. If these issues go unanswered, they have the potential to undermine interventions at any level and stage of development (Blum, 1990). First, macrolevel concerns that directly or indirectly affect the vulnerability of African American men to prostate cancer are presented. These include (a) ways to educate African American men about prostate cancer, (b) ways to target and support participation of African American men in PSA screening, and (c) ways to advocate for better service delivery for African American prostate cancer patients. Second, microlevel concerns are presented. These include (a) communication issues and (b) self-esteem/sexuality concerns.

Macro Interventions

Education

Because prostate cancer is a male-only disease, each man must assume individual responsibility for educating himself about prostate cancer. This includes knowledge about prevention and the course and consequences of the disease. Most important is the need for African American men, particularly those age 40 and older, to become more knowledgeable about and sensitive to symptoms of prostate cancer. Making a commitment to have an annual physical exam, including a PSA test, is critically important. For example, Henry's vigilance and commitment to having an annual physical actually paid off, in that his cancer was detected at an early stage when survival is more likely. Effective efforts to reach men about this sensitive topic require considerable patience. Reaching out to black men, particularly low income men, will be difficult and time consuming. Thus, staff expectations must be in sync with the realities of clients' situations to prevent unnecessary delays.

Key organizations at local, state, and national levels should also assume responsibility for reaching out to educate vulnerable men. In light of the vulnerability of these men, organizations should educate and train their staff about circumstances of African American men and this disease. For example, staff cannot assume that all black men are aware of and understand their susceptibility to prostate cancer. Despite Henry's numerous visits to his internist and urologist, he was only slightly knowledgeable about his vulnerability to this disease. He did not know, for example, that black men in their 60s were 30% to 40% more likely than a white man of similar age to contract prostate cancer, nor did he realize that black men were twice as likely as white men to die from the disease (Clayton & Byrd, 1993). In addition, Henry was completely naive about the emotional and financial cost of this disease to himself and his family. Throughout the experience, Henry recalled very few instances when a helping professional actually inquired about his ability to effectively cope with the disease. According to Henry, "after the surgery, they left me alone." Why? It is clear that men recovering from prostate cancer need time to heal emotionally as well as physically, and health care professionals can facilitate this healing by using a more holistic approach to patient recovery and rehabilitation.

Another organizational responsibility is the need to reassess the costs involved in treating patients with prostate cancer. Because a significant number of black men are among the 37 million Americans who either are underinsured or lack any form of insurance, this disease is connected to their inability to afford the cost of treatment. Although the American Cancer Society (1994) recommends early detection, financial costs prohibit many African American men from accessing and receiving quality care. For example, the cost of Henry's surgery and associated medical services exceeded $12,000, all of which was covered by his insurance. Expenses like this prevent too many African American men from receiving proper medical care. As a result, many black men may ignore critical warning signs and end up having a disease that has spread to other parts of their body. The combined effect of this dilemma and the ever-changing status of welfare reform on health services to lower socioeconomic men suggests that controlling costs would allow the opportunity for more men with the disease to be treated in well-equipped hospitals with skilled physicians. This clearly calls for more cooperative/collaborative relationships between public and private health care systems. Joint ventures like this have the advantage of spreading cost and workload and demonstrating a more visible commitment to the community and its residents.

Screening Issues

It is not surprising that although prostate cancer disproportionately affects African American males, few African American men actually participate in screening opportunities. Debates about the merit of screening are confusing because they reflect a range of opinions about the advantages or disadvantages of engaging in screening opportunities for both white and black participants. For example, a 1995 study examined prior screening behaviors of a stratified sample of 1,504 men, 20% of whom were African American (and 80% white Americans; Demark-Wahnefried et al., 1995). Respondents were asked questions about why some black men resist participating in screening events. Results show that (a) black men, more than white men, resist participating in screening because they view the illness as a death sentence, and (b) fewer physicians were willing to refer black patients. Interestingly however, only slightly more than one third (35%) of black patients had no regular physician. Most surprising was that only 28% of each racial group reported having talked with their doctor about screening. Perhaps this lack of input from physicians explains in part why black respondents were significantly less likely than whites to agree that men with prostate cancer could lead normal lives (62% vs. 72%, respectively). As the authors note, "these perceptions may constitute barriers to screening, which will have to be overcome if participation by blacks in prostate cancer screening is to be accomplished" (p. 350). Drawing on Rabin's (1994) work, the following points should be considered when developing strategies to increase participation of African American men in screening events:

- Make an effort to understand the cultural values and media behaviors of African American males in the targeted area, but be sure to stay away from stereotypes.

- Be sure to choose the right message and use culturally specific methods of communication.

- Be sure to talk "to" rather than "at" potential participants.

- Develop the approach from solid research rather than through stereotypical perceptions of what African American males must be like.

- Use high-profile individuals and specialized mass media approaches to get the message out to African American males.

- Develop the approach so that it appeals to multiple senses.

- Remember, some cultures respond to oral traditions, whereas others are more comfortable with written words.

- Get permission to relay sensitive messages to your group.

Stoy, Curtis, and Dameworth, (1995) suggest that church-based rather than media-based screening strategies worked best in their efforts to increase participation of African Americans in a cholesterol-reduction program for seniors. Their success clearly underscores the pivotal role churches play in

African American communities. The authors note, however, that the approach requires considerable time, resources, and knowledge of the identified community, its residents, and their problems.

Advocacy

Successful intervention on behalf of African American prostate cancer patients will depend on professional staff's ability to engage in a certain amount of advocacy work. Policymakers and service providers must be informed about the extreme vulnerability of black men to prostate cancer. The debilitating effect of this disease on black men must be brought to the attention of the public. A prime objective of helping professions is to connect people with much needed resources. To accomplish this goal, workers must at times serve as brokers (connecting clients to services), mediators (mediating between clients and the needed resources), and/or advocates (representing, or defending clients). The fact that African American men generally receive culturally irrelevant prevention information about the disease, and often receive a lower quality of health care, suggests that professional roles must become more active. For example, health care professionals should find ways to increase African American males' access to needed social services. This might be done by targeting communities with high concentrations of African American males and then developing and implementing strategies that ensure their participation. Participation is not guaranteed, however. Because of the high mistrust of outsiders in some black communities, it will be essential that all interactions and services be implemented with the highest level of expertise and cultural sensitivity. Service delivery models that do not promote the dignity and self-worth of clients should not be used. In addition, it is important that professional staff evaluate and monitor their own practice to ensure that services are delivered free of stereotypes and unconscious biases.

Micro Intervention

Henry's disclosure about his experience with prostate cancer posed an obvious risk to himself and his family. Yet, Henry felt it was important that he share his story, hoping that other African American men and health care providers would benefit after reading about the complexities of his attempt to cope with the experience. The story reveals a rage of clinical issues that bear on clinical work with prostate cancer patients and their families. Of these, three have been singled out (issues with communication, self-esteem issues, and concerns about sexuality); because they seem to be central to Henry's immediate needs.

Communication Issues

Accurately assessing families after a member has been diagnosed with a life-threatening illness is difficult yet necessary. The task is difficult because families will vary in terms of how the unit, and each member, manages to come to grips with the impact of the illness. If the patient "bears his loss well" (Shapiro, 1993, p. 3), quickly attempts to resume normal activities, makes few demands (particularly emotional demands) or tries not to disconcert others, the patient is presumed to be coping successfully with illness and its attending problems (Shapiro, 1993). Through the assessment process, professionals are able to determine whether or not patients or their families are indeed able to adjust to the dynamics of the illness. Under ideal circumstances, if the patient bears the illness well, and family members are able to communicate openly and honestly about the illness and its impact, the adjustment will be less difficult for patients and their families. Conversely, if family members are unable to communicate with each other about the illness and its impact, the adjustment (the patient's and the family's) will be more problematic and require more time. To understand and respond effectively to each family's unique style of communicating, professionals must often suspend advice giving in exchange for active listening, so that they fully comprehend each member's views, feelings, and experiences with the illness. Professionals will need to assess feelings of fear, anger, remorse, and hope and determine how each family member expresses the struggle to incorporate these feelings into his or her life experiences. For example, the inability to communicate was clearly a problem in Henry's family. Despite his fear and anguish about his condition, he consciously chose not to share the information with his wife or children. He actually anticipated that if he had shared the information, he would not receive the support he wanted and needed from them. Understandably, Henry was terribly frightened by the diagnosis, afraid of the unknown, and like other men, he anticipated the worst. He had no idea what would happen to his family, his job, or his friends. But Henry's fear of the unknown and subsequent withdrawal from his family played a significant role in silencing rather than opening up channels of communication within his family. Instead, Henry sought advice and understanding from a friend.

Professional intervention with Henry should first acknowledge and respect Henry's feelings. Beyond this, interventions should focus on helping Henry identify and express his needs "clearly and assertively to other family members" (Shapiro, 1993, p. 234). Additional work should not ignore the impact of the social context on health beliefs and behaviors. As Sussman (1996) noted, the way decisions are made about how and where to seek care occur within a medical belief system that emerges from the cultural context of the patient, and the way medical symptoms are presented can affect these decisions. This means professionals must be aware of the potential harm that may result when the patient's communication style is different from the worker's. As an African American man, Henry might interpret and respond to his illness quite differently than a white man. Adding this important dimension to the assessment process will require professionals to spend time educating themselves about the health beliefs of African American families, including how these beliefs influence every step of the "health-seeking and maintenance process" (Sussman, 1996, p. 485).

It is important for professionals to keep in mind that children of the critically ill person are often neglected despite their fear and anxieties over their parent's illness. Because of the transgenerational effect of this disease, sons of prostate cancer patients are in need of prevention information. However, in many situations, children are left alone or must turn to a relative to interpret the meaning and implications of their parent having prostate cancer. Professionals should encourage families to bring children into conversations about the cancer and its impact. This applies to African American men who will need help finding ways to tell their sons that they are prime candidates for an illness that may, at some point in their lives, render them impotent. Asking questions about the well-being of children is extremely important. Also, referring parents and their children to a support group may work. However, professionals need to know that minorities typically shy away from support group formats. If the support group is provided through the church, participation may be more attractive.

Self-Esteem/Sexuality Issues

Pearson (1994) recently wrote, "The black male in today's society continues to be at risk on a variety of important sociocultural and health issues, which impact negatively on his life, and on the lives of his family, friends, and the community" (p. 81). Over a decade ago, Staples (1982) wrote,

It is difficult to think of a more controversial role in American society than that of the black male . . . he is a visible figure on the American scene, yet the least understood and studied of all sex-race groups in the United States. (p. 1)

It is frightening that attitudes and perceptions of African American men change very little over time. Thus, black men are confronted with attitudes describing them as lazy, irresponsible, inarticulate, sexually promiscuous, and predictably dangerous. As a result, the therapeutic context in which white therapists interact with black male patients is often constrained by these perceptions, which generate mutual misunderstanding and distrust. Because of this dynamic interplay of perceptions, professionals need to develop skills that convey and create a climate of trust and positive regard. To do this, professionals must see the therapeutic value in allowing black male patients the opportunity to tell their story. This means encouraging patients to share their experience of being ill and how the illness affected their perceptions of what it means to be a black man in this society and what it means to be a husband, father, and worker in a society that seems indifferent to their existence. Using appropriate probes, active listening, and sensitive attending skills, professionals will be able to convey a sense of openness, acceptance, and trust. During this exchange, the professional has an opportunity to examine how and to what degree self-esteem issues figure into the patient's coping strategies, strengths and weaknesses, and the ability to ask for support through his new challenges.

Another treatment consideration worth noting is addressing the question of resuming intimate relationships. Professionals should be prepared to deal with uncertainty, embarrassment, and humiliation. Because some men withdraw during their ordeal with prostate cancer, it is important that professionals attempt to identify individuals within the patient's support system who can help facilitate rebuilding the patient's sense of self-worth. For men who have significant others in their lives, professionals should involve these partners in discussions about how the illness affected their lives and how open and supportive they (the partners) would be to new ways of accomplishing intimate contact. The loss of intimacy affects self-confidence. Thus, focusing on feelings of intimidation and rejection should gradually improve the patient's positive feelings about himself. Although men's support groups offer an excellent opportunity to work on these issues, professionals need to be aware that black men are slow to engage in this type of therapeutic format. Perhaps a smaller, more carefully screened gathering of men would afford black men a more caring and less threatening environment in which to share their experiences. Considering the assault to one's sexuality that occurs after a medical intervention for prostate cancer, any number of the above factors may be evident in the patient's life. Nonetheless, professionals should stress the importance of (a) participating with their partners in couples counseling to uncover feelings that obstruct intimacy; (b) becoming familiar with community resources, such as churches, mental health clinics, or self-help groups that can be used to help individuals and couples sort out ways to achieve their desired level of intimacy; and (c) recognizing the limits of outside interventions. In other words, if the offer of help is not accepted, the professional is obligated to accept that decision.

Professionals should remember that a major contributor to a diminished sense of self-esteem in many men is the impairment of their sexuality and the presumed image the condition projects. Acknowledging publicly that one is being treated for prostate cancer informs everyone that the patient has dealt with incontinence, impaired sexuality, or impotence—the inability to achieve and sustain an erection sufficient to engage in intercourse. Data suggest that the probability of impotence occurring in survivors will vary between a low of 50% (those diagnosed at a younger age) to a high of 90% in men treated by either radical prostatectomy or external beam radiation (Lewis, 1994). Professionals addressing this issue should obtain as much information about the problem as possible; particularly how African American men perceive and deal with this condition. Unfortunately, sexual stereotypes about African American men still exist, and professionals must guard against their use. Nonetheless, patients must be helped to accept and become comfortable with their new sexuality before they can expect others to accept them. This concept is key to reshaping the sexual lives of prostate cancer survivors. Here, professionals will need to help patients and their partners talk about new ways to achieve sexual pleasure. This will require open and honest communication. Helping patients learn to overcome fear of failure and embarrassment is an issue that professionals cannot overlook. Moreover, working collaboratively with the patient's urologist is a must.

A number of devices (noninvasive or invasive) are available to men who seek help for their erectile problem. Specifically, their purpose is to make the penis rigid enough to engage in sexual intercourse, but again, professionals should insist on the inclusion of partners in selecting a device most appropriate for the couple. Noninvasive techniques work on the principal that an erection occurs when the penis is placed in a vacuum pump which forces blood into the penis, thus creating an erection. To sustain the erection, a constricting band, which should not be worn more than 30 minutes, is placed over the penis down to its base. Obviously, there is nothing spontaneous about using this device, and questions such as where to have sex and how often are issues professionals must help couples address. Invasive techniques used to create and sustain an erection include self-injections and penile implants. The self-injection method involves injecting an appropriate amount of papaverine hydrochloride into the neck of the penis. An erection occurs shortly after the shot, which is simple to perform and usually painless. An erection is maintained from 1 to 3 hours and can be repeated in 24 hours. However, each patient must experiment to determine how much of the drug is appropriate for him. If the dose is too strong (which causes considerable pain) or too low (an erection does not occur), their purpose is defeated, which can lead to frustration and further questions about self-esteem from the patient and his partner. The penile implant is a "technique whereby a prosthesis is surgically implanted within the penis resulting in an erection sufficiently rigid to engage in sexual intercourse" (Lewis, 1994, p. 181). Lewis notes that while it may be effective in helping patients regain an acceptable level of sexuality "their safety has recently come into question" (p. 181). Unfortunately, there is a dearth of solid data describing partner satisfaction with any of these devices. Hence, professionals are encouraged to work collaboratively with the patient, his partner, and his urologist. Yet, professionals can be very supportive in helping men and their partners understand that although these devices may serve their purpose, sexual pleasure and gratification can be achieved through means other than an erect penis. However, the decision to engage in the excitement and benefits that derive from exploring other facets of one's sexuality, in safe trusting relationships, is left up to patients and their partners to decide.

RECOMMENDATIONS

Engaging African American men in treatment is not easy. However, when these men are available and psychosocial services are indicated, health professionals need to consider the following recommendations:

1. Professionals must be knowledgeable about prostate cancer, theory and practice, and its consequences. This includes knowledge about the racial disparities in screening, as well as the incidence, survival, and mortality rates of the disease among African American men.

2. Professionals should avoid stereotyping African American men. This means professionals should take time to sort out fact from fiction about these men.

3. Because of the class variations among African Americans, interventions must be tailored to fit the specific context (community/neighborhood) in which services are offered. In other words, health workers need to understand that African Americans are not a monolithic group: Health beliefs and behaviors will vary greatly among African American men and within their families. For example, interventions for black middle-class men may differ considerably from models developed for more disadvantaged black men.

4. Focusing treatment interventions on families of patients provides valuable clues about coping styles and patterns of behaviors that may negatively influence plans to resolve stress or hinder prescribed medical regimes.

5. The religiosity of African Americans cannot be overlooked. A critical illness is often viewed as God's punishment for a transgression (Landrine & Klonoff, 1992; Sussman, 1996). Therefore, the course and outcome of the illness are not changed by medical interventions but through the hand and will of God. This is a common perspective in many African American communities, and professionals must learn to understand and respect its importance in the life experiences of families of men surviving prostate cancer.

6. Professionals should understand the importance of extended families and determine collaboratively how members might be used during the patient's recuperation.

7. Professionals must evaluate the impact of an illness on the attitudes and behaviors of children.

All families, regardless of race or ethnicity, dread the thought of prostate cancer. Yet, patients can be helped to understand that being diagnosed with the disease does not have to be a death sentence. Good medical care combined with skillfully delivered psychosocial interventions will go a long way in helping patients develop a hopeful and healthier outlook on life.

CHAPTER 7

Working With African American Males With Diabetes

LEO E. HENDRICKS

Despite numerous and piercing cries to stem the rising tide of diabetes and its complications in African Americans, efforts to document strategies to assist practitioners in working with this population group have been few (National Diabetes Information Clearinghouse [NDIC], 1990; U.S. Department of Health and Human Services, 1989). Suggestions on how to work with African American males with diabetes have been rarer. Therefore, it is no small wonder that nagging discomfort on the part of health care workers has been noted in their attempts to address the diabetes problem, which Dr. James R. Gavin III, chair of the American Diabetes Association's African American Program, has said is "ravaging the black population" (NDIC, 1989). This uneasiness has stemmed, in part, from such unanswered questions as: Why is diabetes on the increase among African American men? Why are African American men often fatalistic about diabetes and its complications? What things motivate African American men to adhere to their diabetes treatment regimen? What skills are necessary for a clinician to have in working with African American males with diabetes?

As a first step toward answering these questions, and to quell the compelling pleas to stem the increase of diabetes and its complications among African American men, this chapter suggests a practical guide for working

AUTHOR'S NOTE: I want to thank my God for His Grace, through Jesus Christ my Lord, and my lovely wife of 34 years for their invaluable assistance in writing this chapter.

with them. In setting forth this guide, I draw on existing literature, clinical experience, and anecdotal accounts of practitioners working with African American males with diabetes. Because of the misunderstanding that sometimes exist as to what diabetes is, it is important that practitioners know the commonly accepted definition when working with African American males with diabetes.

WHAT IS DIABETES?

Diabetes mellitus, commonly referred to by many African American males as "sugar," comprises a heterogeneous group of disorders characterized by high blood sugar levels. Diabetes occurs when the body cannot properly metabolize carbohydrates, fats, and proteins, resulting in abnormally high levels of glucose in the blood. Diabetes is a chronic disease that may develop slowly or as an acute metabolic crisis. Four major types have been defined by the National Diabetes Data Group (NDDG) and World Health Organization (WHO) (Harris, 1995). However, for purposes of this chapter only two types are considered: insulin-dependent diabetes mellitus (IDDM) and non-insulin-dependent diabetes mellitus (NIDDM). Insulin-dependent diabetes mellitus, or Type I diabetes, is less common than NIDDM and usually develops in children and young adults. People with IDDM must have daily insulin injections to sustain life. (Santiago, 1994; U.S. Department of Health & Human Services, 1986).

Unless an African American male is diagnosed and receives proper treatment, his diabetes can be an overwhelmingly serious disease. For example, African Americans experience higher rates of at least three of the serious complications of diabetes: blindness, amputations, and end-stage renal disease (ESRD). Rates of severe visual impairment are 40% higher in African American patients with diabetes than in white patients. Compared to whites, African American men have 30% higher rates of blindness. African Americans with diabetes undergo twice as many amputations as do whites, and studies in Michigan and Texas found that the rate of ESRD was at least four times higher in African Americans with diabetes. Moreover, diabetes is now the sixth leading cause of death by disease among African American men (NDIC, 1992).

Diagnostic tests for diabetes are recommended if a patient has a positive screening test or obvious signs and symptoms of diabetes, for example, increased thirst, increased urination, increased hunger, or weight loss. A diagnosis can be made on the basis of a random plasma glucose concentration

TABLE 7.1 Diagnosis of Diabetes

Unequivocal

Fasting plasma glucose (PG) ≥ 126 mg/dL on one separate occasion	or	Random PG ≥ 200 mg/dL plus classic symptoms

Equivocal

Random PG > 200 mg/dL no symptoms	Fasting PG ≥ 110 and < 126 mg/dL
Fasting PG < 126 mg/dL but family history of non-insulin-dependent diabetes mellitus and possible symptoms	

plus signs and symptoms of diabetes, a fasting plasma glucose concentration, or a properly performed oral glucose tolerance test (OGTT) (Raskin, 1994). In African American men, the diagnosis of diabetes mellitus is restricted to those who have the symptoms listed in Table 7.1.

The most common kind of diabetes in African American men is non-insulin-dependent diabetes mellitus, or Type II diabetes (Harris, 1995; Hendricks & Haas, 1991). African American males at highest risk for diabetes include those who

▨ have first-degree relatives with diabetes mellitus

▨ are obese

▨ are older than 40 years of age plus any of the preceding factors

▨ have hypertension or hyperlipidemia

▨ have previously identified impaired glucose tolerance (IGT)—patients with IGT have plasma glucose levels that are higher than normal but not diagnostic for diabetes mellitus (Raskin, 1994)

Moreover, the frequency of diabetes in African American males is influenced by the same factors that are associated with NIDDM in other populations, including obesity, physical inactivity, insulin resistance, and genetic factors (Tull & Roseman, 1995).

In spite of this, Tull and Roseman (1995) point out prevalence of known physician-diagnosed diabetes among African Americans is 3.7% overall, rising from 1.3% at age 0 to 45 years to 17.4% at age 65 to 74 years. What is more, the rate of diabetes in African Americans has tripled during the past 30 years. Prevalence of diagnosed diabetes in adults is now 1.4 times as frequent in African Americans as in whites. This excess occurs for both African American women and men. Added to this irksome state of affairs, Gavin (1996) notes, African Americans often display a fatalistic attitude about diabetes, seeming to believe there is nothing they can do about it.

Why this attitude? In part, the answer may be lack of optimum treatment strategies for the complications of diabetes and lack of educational resources that are relevant to concerns of African American males and their lifestyles (NDIC, 1989); there is also a lack of awareness among physicians and other health care providers that diabetes is a serious disease, especially for African American men. Furthermore, clinical experience reveals a number of African American men may have this attitude because their doctors have informed them that "no matter what you do, you'll get the complications from diabetes." This picture is clouded further by the fact that half of African American men with diabetes "don't even know that they are seriously ill" (Gavin, 1996). More important, perhaps, this no-helping-it attitude may be accompanied by a lack of education among African American males in modern diabetes self-management techniques (NDIC, 1990). Whatever the reasons, there are no easy answers to why African American men often harbor fatalistic attitudes about diabetes or why diabetes is on the increase among them.

Even so, Lipson et al. (1988) argue that the reason for the increase in diabetes among African American males probably lies in a complex combination of genetic, environmental, and nutritional factors. They state that there is no doubt that certain lifestyle factors are linked with diabetes among African American men. Indeed, African American males who eat a diet high in fats and simple sugars find themselves at greater risk for obesity. Pi-Sunyer (1990) points out, as well, that obesity goes hand in hand with Type II diabetes.

Stress is also important. For poorer African American men, the stress of day-to-day life is great and may worsen blood glucose control or bring on diabetes more quickly in those at risk for the disease (Lipson et al., 1988). Other factors that may be identified with the increase in diabetes prevalence among African American men include lifestyle changes associated with the improving economic conditions of African American males, such as changes in eating habits, levels of physical activity, and patterns of obesity, together with longer life expectancy and increased genetic susceptibility. Nevertheless, little is known about the changes in risk factors or diagnostic methods that may have precipitated the dramatic increase in the prevalence of NIDDM among African American men (Tull & Roseman, 1995).

Amid these speculations and observations, the good news is that treatment for NIDDM or Type II diabetes is much the same among African American men as among all Americans. Health care providers try first to control diabetes with dietary changes, replacing foods high in sugar and fat with lean meats and fresh fruits and vegetables. Men who are obese are urged to lose weight (Lipson et al., 1988). In fact, moderate weight loss (10 to 20 pounds), whatever the starting weight, has been shown to reduce high blood-sugar levels, high blood pressure, and dyslipidemia (Watts et al., 1990; Wing et al., 1987). For many African American males, this treatment is successful (Franz, 1994; Lipson et al., 1988).

However, many African American males have more difficulty changing eating habits, and their health care providers are often not successful in helping their patients to lose weight. If changing diet is difficult, reducing stress is almost impossible for some African American men. These matters are compounded by the few physical fitness resources available to African American males who live and exercise in urban areas. In some areas, it may be difficult or even dangerous to go outside and exercise, especially in poorer communities. Moreover, men who have other health problems, such as high blood pressure or diabetic nerve or eye damage, may not know how to exercise safely. When diet and exercise fail to control diabetes among African American men, oral agents or insulin may be added to the treatment regimen. Unfortunately, many African American men with diabetes do not receive education necessary to convince them of the value of their medication (Lipson et al., 1988).

Other factors in addition to inadequate diabetes self-management education can interfere with care. Poverty or limited education can make it difficult for African American men to follow a diabetic meal plan or to buy diabetes pills or insulin (Lipson et al., 1988). Also, the literature and clinical experience have shown some of the existing barriers to diabetes care for African American male include

▨ the cost of diabetes care and supplies

▨ the complexity of the diabetes treatment regimen

▨ the lack of understanding of diabetes food exchange list

▨ the lack of involvement in deciding diabetes educational goals and outcomes (Hendricks & Hendricks, 1994)

In addition, Anderson et al. (1991) have pointed out that potential barriers to improved health care and health for African American men with diabetes include racism, lack of knowledge, incorrect beliefs, lack of access to health care, differing cultural values and priorities, and poverty. Given this host of problems facing African American males with diabetes, what is a practitioner to do?

MEETING THE CHALLENGE OF DIABETES AMONG AFRICAN AMERICAN MEN

An initial step for health care providers concerned about working with African American males with diabetes is to obtain knowledge and understanding of how diabetes affects their lives and of their needs as people with diabetes mellitus. The second step is for practitioners to acquire diabetes wisdom, forming and maintaining a viable relationship with African American men with diabetes.

Inherent in effective use of diabetes wisdom is the ability of health care providers to apply their knowledge of diabetes to the specific beliefs, experiences, food patterns, and health care practices of a given African American male to help him formulate a practical and beneficial treatment regimen for himself. In short, efficacious treatment of African American males with diabetes requires practical application of sensitivity to and recognition of their unique cultural values and needs (Raymond & D'Eramo-Melkus, 1993). Culturally sensitive diabetes care can foster empowerment by enabling African American men with diabetes to take care of their health through the recognition and promotion of individual strengths and personal goals (Anderson et al., 1991).

Practitioners should be aware of a major strength of African American men: their religious conviction. Whether they are active or passive in their religious practice, most African American males seem to be influenced by some moral or religious upbringing. Thus, a practitioner may use their susceptibility to religious influence to help them solve assorted problems related to management of their diabetes. A workable approach is to ask the patient, "Who will you turn to for help in managing your diabetes?" Their response, not infrequently, may be summed up in the reply, "Since there is no cure, only God can help me. My friends try to help, but they don't understand." A follow-up question to this reply would be along the lines of, "How do you think God will help you with your diabetes?" Depending on the patient's response, a practitioner will tailor his or her assistance to the patient's lifestyle and religious orientation.

Optimal self-management of diabetes for the African American male will require his changing some existing behaviors as well as adopting new ones. A successful program for behavior change requires comprehensive patient education, skill development, and motivation. This is best accomplished through a team effort. Physicians, dietitians, nurses, social workers, and other professionals—that is, the health care team—should use their expertise to design a therapeutic regimen that encourages active patient participation in achieving the best blood sugar control possible (Raskin, 1994).

The knowledge and skills necessary to implement a diabetes treatment regimen for an African American male cannot be acquired during a single brief encounter on the day of diagnosis or during a short series of diabetes self-management skills training classes. Change occurs gradually over time and generally occurs in small increments. It is not uncommon for African American men with diabetes to experience periodic setbacks when motivation wanes and barriers to implementing a behavior interfere with self-management of diabetes. This is when the African American male benefits from the experience and availability of a multidisciplinary health care team, which can provide not only specific problem-solving skills but also necessary support from clinicians who genuinely care about him (Raskin, 1994).

The literature suggests that African American men with diabetes need not just a clinician-patient relationship but an amiable sustained partnership with their health care provider (Leopold, Cooper, & Clancy, 1996; Lipson et al., 1988). A sustained partnership facilitates tailoring a specific intervention or specific advice to the needs and circumstances of a particular African American male with diabetes. In this relationship, the clinician knows not just the patient's medical history, but his personal history and family, work, community, and cultural context, as well as his preferences, values, beliefs, and ideals about health care, including preferences for information and participation in clinical decision making. The clinician expresses humaneness toward the patient through such qualities as interest, concern, compassion, sympathy, empathy, attentiveness, sensitivity, and consideration (Leopold et al., 1996). If optimal diabetes control and subsequent improvements in an African American male's health outcomes are to occur, a health care provider must engage himself or herself in this kind of clinician-patient relationship.

WHAT MOTIVATES AFRICAN AMERICAN MEN TO ADHERE TO THEIR DIABETES TREATMENT REGIMEN

Yet, one to the most formidable tasks for practitioners working with African American males with diabetes is patient nonadherence, which results from a lack of understanding, lack of reinforcement, and wavering commitment to the treatment plan (Stolar, 1995). Strategies to improve and maintain adherence can take many forms. Clinicians need to be sensitive to factors that influence whether a patient is ready and willing to make changes and then devise a plan to facilitate the desired change. The behavior change process is similar to the education process and involves assessment, planning, implementation, documentation, and evaluation (Raskin, 1994).

Increased motivation for African American men to adhere to their diabetes treatment regimen is enhanced when a practitioner is genuinely caring and is skilled in helping a patient, in his own way, to identify some altruistic reason for adhering to his diabetes regimen; is able to tell the patient what's in it for him, in a way that is real to him, if he sticks to his diabetes regimen; and has the wherewithal to communicate with the patient one or more times a week concerning his diabetes (see Table 7.2).

WHAT CLINICAL EXPERIENCE HAS TAUGHT

Health care workers who meet the challenge of working with African American men with diabetes will need to take into consideration what has been learned through clinical experience. Clinical work has shown the way to get off on the right foot in building a viable working diabetes relationship with African American men is to give them a working definition of diabetes that fits their frame of reference. They need to know what diabetes is. The clinician must tell them how they got this disease. They want to know who or what is responsible for their diabetes.

In a like manner, they want to know what is going to happen to them, as far as the diabetes is concerned. They want to know about the complications associated with diabetes. Invariably, they ask, "Am I going to lose my legs?" This question is often followed by the question, "Am I going to lose my eyes?"

Many African American men with diabetes have the fear of injecting insulin, too. They do not want to stick themselves. However, when the health care practitioner does a demonstration of injecting insulin and has the patient to do a return demonstration, this tends to alleviate the patient's fear. In addition to fear of "the needle," many African American males with diabetes have a manifest fear of experiencing a low blood sugar reaction. People who have low blood sugar reactions experience any number of adverse events, for example, crabbiness, light-headedness, trembling, slurred speech, and confusion ("Diabetes in the Elderly," 1994). Sometimes, they have such bad

TABLE 7.2 Principal Ingredients That Contribute to African American Men's Motivation to Adhere to Their Diabetes Treatment Regimen

Care and Concern†	Altruistic Reason(s)	What's in It for the Patient	Frequent Patient Communication
Caring concern on the part of the practitioner for the patient and his diabetes.	Practitioner skilled in helping patient to identify some altruistic reason(s) for adhering to his diabetes treatment regimen (e.g., spouse, grandchildren, people who depend on him, his place of worship). It is crucial that a patient identify some reason(s) other than his own welfare for maintaining adherence to his diabetes treatment regimen. It is important for the patient's self-esteem to feel needed by some one else.	Practitioner telling the patient "what's in it for him," personally, if he were to be consistent in adhering to his diabetes regimen. If the patient is able to perceive some immediate benefit—if he functions better and has better mental health—he is much more likely to adhere to his diabetes regimen as negotiated with his health care provider.	Practitioner's wherewithal to communicate with the patient one or more times a week. The Diabetes Control and Complications Trial (DCCT, 1993) found that intensive patient follow-up contributed to improved metabolic control.

†Care and Concern + Altruistic Reason(s) + What's in It for the Patient + Frequent Patient Communication = Increased Patient's Motivation to Adhere to His Diabetes Treatment Regimen.

reactions they pass out. When educated about the causes, signs, symptoms, treatment, and prevention of low blood sugars, patients tend to be less fearful.

Another chief concern of African American men with diabetes, observed through clinical experience, is impotence or erectile dysfunction (Ackerman, Montague, & Morganstern, 1994; Silverberg, 1989). Patients want to know what can be done for it. Moreover, they may have depression or anxiety along with their impotence because they have not been able to talk openly with anyone about their erectile dysfunction. African American men are aided immensely in coming to grips with their impotence by practitioners who educate them about the disorder and its treatment, adjusting the amount and complexity of information to the patient's clinical state, being clear about what the patient can expect from treatment and when he can expect it, and encouraging the patient's active participation in the treatment process (Leopold et al., 1996).

Eating, drinking, smoking, and lack of money are problem areas that also contribute to the web of concerns of African American men with diabetes. In attending to these matters, a practitioner must see to it that African American males are educated about proper dietary management and associated risk factors, tell them why they cannot smoke, explain how smoking affects diabetes, and make it known to them that alcohol has no nutritional value. They should know, as well, that alcohol contributes to low blood sugar reactions and high triglyceride levels. In addition, diabetes patients should be informed that alcohol worsens neuropathy and, at the same time, may interfere with their sexual functioning. Not unexpectedly, lack of money contributes to the worries of African American men with diabetes. It is not uncommon for the diabetes clinician to hear them say, " I don't eat right because I can't afford it."

Early in the clinician-patient relationship it is evident that African American men with diabetes need close follow-up regarding their diabetes care. Frequent contacts, either in person or by telephone, one or more times a week, to review goals they have set, discuss problem areas, or talk about their general well-being, contribute in no small way to positive adherence to the diabetes regimen. African American male patients need a social support system.

Why is this true? Because they do not have a lot of support in their homes. A sizable number of African American males seen in the clinical situation do not have family members who are interested in their diabetes. Not unlike others, African American males need and want to have a sense of belonging. They need to feel that someone cares about them. Positive feedback or encouraging words to patients about achieving their diabetes goals is an important way that a health care provider can demonstrate that he or she cares about the African American male who has diabetes.

WHAT AFRICAN AMERICAN MEN WITH DIABETES LOOK FOR IN THE CLINICIAN-PATIENT RELATIONSHIP

In addition to the foregoing, practitioner's characteristics deemed desirable by African American men with diabetes include the following:

◆ Compassion: When African American men sense their health care provider is genuinely concerned and desires to alleviate or solve their diabetes self- management problem, they make positive steps in managing their diabetes more effectively.

◆ Patience: African American males do not like to be rushed; therefore the health care provider who exercises patience with these patients gives these men the time they need to work through some of their defense mechanisms—for example, denial, anger, anxiety, fear, frustration, and helplessness.

◆ Active listening: This means listening that includes giving verbal feedback, questioning, offering suggestions and recommendations, and nodding of the head during the interview or clinic visit. This is another way of letting an African American male know that you are concerned about him and his diabetes. This kind of active listening communicates to the African American man that the practitioner is interested and is there to help.

◆ Knowledge about diabetes and its complications: African American males like to know that their diabetes specialist is a person "in the know" about the latest in diabetes care. Moreover, when an African American male patient has been told that he has a chronic disease that carries with it numerous complications if not managed properly, he wants to know the answers to questions such as, How did it happen? Why me? Did I do anything to cause it? How will it affect my lifestyle? Will it affect my children? Will I be able to work? I lose my job if I have to take insulin; will I have to take insulin? Will I lose my legs like my neighbor who has diabetes? To answer such questions, the health care provider must be knowledgeable about diabetes, the importance of diabetes education and treatment, and the benefits of blood glucose control.

◆ Ability to use the Socratic lecture method in educating patients about diabetes: This means the use of questions, in an exchange with the patient, to get across diabetes information that will empower the patient to take charge of his diabetes.

◆ Cultural sensitivity: To avoid "throwing the baby out with the bath water," the practitioner must be aware of the cultural behaviors that are capable of fitting into the African American male patient's diabetes treatment plan. For example, when it comes to discussing nutritious meal plans, the African American male may be accustomed to eating "soul food." Many of the foods termed soul food are very good sources of high fiber. Therefore, the food itself could very well be included in the meal plan, but perhaps the preparation of the food would need some modification.

◆ Availability and accessibility: The most disturbing comments heard from African American men in treatment for diabetes today are centered around the inability to reach their health care provider by telephone and the limited time spent with them during their scheduled clinic visits. The automated voice mailbox or the secretary may receive the patient's calls, but return calls to the patient are seldom made. When African American men are given an appointment to see their diabetes health care provider, they report that they are rushed through these visits. Thus, when the African American male patient is not given the chance to discuss his diabetes-related problem with his health care provider, the patient feels that he has not been helped, even though he was seen by the practitioner.

Practitioner accessibility is important to African American males with diabetes because they like to call their health care provider. Invariably, patients hear lots of things via the media concerning diabetes, and they will come and ask the practitioner about what they hear in the news expecting that he or she will give them the "low down" on what has been reported concerning diabetes. They like to talk about their diabetes and any other concerns they may have. It is during these kinds of encounters that the most active level of education and support in the behavior change process occurs. Individualized education and problem solving are the keys to successful behavior change for African American men with diabetes. Success in helping African American men maintain their blood glucose levels as close to normal as possible is enhanced when the practitioner is dedicated to facilitating the healing of his body, mind, and spirit, that is to say, when the practitioner responds to the full human person—his emotional, spiritual, intellectual, and physical needs.

Notwithstanding these things, the future role of the practitioner working with African American males is expected to be as a disease manager. Disease management means taking a much more comprehensive approach to all aspects of diabetes care. Disease management is an ongoing, defined approach that begins the moment the African American male is diagnosed with diabetes. The focus is on preventive care: keeping the patient from developing complications and thus reducing health care costs. Disease management requires a much more long-term approach to the cost of treating African American men with diabetes (Stolar, 1995). As a practitioner would assume the role of a disease manager and make use of the practical guidelines set forth in this chapter, the expectation is that he or she will contribute markedly to the reduction or prevention of the devastating complications that may affect African American men with diabetes.

CHAPTER 8

Reducing Risk Taking Among African American Males

STEVEN SCHINKE
KRISTIN COLE
CHRISTOPHER WILLIAMS
GILBERT BOTVIN

The primary prevention of risk-taking behavior among African American male youth in this country continues to challenge practitioners, scientists, and policymakers. Particularly refractory to preventive intervention efforts are risk-taking problems of violence and drug use. Rates of violence and drug use among African American adolescent males are unacceptably high. Indeed, including violent crime, murder, and forcible rape, reported rates of violence among juveniles in this country are at an all-time high. Despite trends toward decreased substance use among teenagers nationwide, significant numbers of youth in America's large urban areas abuse drugs to their and society's detriment. Adolescents from ethnic-racial minority groups are at highest risk for violence and drug use. Although innovative approaches to preventing violence and drug abuse have emerged in recent years, new intervention approaches are needed for African American male youth. Toward discovering such responsive prevention approaches, this chapter discusses a culturally tailored, youth-oriented program aimed at reducing the incidence of violence and drug abuse in a sample of African American male youth.

CURATIVE HYPOTHESES

Because risk taking is associated with disadvantaged circumstances, preventive interventions that target behaviors and life skills without addressing the larger community circumstances are limited. Yet, many African American male youth from poverty-stricken environments avoid risky behaviors altogether. Studies on resiliency in disadvantaged communities suggest that social skills can help protect African American boys from high-risk behavior (Schinke, Botvin, & Orlandi, 1991; Turner, Norman, & Zunz, 1995).

PREVENTIVE INTERVENTION

Clearly, risk-taking prevention intervention must address personal, behavioral, and environmental factors to effect prevention competence in African American male youth. Problem behaviors in adolescence tend to cluster. Moreover, common underlying factors contribute to many problem behaviors in African American male adolescents. For the purposes of this chapter, we have narrowed our focus to violence and substance abuse prevention intervention for African American adolescent males.

An illustrative drug use and violence prevention intervention for African American male adolescents took place in inner-city community-based organizations and included such cognitive-behavioral skills and components as body awareness, self-protective skills and self-efficacy, relaxation, self-assessment, self-instruction, assertion, problem solving, thinking ahead, coping, conflict resolution, social perspective taking, critical viewing, enhancement of social proficiency and resiliency, and social supports for maintaining personal change. Our experience has shown us that recruiting and retaining high-risk youth is facilitated by basing intervention in community-based organizations, rather than in schools. Community programs are typically perceived as more neutral than are schools, and they also have access to youths who do not attend school.

In our past work with African American male youth, we enhanced the cultural specificity of intervention with mythic stories drawn from ancient African culture. We adapted the stories to highlight a particular life skill; skills illustrated in the stories were subsequently related to the youths' contemporary circumstances in skills sessions. The ancient stories ground the skills in a meaningful context for African American boys. Such a context may increase African American male youths' self-esteem, race consciousness, and cultural pride, factors that are associated with minority risk for problem behavior (Szapocznik & Kurtines, 1980).

We also included stories of historical and contemporary African American heroes. These biographies were adapted to highlight how each hero used skills to overcome obstacles. Many of the obstacles in the heroes' biographies (poverty, discrimination) are similar to those faced by inner-city African American male youth today. The biographies also addressed the sense of hopelessness that plagues so many inner-city boys. Each biography serves as an example of positive options to problem behaviors such as substance use and violence. Because the stories also relate how each hero achieved his goals along conventional pathways, the risk factor of alienation from social institutions is concurrently addressed (Kaplan, Martin, Johnston, & Robbins, 1986). Although there is a lack of evidence for using culturally specific biographies in substance use and violence prevention with African American male youth, such stories have been proven effective in the treatment of anxiety symptoms in Hispanic children (Constantino, Malgady, & Rogler, 1990).

A contemporary rap video was produced for intervention. The video portrays two characters and the situations they encounter growing up in the inner city. As they negotiate the situations, the characters model skills from the curriculum. Youths view distinct episodes of the video during intervention sessions; each segment highlights a different skill.

To enhance the cultural sensitivity of the rap video, peer leaders and school personnel helped develop the script. The purpose in using a videotape was to demonstrate intervention skills in an engaging and meaningful style. Positive identification with characters and the contextual relevance of the modeling incident have been identified as important components of successful observational learning. An example of a contextually relevant modeling incident in our video is a scene involving drug dealing. According to the African American peer leaders involved in script development, such a scene was more relevant to youths than a drug-using situation. These perceptions were echoed in a U.S. General Accounting Office (1990) drug education survey, in which students criticized the drug education they received because it did not address the subject of drug selling, a problem they said was as prevalent as drug use itself. The rap video reflects inner-city African American male risk factors by teaching skills within the context of an environment that has easy access to drugs and strong peer influences. Other video segments teach skills to increase positive peer and adult supports.

African American male peer leaders modeled skills in role-plays and assisted adult leaders. Research has identified peer influence as one of the strongest risk factors for majority and minority culture youth substance abuse (Oetting & Beauvais, 1987). Other research has documented the effectiveness of using peer leaders in problem behavior prevention (Botvin, Baker, Dusenbury, Tortu, & Botvin, 1990). Finally, a "life story" component in the intervention allowed subjects an opportunity to record how each skill related to their own lives. The use of life story as a positive coping technique in dealing with adverse life events has clinical support (Borden, 1992).

The following paragraphs describe in greater detail the particular components of the intervention. Each of these components was delivered sequentially, devoting two or three (depending on available time) 40-minute sessions to each component.

Body Awareness. African American male adolescents may better integrate facts about drug use and violence, or other risk-taking behavior, if they have a schema for understanding the material. Thus, drug use and violence facts will be meaningful as African American youths become attuned to their bodies' need for protection. Initial prevention sessions help youths develop their body awareness through body outlines, height and weight measurements, blood pressure measurements, and still photographs. After building their body awareness, youths are better prepared to receive facts about drug use and violence.

Drug abuse facts focus on tobacco, alcohol, and other drug use. To avoid losing youths' interest, facts are presented through films, demonstrations, lung kits, and role playing. Violence material, similarly presented through films, demonstrations, and role playing, focuses on the disproportionate rates of violence in African American minority groups and the availability of guns.

Self-Protective Skills and Self-Efficacy. Studies find that information-only programs are unsuccessful in changing risk-taking behaviors (Edgar, Freimuth, & Hammond, 1988; Schinke et al., 1991). Without skills to translate knowledge into protective behaviors, young people do not alter their behavior. Presented throughout intervention sessions, self-protective skills and self-efficacy help African American male youths translate facts about drug abuse and violence into behavior change. Following an operant learning model, practitioners reinforce youths whenever they make statements evincing self-efficacy about drug nonuse, nonviolent conflict resolution, or other healthy behaviors.

Relaxation Skills. AfricanAmerican boys can be taught how to recognize physical cues for anger and how to decrease those physical cues through deep breathing, counting, and imagery. Youths learn to take slow, deep breaths when faced with a situation that is making them mad. Youths also learn to pause and count slowly inside their heads to provide a break between what has made them angry and their reaction. Finally, youths learn to use imagery as a distraction from anger-provoking situations.

Self-Assessment. African American boys practice thinking about the triggers for their anger in a given situation, how they respond or behave when angry, and what the consequences were of their behavior. Using behavioral histories and daily logs, youths learn to identify personal triggers (both direct and indirect) for their anger. Once these are identified, youths are encouraged to develop new patterns of behavior that may help them to avoid future conflict situations. In role playing, youths can act out various overt and covert triggers for anger.

Self-Instruction. Youths are shown how to use internal statements to help them guide their behavior. Youths learn how internal statements, or reminders, can prevent them from losing their temper or engaging in drug use. Via role playing, youths practice using reminders to help them to diffuse anger-provoking situations or drug use opportunities.

Assertion. Assertive, aggressive, and passive behavior styles are defined, and training is provided in assertiveness. Role playing demonstrates assertive, aggressive, and passive behavior responses to drug use opportunities or anger-provoking situations. Youths are encouraged to use assertion skills, rather than aggression or passivity, in response to challenging situations,

Problem-Solving. A five-step sequence, SODAS, helps youths reduce drug use risks and delay and control their responses to anger-provoking or other troubling situations. Insufficient problem-solving skills can lead to aggression. Through vignettes, practitioners might demonstrate the five-step sequence of *Stop, Options, Decide, Act,* and *Self-Praise.* In the Stop step, youths pause and define problems and their role in solving them. In the second step, Options, youths consider alternatives to behavioral risks. In the Decide step, youths systematically choose the best solution by ranking their options on costs, benefits, and feasibility. Act, the fourth step, involves planning and rehearsal. After planning thoughts, words, and gestures appropriate to the problems, youths practice how to handle situations related to drug use, violence, or other risk-taking behavior. In the Self-Praise step, youths reward themselves for using problem solving.

Thinking Ahead. Youths are taught to anticipate the negative consequences of their drug use or angry behavior. Impulsivity has long been recognized as an important risk factor for violent behavior and for drug use (Kendall, Ronan, & Epps, 1991). Thinking ahead skills teach youths to pause between anger-provoking stimuli, or drug use opportunities, and their behavior response.

Youths learn that delaying their response to a conflict situation can diffuse the conflict.

Coping. Youths need cognitive and behavioral strategies to adaptively handle stresses that may trigger drug use or violence. Cognitive skills emphasize internal statements of self-praise and affirmation to help adolescents manage their behavior and reduce drug abuse and violence risks. Behavioral coping skills teach youths to reward themselves overtly for successful prevention efforts.

Conflict Resolution. Negotiation and compromise skills help African American youths control conflict situations. Recent studies have found that violence does not typically occur as a sudden, unpredictable event but rather as the result of escalating interpersonal conflict, with both parties playing a role in the failure to resolve the conflict (Hammond & Yung, 1991; Prothrow-Stith, 1991). This research suggests that including conflict resolution skills in prevention interventions for African American male youths could affect rates of violence.

Social Perspective-Taking. Youths learn to read facial expressions; interpret nonverbal behavior, mood, and emotional reactions; make inferences from nonverbal and verbal behavior; recognize how their words and behaviors affect others; and behave in a way that shows respect for the rights and needs of others. Aggressive youth are weak in the areas of social perspective taking and empathy. These youth have difficulty understanding how the other person in a social interaction would see the situation, and they often misunderstand how their own behavior is perceived by others. Preventive interventions designed to strengthen perspective-taking skills have shown promise.

Hostile Attributional Bias. This social perception deficit is common in aggressive youth. These youth tend to perceive more hostility in other people's behavior than was actually directed at them. Toward addressing social perception deficits, practitioners initially (and youths subsequently) might role-play the antagonist's perspective. Role playing the antagonist can teach youths empathy, increase their accuracy of social perception, and counter hostile attributional bias.

Critical Viewing. African American boys learn how to analyze media portrayals of conflict and drug use. Research has shown that passive consumption of commercial television can lead to attention deficits, nonreflective thinking, and irrational decision making (Keating, 1990). Studies suggest that viewing a great deal of violent content can contribute to aggressive feelings and behavior (Strasburger, 1995). To combat passive viewing of television, youths can analyze media portrayals of drug use and violence for consequences, roles, the degree to which other options besides drug use or violence are explored, and the frequency of nonviolent conflict resolution.

Enhancement of Social Proficiency and Resiliency. In this component, youths acquire and practice interpersonal skills toward increasing their social proficiency and resiliency. Interpersonal skills introduced through vignettes will show youths how other adolescents successfully interacted with peers and others to avoid social triggers for drug use and violence. Youths learn skills to accomplish such different purposes as communicating to achieve an objective, maintain a relationship, and gain self-respect. Through cognitive rehearsal and role-playing situations, youths practice communication skills. Youths refine their skills first in routine situations, then in more challenging interactions.

Social Supports for Maintaining Personal Change. Peer networks influence African American male adolescent drug use and aggressive behavior. Accordingly, to increase African American male youths' positive peer supports and to prevent skills erosion, intervention should build strong and adaptive social networks. Peer leaders who are African American, male, and 2 years older than youths can help deliver intervention (data suggest they are more effective than adults in presenting problem behavior prevention programs). Intervention that requires youths to meet together regularly and frequently will foster the development of positive, healthy clusters among youths. Consequently, peer clusters will further youths' positive social development rather than their deviance.

Intervention that includes skills intervention as well as recreational, artistic, and cultural opportunities can promote African American male peer bonding by providing interactions around behaviors that often require sharing, positive risk taking, and negotiation. Also, these activities expose youths to a variety of positive behavioral alternatives.

Concurrently, because sensation seeking is related to drug use and possibly to aggressive behavior, the intervention should target African American male youths' desire for stimulation. With opportunities to meet individual and social needs, youths may feel less of a need to seek out unsupervised, informal associations that are potential opportunities for drug use or violence.

Parent involvement can strengthen African American male youths' learning through positive family interactions that support anger management and drug abuse risk-reduction efforts. Because family orientation is a strength of African American culture, parent involvement (with parents defined loosely as any significant adult family member) is critical to preventive intervention with African American male youth. Interactive exercises should encourage parent-child communication not only around risk reduction content but also around shared enjoyable activities.

Together, the above components could make a strong preventive intervention for African American males. However, as with any intervention targeted at a specific population, all intervention material should be focus-group tested with a sample of youth and their parents. Skills-based preventive interventions with components similar to those described above have been found to be effective for deterring cigarette smoking with African American youth, for decreasing intentions to drink alcohol and use illicit drugs among African American and Hispanic youth, and for reducing the frequency and amount of alcohol use and episodes of drunkenness.

STRENGTHS

Little attention has been paid to the strengths that protect and motivate African American male youth to mature into productive, healthy, and law-abiding citizens. The tendency to overemphasize pathology and deficiency and de-emphasize strengths and adaptive traits is prevalent in the empirical literature. More research is needed on resiliency in African American males. For the purposes of this discussion, resiliency is the ability to cope with, recover from, or overcome traumatic events and chronic situations.

A first step in understanding strengths in African American male culture is to look at racial socialization. Race socialization, according to Rotherman and Phinney (1987), is the "developmental process by which children acquire the behaviors, perceptions, values, and attitudes of an ethnic group, and come to see themselves and others as members of such groups" (p. 25). Parents of all races engage in race socialization, either actively or passively.

Racial socialization can provide young inner-city African American males with strengths to draw upon as they negotiate their way through the obstacles of urban environments. At its best, racial socialization teaches African American males (a) to attribute negative appraisals by the majority culture to that culture, rather than internalizing such appraisals; (b) to measure themselves against their black peers, rather than against their majority culture peers, which may result in fewer negative standards of evaluation; and (c) to value the domains that their culture considers important, rather than the domains that the majority culture group deems important. Intervention described earlier includes principles of race socialization.

Hill (1972) describes five key strengths that are commonly held within African American family life. These strengths include strong kinship bonds, strong work orientation, adaptability of family roles, strong achievement orientation, and strong religious orientations. Other researchers identify such variables as kin-structured networks, elastic households, and unwavering optimism as strengths that are characteristic of African American families. Given the emphasis on extended family in African American culture, preventive intervention for black male youth needs to target not only immediate family members but also aunts, uncles, cousins, and other significant relatives. McAdoo (1992) found that extended family members are viewed as helpful by parents of African American youths. In sum, family bonds, religiosity, and race socialization are common strengths that African American males can draw on as they attempt to avoid engaging in risky behaviors. Building these elements into a prevention effort will likely produce more reliable effects.

RESOURCES

Because common sources of resiliency for African American males are the family, community programs, and the church, it is advisable to include them in a preventive intervention. Yet, African American males often experience a type of double jeopardy in relation to social service institutions. Not only are African American males likely to mistrust social service personnel, they are also frequently frustrated by agency practices and expectations that are incompatible with their culture. Service agencies and intervention and prevention programs generally expect their clientele to be motivated to seek help, express weaknesses, and openly display emotions. Yet, African American males are socialized to be tough and stoic and therefore may avoid social service agencies that encourage them to be otherwise.

Practitioners working with African American male youth would benefit by collaborating with existing community programs (churches, afterschool program, civic organizations) that have among their goals the empowerment of their constituents. The major goal of empowerment practice is to help individuals and communities modify situations that contribute to the persistence of problems. Rather than focusing on individual change and deficiencies, the potential outcome of empowerment practice includes a combination of personal, interpersonal, and social change.

CONCLUSION

Growing rates of violence, drug use, and other problem behaviors among African American male youth are alarming. Clearly, there is a need for responsive, effective problem behavior prevention for African American male youth. Yet, most prevention efforts to date have neglected the particular strengths and weaknesses of this population in their delivery methods and content. Perhaps future risk reduction efforts will be more successful as practitioners and researchers alike grow increasingly aware of the importance of grounding intervention in the target population's unique cultural experiences.

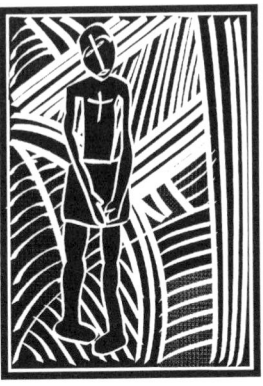

PART III

Education

It is imperative that African American males increase their educational achievements, if they are to prosper in the 21st century. This is true, even though they have made dramatic educational gains since World War II. Their high school completion rates rose steadily from the 1940s into the 1970s (Wetzel, 1989), and the proportion of African American high school and college students has risen sevenfold since the 1940s. This achievement is to be lauded: Absence of a high school diploma—at least—is the frequent harbinger of high unemployment, substance abuse, crime, and a free fall into the underclass.

Still, African American males suffer from a higher dropout rate than the national average. Moreover, the dropout rate in some inner-city schools is believed to be as high as 40% to 50% (LeCompte & Goebel, 1987). Hence, it is estimated that 36% of all African Americans who are 25 years and older do not possess a high school diploma, compared to 22% of whites (U.S. Bureau of the Census, 1998). A wealth of explanations have been put forth to explain the educational difficulties of African American males: a decline in parental involvement, an increase in peer pressure, a decline in nurturance and an increase in discipline problems, a decline in teacher expectations, a lack of understanding about students' preferred learning styles, and a lack of male teachers (Kunjufu, 1986). It has also been argued that some African American youth have adopted an oppositional frame of reference to academics, specifically perceiving academic success as "acting white" (Fordham & Ogbu, 1986), or have themselves succumbed to the myth that African American males are intellectually inferior (McDavis & Parker, 1988; see Howard-

Hamilton, 1995). It is likely that each of these explanations has its unique truth. Yet, while too much time has been devoted to discussing the educational plight of African American males, not enough time has been devoted to developing potential strategies to improve their educational and career statuses (Garibaldi, 1992).

Prisons are now competing with schools to be the primary educator of African American males (Rivera, Jackson, & Jackson, 1993, p. 1). This is occurring as African American college enrollments have ebbed and flowed over the past 30 years. In the late 1960s, enrollment increased substantially but fell in the mid to late 1970s and increased again at the end of the 1980s and into the 1990s. At present, African American males account for only 3.5% of the total enrollment in U.S. colleges and universities (U.S. Bureau of the Census, 1998). Only 29.7% of African American males who graduated from high school in 1992 enrolled in an institution of higher learning. This is a reduction from the 32.2% in 1991and the 34.4% in 1990 (Davis, 1994). And the small number of African American males who do enroll have a significant risk of failing to complete college (Allen, Epps, & Haniff, 1991; Fleming, 1984).

The goal of the authors of this section is to enhance the educational and career outcomes of African American males. Fortunately, the importance of cultural sensitivity has increasingly been presented in models developed to motivate and direct these African American youth (Atkinson, Morton, & Sue, 1989; Kunjufu, 1986; D'Andrea & Daniels, 1992). In keeping with this trend, it will be apparent from most of the readings here that any effort to help educate African American youth must include an awareness of and sensitivity to their unique cultural characteristics.

CHAPTER 9

African American Males: Their Status, Educational Plight, and the Possibilities for Their Future

PAULA ALLEN-MEARES

The literature provides no best educational approach or model of intervention to assist African American males to improve their academic performance. In the author's opinion, too few programs address the totality of factors and institutions that cause this dreadful waste of human potential. It would appear that historical events and institutional racism have singled out the African American male as one of the least deserving members of our society. Informal discussions with African American school-age males and those who have now reached young adulthood attest to this race-gender bias. African American males' abilities to plan productive futures are hampered by memories of how teachers and schools ignored their academic and creative potential, assigned them to the lowest ability grouping in the school, and saw them as physically threatening. This group appears to be the last to be educated, and thus their employability and self-sufficiency are limited.

This chapter addresses the current academic and school status of African American males, the theories and points of view that attempt to explain their poor educational outcome, and select educational interventions that appear to be promising and/or that have some empirical validation.

Numerous reports confirm that African American males consistently lag behind their white male and African American female counterparts (Slaughter-Defoe & Richards, 1995) in both school completion rates and employment. They are less prepared academically and thus less able to compete in the employment market. More specifically, they often fail to meet the three types of literacy skills (i.e., prose, document, and quantitative) that are required for successful employment. For example, a study by Garibaldi (1992) revealed that only 21.3% of African American males were able to locate information in an article, compared with 63% of white males; even fewer were able to synthesize information from a newspaper article or determine the amount of a tip when given an exact percentage. In an urban school system where 87% of the 86,000 students were African American, 58% of the nonpromotions, 65% of the suspensions, 80% of the expulsions, and 45% of the dropouts involved African American males—even though these young men represented 43% of the school population.

The data concerning achievement are even more depressing. For example, in the New Orleans public schools, African American males scored in the lowest quartile on the reading and mathematics section of the California Test of Basic Skills (Garibaldi, 1992). In Milwaukee, during the 1988-1989 academic year, the percentage of African American males scoring at or above the national average on the norm-referenced reading test dropped from 28% in Grade 2 to 24% in Grades 5 and 7. About 40% of all adult African Americans are functionally illiterate (Jaynes & Williams, 1989). Nationally, one fifth of all African American males drop out of high school. Furthermore, these youth are more likely to be misplaced in classes for slow learners than their white male counterparts. Although there is much debate about the cultural sensitivity and white Anglo Saxon bias of psychometric tests used to place pupils in special education and remedial programs (Mercer, 1979), these devices are still heavily relied on in making educational decisions.

THEORETICAL EXPLANATIONS OF ACADEMIC FAILURE

The current literature on this topic affords a number of theoretical explanations for academic failure.

1. *Cultural contradiction.* This perspective suggests that African American students are expected to learn in an environment that negates their home language, denies their unique history and transportation to America as slaves, and demeans their culture (Leake & Leake, 1992). It is this incongruency that leads to poor educational outcome.

2. *Fourth-grade failure syndrome.* Kunjufu (1988) believes that in the fourth grade many previously successful students begin to flag and fail. Furthermore, he believes that boys are particularly at risk if they neither are

involved in a team sport nor come from an academic household and if they demonstrate macho behavior, are exposed to negative peer group influence, have teachers who hold low expectations for their performance, and have no role models or societal social skills. He attributes the decline in male performance to incompetent teaching at the primary level, too few male teachers, parental apathy, increased peer pressure, and greater emphasis on mass media.

3. *Conditioned failure model.* This perspective suggests that African Americans are intellectually inferior to whites (Jones, 1989). This thinking then becomes the basis for the overt and covert legitimization of negative expectations and teacher interaction. It is the classic self-fulfilling prophecy in which the student becomes the reason for his or her own failure. In formulating interventions, proponents of this theory ignore the deleterious role of the teacher, institutional racism, and other contributing societal and family factors that are beyond the control of the youths.

4. *Culture of power theory.* Another explanation for African American male academic performance centers around the notion that a "culture of power" exists in classrooms (and society as well). Those who possess this power are unaware of it and pretend that differential employment of it does not exist (Delpit, 1988). When students, such as African American males or poor white children, do not know the culturally specific clues and appropriate response sets and thus operate from a different cultural perspective, they are disempowered and misunderstood.

This notion of a culture of power in the classroom would suggest that we must teach African American males and others to decode messages so they can participate in the classroom. Teachers need to be made aware of how they undermine their primary objective of educating students through the manipulation of this culture of power. Communicating across cultures has not been an integral component of the educational preparation of those who serve students in our nation's schools, but it needs to become one. Another possible solution is to diversify the educational staff.

5. *Structural and contextual theories.* Much critical attention has focused on the pupil, the African American male student and his so-called deficits. Much more empirical study needs to be devoted to understanding the structural and contextual variables that affect student achievement and development. Davis and Jordan (1994) examined the effects of school context, structure, and experiences on the achievement, locus of control, grades, and engagement of African American males in middle and high school. Drawing on data from the National Educational Longitudinal Study (NELS), they found that middle school students in urban schools performed less well in composite achievement than did those in suburban and rural schools. Also,

achievement at the eighth-grade level was found to be lower in schools where discipline was stressed and where teachers had difficulty motivating students and were often absent. Academic workload was the only variable found to influence school grades. For high school students, only their teachers' loci of control, or the degree to which teachers felt a sense of accountability and responsibility for the success of their students, proved to influence achievement significantly. Tenth graders attending urban schools were less engaged than their counterparts in suburban and rural schools. African American males were more engaged in smaller schools. Perhaps large urban schools are not environmentally suited for these students to excel.

Tobias (1989) questioned whether the urban context was beneficial, regardless of gender, citing several contemporary issues unique to the urban secondary public schools that affect the educational outcome of African American students. These issues included the relevance of the curriculum, teacher competence, parental involvement, and skillful guidance and counseling.

6. *Contextualized model of African American identity.* This point of view is related to the previous discussion concerning structural and contextual explanations. It suggests that the social construction of self relies on the support of others found in the youth's immediate social environment. These people provide a role model of what one can become and how to behave in a specific way (Oyserman, Gant, & Ager, 1995). This theory acknowledges that the student's context also contains institutions and groups—such as the family, community, school, and peers—that provide opportunities for the development of self. These institutions/groups can also be a source of conflict and mixed messages for youth. African American youths may experience a social context that does not lead to the positive construction of self in a healthy and helpful way. Furthermore, they have to face a socially constructed self that is defined by society and a contextual self that is defined by their immediate environment, as well as their African American culture and history. For example, society at large often views African American males as violent and hostile. Teachers in schools may adopt these views and respond to these students based on stereotypes—diminishing their opportunities in the classroom and sending messages to them that they are inferior or less important. Individualism is highly valued in hegemonic culture and thus in the classroom, whereas African American culture tends to emphasize collectivism, creating another source of conflict for youth. We need to consider the strengths and capabilities of these youths, including their leadership, their sense of community, their participation in religious/spiritual organizations, their extended family relations, and their desire to belong.

INTERVENTIONS

After contacting leading researchers on this topic and surveying the current literature, I concluded that although there are a growing number of school- and community-based experiments and programs that specifically target African American males, only a few of these programs offer empirical validation. Some programs that do not specifically target African American males focus instead on ways to increase the achievement (reduce inequalities) of disadvantaged, poor, and minority children in general. The successes and failures of such broader programs hold implications for the population at hand; the best known of these programs are the "big three": James Comer's School Development Model, Yale University; Robert Slavin's Success for All Program, Johns Hopkins University; and Henry Levin's Accelerated Schools Program, Stanford University. Each of these programs has unique theoretical, instructional, and empirical grounds; practice principles; and interventions. Other school-, community-, and family-focused programs—including the immersion model—are also discussed, followed by a survey of various classroom and individual interventions.

Schoolwide Approaches

1. *Comer's School Development Model.* Comer (1988) makes the case that poor African American children who live in an alienated society require special attention beyond the instruction and curriculum offered by most schools. A successful outcome for this group of pupils depends on applying our knowledge of childhood development to change school climate and to create a consensus between parents and educators on the direction of schooling. All children can be successful if this set of circumstances is achieved. The primary intervention is to use teacher and parent consensus building and involvement to provide a supportive climate for learning; this critical home-school partnership thus fosters change in educational achievement. For Comer, poor academic performance is caused by the weak link that exists between home and school. Thus, school-based management, social skill development of pupils, parental involvement, and a no-fault approach to problem solving are integral components of the intervention. Evaluation of the Comer model found that under it pupils gained in elementary reading and math, experienced a positive change in self-concept, encountered an improved school climate, and showed a decline in suspensions and days absent. One of the advantages of this model is that strengthening the link between

home and school enables the African American student to draw on a united support system.

The Comer approach is consistent with what school social workers have always advocated: The educational success of our children is determined by teacher and parent involvement, school climate, and engagement of the school as a part of the community (Allen-Meares, Washington, & Welsh, 1996).

2. *Slavin's Success for All Program.* The emphasis of this approach is preventing rather than fixing problems (Slavin et al., 1994). This approach uses every potential intervention to prevent the educational failure of children. The basic goal is to have every child reach Grade 3 at or near grade level. The following programmatic interventions are used: reading tutors (certified teachers working one-on-one with pupils); heterogeneous and homogeneous age-grouped classes into which pupils are sorted by reading levels; intense reading assessments; school teams that include parents so that they can become active supporters of their children's learning; school teams that include supplemental tutors; a strong effort to keep all students in regular classrooms; certification of all teachers and provision of special in-service preparation in reading; and periodic meetings of a broad-based advisory group to discuss problems and to help identify appropriate next steps. The family support teams consist of social workers, parent liaisons, counselors, and others.

This approach has two essential principles: prevention and immediate intensive intervention. It is assumed that no new resources are needed to operationalize this approach; current resources are shifted from such areas as special education, reading programs, and related personnel to others. Evaluations show large effects on students' reading scores (Slavin et al., 1994). The results show a minimum of a .5 standard deviation increase over the control schools and a maximum of a 1.5 standard deviation increase for the bottom quartile of students. The effects not only are maintained but actually increase over time. As stated, African American males experience considerable difficulty with literacy (reading in particular), and interventions abstracted from this approach hold promise when combined with other empowerment interventions.

To achieve these results, a school system must make a commitment to restructure its elementary schools and to reconfigure the uses of Title I/ Chapter 1, special education, and other funds to emphasize prevention and early intervention. The program also requires a favorable vote by at least 80% of teachers. Helping professionals can play a meaningful role in the formulation of teacher and parent groups and can assist in restructuring the school and adopting a prevention orientation.

3. *Levin's Accelerated Schools Program.* This program emphasizes accelerated educational programming for at-risk students over the historical approach of remediation (Levin & Hopfenberg, 1991). It was established at Stanford University after a study found that remedial programs for at-risk pupils only slowed them down—students ended up farther behind their peers. Accelerated schools operate on the premise that at-risk students must learn faster than privileged students. Thus, if status differences (sometimes based on skin color, gender, learning rate/achievement, physical size) can be minimized, low-status children will increase their participation and subsequently their achievement levels.

Low-status children are prepared through enhancement of social skills and competency development activities (Cohen, Rachel, & Lotean, 1994). In other words, through group work, these children are empowered to feel good about themselves, eventually leading to change in social status within the classroom. We know from reports in the literature that African American males are often assigned low social status in a variety of group settings, which results in alienation and the development of socially unacceptable behaviors to gain status. The Accelerated Schools approach attempts to be inclusive, treating all students as if they have equal promise and building on their strengths. Contrary to the deficit-remediation model, it intensifies the pace of learning. High expectations are set and site-based management and task forces work to achieve objectives. A primary value undergirding the approach is equal rights to high quality education. Presently, many African American males do not experience a quality learning environment in their classrooms, and the teachers' primary approach is remediation.

4. *School-, community-, and family-focused collaboration.* I recently had the pleasure of learning about an innovative program called Project Kofi for African American males in St. Paul, Minnesota. This is a collaboration of the school system, county social services, and a nonprofit community agency (Rosseau, 1995). It is a school-based, family-focused, community-supported collaboration with an Afrocentric cultural ideology at the core of the program. A student meeting the admissions criteria of the program must be a male of African American ancestry who resides in the area, attends Grades 3 to 6 in a designated school, and has parental permission and a family agreement to participate. Goals of the program include increasing the African American male's positive functioning in home, school, and community, developing self-confidence and an awareness of the rich history and culture of African Americans, and supporting the African American family as a resource.

The program provides the family with community-support services, such as parent support and education for parenting assistance in the acquisition of culturally and developmentally reasonable life skills. Crisis assistance is available for family and student. Recreational activities are organized, and there is an array of evening services offering transportation, food, and parent support groups. In a rite-of-passage program, students actually participate in a graduation exercise. Students are also assigned a case manager. The goal of the program is to provide an abundance of excellent role models for young African American males. The program founder (Rosseau III) views it as an initiative to develop manhood and more responsibility.

An outcome evaluation of the program, using standardized measures, grades, attendance, and family perceptions, found improvement in behavior and a decrease in the incidence of disruptive behavior as well as a decrease in the number of days absent from school.

5. *African American immersion school.* A related approach—which is gaining national attention and creating considerable controversy—is the development of a total learning environment, one designed specifically to respond to the unique needs and strengths of the young African American male (although in some instances females are included). Traditional skills are stressed (reading, communication skills, etc.) and are complemented by unique experiences that enhance and empower students (Leake & Leake, 1992).

The objective is to raise the social, communication, problem-solving, critical thinking, and citizenship skills of African American males and to promote special programs. This educational intervention includes culturally specific group experiences and attention to adolescent male development and the competencies required to move to the next stage of development.

The Milwaukee school system has adopted this approach, and teachers, parents, and other community groups have built a consensus around this concept. However, this program has come under attack from critics, who argue that the isolation of African American males further stigmatizes them and that their future depends on their functioning in an integrated environment. In addition, some programs exclude females, which only adds to the segregation experienced by African American males.

The next group of interventions are those that target the classroom and individual students.

Classroom and Individual Interventions

1. *Direct instruction.* Reports in the literature support the efficacy of direct instruction (teacher-led), with the teacher serving as the vehicle of instruction. Brophy and Good (1986) found consistent positive correlations

between certain teacher behavior and achievement gains by students. These behaviors included

- amount of instruction (including covering more pages, lengthening the amount of time students are in school, institutional engagement time, and time being taught by the teacher) and

- quality of instruction (including greater effectiveness of teacher-led compared with individualized instruction, redundancy and sequencing, teacher enthusiasm, apparent superiority of fast-moving instruction, and avoidance of personal criticism of the student).

It is recognized that these areas are not mutually exclusive. Student achievement increased with increased effectiveness of teacher behaviors in such areas as content covered, role expectations, student engagement time, active teaching, structure of information, and pace and reaction to student responses.

According to this approach, to maximize learning, students of lower socioeconomic status require more structure (more active instruction, more frequent feedback, smaller steps with higher levels of student success). These students also require from their teachers more expressions of warmth and encouragement—characteristics of effective teachers. Murrell (1994) studied the responsiveness of teachers to African American males through observing discourse patterns and speech events. Although no data were collected on females or non-African American pupils (i.e., the study lacked a comparison group), Murrell concluded that teachers systematically underserve African American male students in the classroom. Unfortunately, the methodological shortcomings of the study minimize the generalizability of the findings and undermine any claim to differential treatment. However, the general supposition on which the study was based offers an important line of inquiry.

2. *Cognitive modeling and self-instruction.* An empirical study by Tucker and colleagues (1995) employed a program designed to enhance the educational achievement of low-income African American elementary and high school students—cognitive modeling and self-instruction. This study included 148 students and their parents. Known as the Partnership Education Program, it taught self-instruction learning methods, success behavior, and skills to self-manage emotions (e.g., how to constructively handle and express one's anger). This program involved a partnership of parents, community public schools, and a university. Results indicated that participants

experienced some gradual but significant beneficial effects on school-reported deviance and predictors of grade point average (GPA). Parent training and involvement in the education of their children were essential elements of this 2-year afterschool intervention. Specifically, the program helped to minimize the documented decrease in math GPA and had a beneficial effect on the mean reading GPA.

African American students need cognitive strategies that help them to negotiate the educational system as well as to increase their sense of confidence and competence. These internal mechanisms or ways of coping must be developed within the reality that African American students will probably not receive the same intensity of reinforcement and incentives enjoyed by other groups. Their internal locus of control must be strengthened within this context.

3. *Responsibility training.* Developing into a responsible individual begins in the home early on in the child's development when parents set limits, define expectations, and ask children to contribute by assigning chores. An intervention that needs to be considered is the development of home-based responsibility training. Age-appropriate training should include attention to academic studies, sexual behavior, family membership, role differentiation, and societal survival skills (Kunjufu, 1988). Because some parents are more apt to set limits, clarify expectations, and act on negative behaviors than others, in some instances, other institutions—such as a church or recreational center—could contribute to parental efforts by setting limitations and by requesting youths to perform age-appropriate tasks.

4. *Other interventions.* Schools must recruit competent teachers and administrators who embrace a multicultural perspective. Too many of our teachers approach the education of African Americans in general, and males in particular, with fear and trepidation. They set low expectations and do not instill a sense of hope and pride. The educational preparation of teachers and professionals from related disciplines must address the diversity of school-age children, their unique learning needs, and their life circumstances.

It is important to experiment with various educational alternatives. One should not assume that all African American male pupils will respond to the same intervention or educational program in the same way. They need to be treated as a heterogeneous group, with varying needs and life experiences that determine the kind of educational intervention that will enhance their achievement and academic success. Our approach must emphasize the significant diversity among African American males—the current research assumes homogeneity.

Educators and practitioners who are a part of integrated service teams or community-based agencies need to assist schools in analyzing data regarding differential experiences (e.g., the rates of suspension, expulsion, academic failure, and noncompliance behavior problems) of vulnerable groups of pupils. We know that many African American males are not achieving in the current educational environment. Although the school cannot be held solely accountable for this sad state of affairs, it *is* the institution that influences students most throughout their school-age years. Racism and adverse policies do exist within this institution. Community conditions such as poverty and other environmental deprivation factors contribute to the erosion of support and the lowered quality of life that adversely affects African American males' school achievement and aspiration.

SUMMARY

The dilemma of the African American males is as follows: "What happens to an individual who perceives the larger society as hostile, intolerant, and uncaring; that opportunities for survival and advancement are limited; and that there is little hope of rising above the status quo?" (Allen-Meares & Burman, 1995, p. 270). The outcomes are clear: frustration, anger, a pessimistic view about the future, lower self-esteem and self-worth, a sense of powerlessness, and a host of physical and mental health problems. The target of intervention must be the policies and practices of significant institutions that deny this group equal access to the various opportunity structures.

It is well documented in the literature that African Americans in general hold education in high esteem and have consistently expressed their faith that it is the key to economic independence (Mickelson, 1990). However, for some, the academic performance record has been dismal—consistently underachieving. What causes this paradox? Data suggest the potential explanation that although these students express an appreciation of the value and importance of an education they may not link education to future opportunities or view it as having a positive return (Mickelson, 1990). They see the underemployment of those who have achieved academically and the devaluation of their talents and skills in the labor market.

These are only partial explanations. They are united by their tendencies to blame the victim and to ignore other social, political, and institutional barriers. It is predicted that African Americans and other minority groups will constitute from 20% to 30% of the youth and young adult population by the year 2010. If these individuals are not educated adequately, they will not be competitive with their highly skilled peers for the information technology age (Ozawa, 1986). This potential outcome is both tragic and dangerous.

Our approaches to the education of this group have been too driven by a preoccupation with pathology. Some African American males are rising above the social and contextual issues that undermine achievement and educational process. We need to examine more closely those young men who are victorious in their pursuit of an education: their survival skills, their resiliency, and the characteristics of their social supports. Research on these phenomena would lead to programmatic interventions on a variety of levels. More important, we should not adopt a cookie-cutter approach, where one intervention is expected to fit all individuals. Instead, we should recognize the heterogeneity of African American males and should embrace situation-specific interventions. We also need to undertake a closer examination of schools and how they perform their primary task for different groups.

In conclusion, if African American male students are to have better educational success/outcomes, societal conditions that isolate and stigmatize them must be dealt with. In terms of specific school conditions and programs, it is very clear to me from the review of different theoretical essays, research reports, and special programs to address their learning needs that there is "no one approach" or "quick fix" that will address the diverse needs within this group. We must experiment with different educational structures as well as curricular and personnel configurations that are not founded on preconceived perceptions/assumptions about their capability, or the traditional educational model. We are losing a generation of men who have unlimited potential to contribute to the shaping of our society. We need to act now, both for their sake and for our own.

CHAPTER 10

Mapping School Violence With Students, Teachers, and Administrators

RON AVI ASTOR
HEATHER ANN MEYER
RONALD PITNER

Given that African American male youth are at an increased risk for becoming the victims and perpetrators of violent crime, many researchers have proposed that preventive interventions be aimed specifically at this vulnerable group (Ash, Kellermann, Fuqua-Whitley, & Johnson, 1996; Dohrn, 1995; Hammond & Yung, 1994; Hausman, Spivak, & Prothrow-Stith, 1994; Kachur et al., 1996; Sautter, 1995). However, designing intervention programs solely for young African American males presents an ethical dilemma. On the one hand, an emphasis on African American males may distract from other powerful social or environmental factors that contribute to a higher prevalence of violence among this group. Interventions created only for African American males may unintentionally predispose well-intentioned practitioners to stigmatize this group rather than focusing on other factors that may contribute to the higher rates of violence within these groups. Second, focusing exclusively on violent African American male

AUTHORS' NOTE: This chapter was supported, in part, through a National Academy of Education/Spencer grant and a National Institute of Mental Health grant to the first author.

youth may minimize the reality that youth violence is a serious social problem for young people in general. On the other hand, the mountain of statistical evidence suggests that catered interventions need to be designed to stem the prevalence of violence among African American male youth (Christoffel, 1990; Gray, 1991; Hammond & Yung, 1993; Harlow, 1989; Issacs, 1992; National Center for Health Statistics, 1992; Prothrow-Stith & Weissman, 1991; Shakoor & Chalmers, 1991).

One strategy that may yield a solution to this ethical dilemma is to focus interventions on the physical and social settings in which youth develop rather than concentrating solely on the individual or problematic youth themselves. Consequently, a challenge for practitioners and researchers is to develop primary preventive interventions and assessment strategies that target entire settings and whole populations of youth before they engage in violent behavior. Interventions that focus on non-native developmental settings (such as schools with large populations of African American males) may be a form of primary prevention that does not stigmatize a particular individual or group "at risk." Moreover, this approach may be more pragmatic and effective than current strategies. If one carefully examines the research on youth violence, it becomes clear that violence is occurring in very specific and predictable locations and times and between very specific age groups of children. Focusing interventions toward the contexts where violence is most predictable has a greater potential for reducing the overall incidence of violent events. Because the majority of African American male adolescents spend a good proportion of their time in school, and because assaultive violence at school is a serious social problem, the authors of this chapter have chosen to focus on middle and high schools that have high rates of violence.

SCHOOL VIOLENCE

Many forms of violence between youths are associated with the school's social or physical context. Dating back to 1978, the Safe School Study for the U.S. Congress suggested that schools may be the most violent setting for American youths. Currently, 92% of the general public also believes that school violence is a serious problem in U.S. schools (Elam, Rose, & Gallup, 1994). Kachur et al. (1996) estimated that ethnic minorities in urban schools were at greatest risk. In particular, African American students (all grades) in urban schools had the highest estimated rate for school-associated violent deaths. Practitioners working in schools are likely to encounter potentially lethal or lethal events in the schools they serve. In a recent national survey on school violence, 71% of school social workers reported a potentially lethal or lethal event in the schools they served during the past academic year (Astor, Behre, Fravil, & Wallace, 1997).

Previous studies have underscored the importance of documenting where and when school violence occurs. For example, the landmark Safe School Study found that the "locus of much violence and disruption" was usually in areas such as stairways, hallways, and cafeterias and that the risk of violent encounters was greatest during transitions between classes. In that study, 80% of the violent crimes committed against people occurred during regular school hours; of all secondary school assaults and robberies, 32% occurred between class periods, and 26% occurred during lunch (National Institute of Education, 1978). Since then, many articles and important policy reports have implicated these and other dangerous school locations (Carnegie Council on Adolescent Development, 1993; Goldstein, 1994; Gottfredson, 1985, 1995; Kachur et al., 1996; Olweus, 1991; Slaby, Barham, Eron, & Wilcox, 1994). However, very few studies have systematically explored *why* violence occurs in schools, *when* it does, and *how* these times and spaces interact with the prescribed social structure of the school (e.g., teacher roles, administrator roles, etc.). Even fewer studies have examined teachers' and students' perceptions of the combined physical and social structure of the school as it relates to violence. The proposed mapping procedure has the potential for addressing these issues (Astor, Meyer, & Behre, in press).

SCHOOL-BASED VIOLENCE INTERVENTION PROGRAMS

A major problem with most current school violence interventions is that they rarely incorporate the beliefs of teachers, students, administrators, and support staff regarding the reasons why violence is occurring in their school. However, research on school reform and implementation of programs/ interventions in schools suggests that successful interventions tend to emerge directly from the school community and actively integrate school personnel in their implementation. A more significant problem with many current interventions is that they are unidimensional in focus and usually address a singular aspect (either psychological, social, or environmental) that contributes to violence between youth in schools. Such a focus often ignores the inseparable linkage between the social and physical context of the school. As a result, some approaches have addressed the problem of school violence solely from an interpersonal/psychological perspective, some have discussed the influence of more global school variables, and some have focused on security measures or on changing the physical structure of the school building.

Psychological Interventions. Interventions based on psychological theories such as problem solving, social skills training, modeling, and traditional counseling are employed in many U.S. school settings (e.g., Alexander & Curtis, 1995; Astor, Behre, Wallace, & Fravil, 1998; Goldstein, 1994; Guerra, Tolan, & Hammond, 1994; Hammond & Yung, 1993, 1994; Larson, 1994; Prothrow-Stith & Weissman, 1991). In fact, they are part of our national policy related to school violence (National Education Goals Panel, 1995). These and other psychological interventions are based on the assumption that the individuals within the school lack social, psychological, communication, or behavioral skills and therefore need to be trained to handle conflict peacefully. Several programs have taken these widely used clinical techniques and shaped them to be used specifically with African American male students (Bell & Jenkins, 1991; Hammond, Kadis, & Yung, 1990; Prothrow-Stith & Weissman, 1991). These interventions, however, do not explain, incorporate, or address school violence dynamics associated with the physical and social structure of the school (Astor, Pitner, & Duncan, 1996).

Because psychological interventions conceptualize violent behavior as stemming from an interpersonal skill or cognitive behavioral deficit, they fail to address school contextual variables (Cairns & Cairns, 1991; Coie, Underwood, & Lochman, 1991; Dodge, 1991; Guerra et al., 1994; Olweus, 1991; Pepler, King, & Byrd, 1991). In fact, the school itself is rarely described as a significant contributing factor to the violence. However, the research on where violence occurs suggests that children are highly selective about where and when they engage in violence. Research indicates that violence occurs in places and times where there are few adults and/or adults do not define those times or places as part of their official role within the school. Incorporation of the specific organizational and social dynamics may strengthen these more psychologically oriented methods.

School Organizational Programs. Sociological and organizational variables have also been identified as potential contributors to school violence. For example, poor teacher/student relationships, sometimes referred to as "teacher care" (Lee & Croninger, 1995; Noddings, 1992, 1995), urban schools with high concentrations of low-income students (Comer, 1980; Kantor & Brenzel, 1992; Kozol, 1991; Lee & Croninger, 1995), very large and impersonal school settings (Alexander & Curtis, 1995; Meier, 1995), and poor school social climate or organization (Astor, 1998; Morrison, Furlong, & Morrison, 1994; Noguera, 1995; Rowan, 1990; Schorr, 1988; Strike & Soltis, 1985; Zeldin & Price, 1995) have all been associated with school violence. From the perspective of these literatures, school violence is a symptom of a deficit within the functioning of the school organization. Consequently, common suggestions to decrease school violence have included such global prescriptions as improving the relationships between teachers and students; making schools smaller and more personal; strengthening relationships between the school, home, and community; and creating a clear organizational violence policy.

Solutions from these literatures do not address the specificity of the social organizational structure of the school within select times and locations that tend to be uniquely problematic. For example, if violence tends to occur during times when most teachers are not with the students (e.g., taking a break or eating lunch in a separate location), it could be argued that improving the teacher/child relationships in class would not significantly affect student behaviors in areas outside the classroom (e.g., the playground, cafeteria, routes to and from school).

Security and Physical Facility Changes. In an effort to make high schools safer, many school districts have resorted to interventions adopted from correctional systems. These include security guards, metal detectors, video cameras, electronic monitoring of school doors, auditory monitoring of classrooms, and physical changes to the school structure (e.g., eliminating first-floor windows and increasing lighting in dangerous areas; see Goldstein, 1994, for a review; S. Sutton, 1996). These interventions are designed to address the physical locations where violence occurs. However, they are rarely incorporated into the formal social structure or purpose of the school. Some have argued that these interventions make the school climate more "prison-like" and create an atmosphere incompatible with learning (Goldstein, 1994; Noguera, 1995). Conversely, others have argued that these "get tough" interventions are needed in some schools to maintain safety and stability (see Noguera, 1995, for a critical discussion). Nevertheless, no one is arguing that all schools should be transformed into prisonlike settings. These measures appear to be encouraged in unsafe schools where violence has become uncontrollable. Ironically, students', teachers', and administrators' perceptions of security interventions have gone virtually unexplored in the empirical literature.

In contrast to these three approaches, the proposed mapping strategy begins with the premise that an understanding of social dynamics combined within specific physical locations is necessary for the creation of more effective school violence interventions.

MAPPING VIOLENCE WITHIN THE SCHOOL

This procedure is designed to aid practitioners in better understanding how violence within a school building interacts with locations, patterns of the school day, and social organizational variables (e.g., teacher/student relationships, teachers' professional roles, and the school's organizational response to violence). An important goal of this procedure is to allow students and teachers to convey their personal theories about why specific locations and times in their schools are more dangerous. This approach assumes that students, teachers, school staff, and administrators have important information that should be the foundation for setting specific interventions. Interventions should emerge from the information presented by the students, teachers, staff, and administrators in each school.

This process is designed to document (a) the locations and times within each school where violence occurred for that school term/year and (b) the perspectives of students, teachers, staff, and administrators on the school's organizational response (or nonresponse) to violent events in these locations. In particular, this assessment process is sensitive to areas that are "unowned" by adults in the school. By unowned, we refer to times and places that are not perceived to be the responsibility of any adults in the school. Prior research indicates that these unowned spaces are the same locations where most school violence occurs (Astor, Meyer, & Behre, in press).

Who to Include in Focus Groups

We recommend that students, teachers, and staff (e.g., administrators, hall monitors, cafeteria workers) be interviewed in four to five separate focus groups about the physical spaces where violence has been committed, and what time of day the violence has occurred. Students, teachers, and staff should represent various constituencies of the school organization, as well as locations within the school. For the assessment focus groups, we recommend that administrators (e.g., vice principals, principals, district-level officials), teachers, staff, and students be interviewed in separate focus groups. This should be done because students may fear repercussions from teachers, and likewise, teachers may not want to openly discuss issues in front of administrators. It is important that focus group members be assured anonymity, especially with regard to comments about the school's response to violence. To allow for in-depth discussion and responses to questions, we recommend that there be between six and eight individuals per each focus group. The entire focus group process should take about an hour. Using this procedure, practitioners can conduct an ecological assessment of violence within the school in about 6 hours of interview time.

Composition of Focus Groups

Students. Student focus groups could be composed in a variety of ways. Clearly, the nature of the violence may suggest a specific group composition. For example, in a school that has a problem with sexual assaults, some focus groups could be homogeneously composed of girls, whereas other groups may be homogeneously composed of boys. However, in most schools (unless the problem indicates otherwise), we suggest a group of both male and female students. In the past, we have organized students into older (11th and 12th graders) and younger (9th and 10th graders) focus groups with an equal number of males and females in each focus group. However, depending on the nature of the violence within the schools, focus groups could be organized by gender, age, or other relevant characteristics.

Teachers and Staff. Teachers, administrators, and other important school staff members (e.g., security guards, vice principals, hall monitors) are almost never included in research or interventions related to school violence. These individuals often have valuable knowledge about where and when violence occurs, and this information may be critical when structuring interventions to secure spaces within school grounds. Nevertheless, it is not necessary to interview large numbers of school personnel to gain an understanding of where, when, and why violence occurs. Our research suggests that interviews with four to five teachers per school is sufficient to gain an initial and fairly accurate range of teachers' perspectives. In addition, only a handful of cafeteria workers, yard aides, bus drivers, and security guards need to be interviewed in each school to gain an initial understanding of how school personnel are responding (or not responding) to aggression. Based on prior interviews with school staff, practitioners can anticipate themes, which include a sense of "being caught in the middle." Some teachers have expressed a personal desire to prevent violence yet may not possess the skills or knowledge of how to intervene. We have also found that many staff members are unclear about their professional role in nonclassroom locations (see Astor, Meyer, & Behre, in press, for a more detailed description of what types of themes can be anticipated from each group).

In prior interviews, nonteaching staff suggested very specific interventions associated with their area of the school. For example, cafeteria workers in one school revealed that only two or three adults were expected to supervise over 1,000 children during the lunch period. Also, in several schools, secretaries offered very clear suggestions for interventions regarding children who were sent to the office for fighting during less supervised periods (such as recess, lunch, or transitions between classes).

Materials and Procedure

Obtaining School Maps

The first step in this assessment procedure is obtaining a map of the school. It is not necessary to obtain a detailed blueprint. Usually, the school office has a small (8 × 11) map of the school, which is required by fire marshals. Ideally, the map should contain all internal school territory including the areas surrounding the school and playground facilities. Schools with several floors may require two or more pages, one representing each floor. In some communities where the routes to and from school are dangerous, a simple map of the surrounding neighborhood may be added to the assessment process.

The maps are an essential part of the interview process. They tend to anchor discussions to places and times in ways that interviews on issues alone cannot. Two sets of school maps should be photocopied for each participant in the focus groups (one marked A and the other marked B at the upper corner). In addition to the maps, each interviewee should have a pencil or pen and a set of eight circular colored stickers (about an eighth of an inch in diameter). The circular stickers should be used to mark violent events on the map (described in the following section). These materials can be found in most schools/agencies or purchased for a few dollars. The focus groups should be conducted in a room that affords privacy to ensure confidentiality from teachers, administrators, or other students. Therefore, securing a room or unused classroom space would be important for the success of this assessment strategy.

Maps Procedure

The focus groups should begin with the facilitator distributing two sets of identical maps to each individual. The facilitator should orient the group to the different areas of the school as they are represented on the map. Also, participants should be encouraged not to identify any individual's name who may have been involved in violence. The purpose of the discussion is to identify locations rather than individuals. Some groups may need gentle reminders such as "remember, don't use individuals' names." We have found that talking about places rather than people provides the freedom to discuss events without fear of repercussions or revealing personal information about specific friends or colleagues.

Map A: Three Most Violent Events. The first map should be used to determine the location of the most violent events in or around the school building. Using the stickers, participants should be asked to identify the locations (on the maps) of up to three violent events that occurred within the past academic year. In some schools, the "most violent" event may be a lethal shooting, whereas in other schools, fights may be the most violent events. In any case, the participant is free to interpret "most violent" subjectively. Our research suggests that students and school personnel take this task seriously and tend to report fairly severe events. Next to each event (marked by a circular sticker on the map), participants are asked to write directly on the map the following information: (a) the general time frame of the event (e.g., before school, after school, morning period, afternoon period, evening sports event, between classes, etc.), (b) the grade and gender of those involved in the violence, and (c) their knowledge of any organizational response to the event (e.g., sent to principal's office, suspended, sent to peer counselor, nothing, etc.). For the first part of the interview, participants should be encouraged to work on their own recollections and not to discuss locations and times until both maps are completed.

Map B: Dangerous Areas in and Around School. Once the first set of maps is completed, participants can then be given a second map (or set of maps) of their school. On the second map, using a pencil or pen, group members should be asked to circle areas or territories that they perceive to be unsafe or potentially dangerous. We have found that asking about unsafe places reveals different information than asking for events alone. This second map provides information about areas within the school that participants avoid even though they may not possess knowledge of a particular violent event. Participants should then be asked to explain in a few sentences (on the second set of maps) why they believe this particular area or time is prone to violence or should be avoided. Both sets of maps will consume about 10 minutes of focus group time.

When group members are finished with both maps, the facilitator can begin the discussion portion of the interview. The interviews should be tape-recorded so that the practitioner can listen to the interview and examine themes at a later time. In the past, we have transcribed the interviews for ease of reference, as this will allow multiple staff members who are interested in school violence to read and discuss the interviews.

Map Violent Events/Areas Discussion. The first part of the group discussion should center on the specific violent events and the areas marked as unsafe/dangerous on their personal maps. We have asked questions such as, Are there times when those places you've marked on the maps are less safe? Is there a particular group of students that is more likely to get hurt there?

Why do you think that area has so many violent events? The locations marked on both maps will be extremely helpful in identifying specific areas and times within the given school that are at risk for violence.

The overall purpose of the group interviews is to explore why violence is occurring where and when it is. Consequently, the interviews should also focus on gathering information regarding the organizational response to the event (e.g., What happened to the two students who fought? or Did the hall monitors intervene when they saw the fight?), procedures (e.g., What happens when someone is sent to the office after a fight?), follow-up (e.g., Do the teachers, hall monitors, and/or administrators follow up on any consequences given the students? or Did anyone check on the welfare of the victim?), and clarity of procedures (e.g., Does it matter who stops the fight? e.g., a volunteer, security guard, teacher, principal).

Interviewers should also explore participants' ideas for solutions to the specific problems (e.g., Can you think of ways to avoid this type of violence in that place? or If you were the principal, what would you do to make that place safer?). In addition, the interviewer should explore any obstacles participants foresee with implementation (e.g., Do you think that type of plan is realistic? Has that been tried before? What happened? Do you think that plan would work?). Such obstacles could range from issues related to roles (e.g., "It's not my job to monitor students during lunch") to discipline policy and issues of personal safety (e.g., "I don't want to intervene because I may get hurt").

In schools that already have programs designed to address school violence, specific questions should be asked about the effectiveness of those interventions, why they work or do not work, and what could be done to make the current measures more effective. We recommend that the interviewer ask both subjective questions (e.g., Do you like the conflict management program?) and specific questions related to the reduction of violence (e.g., Do you believe the conflict management program has reduced the number of fights on the playground? Why, or why not?).

Assembling the Data

Maps. The information from the individual maps should be transferred to an enlarged poster-size map. Enlarging the small map to a poster is relatively inexpensive ($6) and can be done fairly quickly at most photocopy stores. We believe such a compilation of information is a powerful visual representation that helps school personnel to identify the areas where violence most frequently occurs. Figure 10.1 is an example of how the information from the individual maps was coded into shapes/shades and then transferred onto one combined map representing all the events.

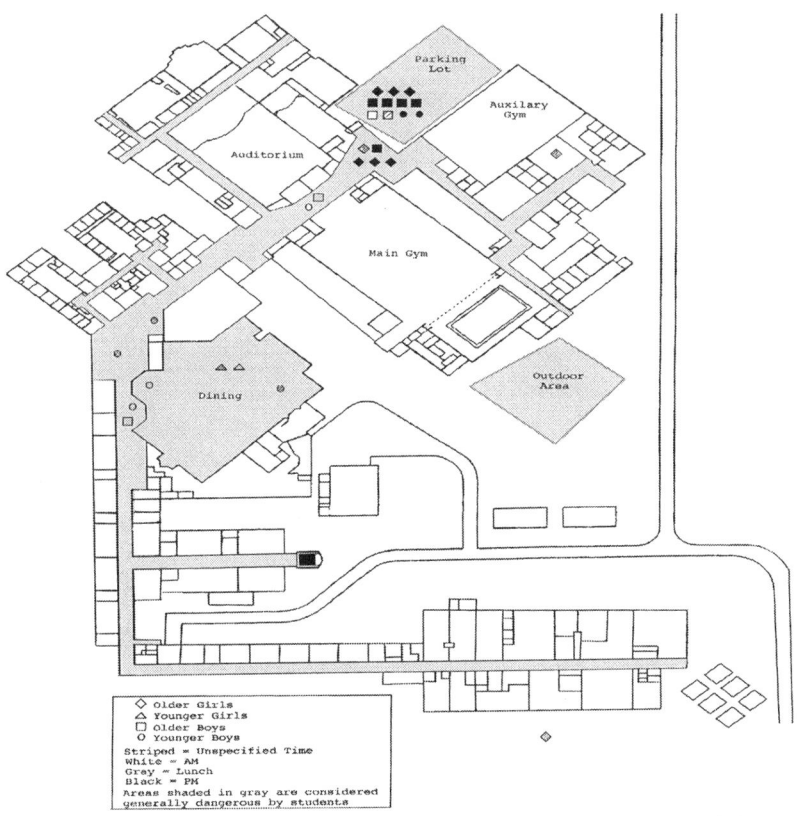

Figure 10.1. Violent Events Marked by Location, Time, Gender, and Age

The events were coded on the poster map by time, age, and gender. This visual depiction of violence as it clusters by age, gender, and time allows school staff to create better specific interventions that include these variables. Unsafe areas from the second maps were also combined and identified by areas shaded in gray.

Transferring all of the reported events onto one large map of the school enables students and staff to locate specific "hot spots" for violence and dangerous time periods within each individual school. As demonstrated by Figure 10.1, the events in that high school were clustered by time, age, gender, and location. In the case of older students (11th and 12th graders), events were clustered in the parking lot outside of the auxiliary gym immediately after school, whereas for younger students (9th and 10th graders), events were reported in the lunchroom and hallways during transition periods. For this school, the map suggests that interventions be geared specifically toward older students, directly after school, by the main entrance, and in the school parking lot. Students and teachers agreed that increasing the visible presence of school staff in and around the parking lot for the 20 minutes after school had great potential for reducing many violent events. Younger students were experiencing violence mainly before, during, and after lunch, near the cafeteria. Many students expressed feelings of being unsafe between classes in the hallways. Again, increased supervision was a common solution for violence in these locations and times.

Interview Data. Compiling all the suggested interventions into a simple readable table is also an important step in creating context-relevant interventions. Students, teachers, and administrators may have differing viewpoints regarding the organizational response of the school when violence happened. Table 10.1 is an example representing the different opinions of the students, teachers, and administrators regarding the organizational response to violence. Relating the diversity of responses to students, teachers, and administrators can provide an opportunity for reflection and may generate ways to remedy violence in certain situations.

We believe this type of format also provides an interesting way to exemplify the different perspectives that may exist within the school in how students, staff, and administrators would deal with violent events. The responses in Table 10.1 pointed to ambivalence about whose role it was to intervene when violence occurred in the school. These contrasting and anonymous viewpoints could (a) function as a vehicle of communication between the various subsystems of the school and (b) lead to the consequent creation of relevant interventions/procedures surrounding violent events.

Organizing the interventions suggested by participants into a table is also recommended. For example, Table 10.2 shows that students had clear opinions about how to make these areas safer.

Depending on the important themes related to violence, comments by the students, teachers, and administrators could be organized in a way to the one presented in Table 10.1. We recommend creating tables for each important theme for the particular school. In the past, we have organized students', teachers', and principals' comments related to race, gender, poverty, community, and religious conflict if it was perceived that these variables were contributing factors to violence with a school. Also, in schools that already have measures to prevent violence we recommend the compilation of tables surrounding those interventions (e.g., metal detectors, security guards, electronic and video monitoring, suspension and expulsion policies). Table 10.3 represents another example of how students', teachers', and administrators'

TABLE 10.1 Core Student, Teacher, and Administrator Comments Related to Organizational Response

Domain	Students	Teachers	Administrators
Organizational response	I wouldn't actually jump in there either because these, like, goons up here they don't care about a teacher and they fight and they not concerned about the teacher. If the teacher gets hit, most likely they going to say they shouldn't be in the way. So it's not they job to break up fights.	Two young ladies were going at it outside of my door, and I went to pull one off. She started punching me . . . and she was swearing. We ended up on the floor. I'll never forget. I looked up and two male teachers were standing there, not doing anything.	We've told the teachers they can take any level of activity they feel comfortable taking. They can intervene physically if they feel they have to. And I've had some teachers do that.
	Because I've seen a lot of people who get suspended and, you know, you see them a few weeks later getting in-school suspension. I mean what's the difference?	I have a call button. . . . They don't answer, they don't respond. I have to run next door and tell my department head. She would pick up the phone and try to locate security. . . . The kid would be back in my class in three days.	If you're in the immediate area, you've got to break that fight up. You're to do what you can. . . . State law requires teachers to be responsible in that situation.
	And she told me to go to the hallway. We went to the hall. The girl came out into the hall. . . . Then you know the teacher is still in the classroom, but she knows all this time that we are arguing and it is going to be a conflict. Why didn't she stop when we were having words?	I can remember a few years back, we had a convicted rapist who was in classes at this school. The teachers were not told that this student was convicted of rape. . . . He was scheduled with a number of young women teachers . . . and the principal never said a word.	There's a liability issue here. It's something that a lot of teachers don't seem to understand. . . . It means that they must at least give a verbal command to stop.
	That's like when the tuition office got held up. Don't you know, I was walking down the hall and I didn't even know what happened. Can you imagine how I felt? I could have got shot for no reason. . . . I think they should let us leave at least when the police came. Evacuated out one of these doors.	I think that some teachers probably would not like to get involved. In fact, I saw one [a fight] about 9 months ago where the teacher walked away from it and didn't want to get involved.	And, many times we would just transfer a student who had one fight. You could say anyone who fights in this building is gone.

TABLE 10.2 Student-Reported Violent Events and Suggested Interventions

Location	Violent Event	Suggested Intervention
Hallway	• pushing • fighting • gun pulled • gang fights • assault	There's so many people that you can understand that the hallways are crowded. That's our number one problem—the hallways are too crowded. Have a rule that if you surround a fight you're helping . . . so you would get the same punishment as the people fighting because you're helping people fight. They [security] should know what is going on in their hallway instead of like two or three of them going down the same way.
Parking lot	• physical fights • weapons • shooting • stabbing • physical threats • racially motivated fights	Well, where there's not supervision [parking lot] there's always going to be trouble. . . . The principal, he should be out there.
Abandoned/ unmonitored spaces	• physical fights/assault • sexual assault/rape • strangers entering • weapons • robbery	Maybe if we had regular security guards. Like they had a 70-year-old man security guard, and like that guy can't even move. People walk in at like 7 o'clock. No guards anywhere. It's just quiet—nobody anywhere. When we have a weapon search, they supposed to check you. There's some people they don't check. More lights . . . or have a monitor. Have somebody down there. I mean lock the school doors. . . . The back door is always open and people come in. I think we need to have IDs to show . . . and then like a speaker at the door.
Cafeteria	• physical fights • food fights • throwing chairs • gang scuffles	They should have at least five teachers in there . . . a minimum of five teachers. Because now there's only two teachers. It's too crowded. Our lunch hour is only 25 minutes. I think you should go basically anywhere during lunch as long as you clean up after yourself because keeping a lot of people together kind of generates fights.

TABLE 10.3 Comments by Students, Teachers, and Administrators on Suspension/Expulsion

Intervention	Students	Teachers	Administrators
Suspension/ Expulsion	No [not useful], because I've seen a lot of people who will get suspended and, you know, you see them a few weeks later getting in-school suspension. I mean what's the difference?	We have kids who are threats. They don't last long around here. They threaten a teacher and they're done. They're gone.	If you are caught with a weapon in school, or if you're caught selling drugs it's expulsion. There's not even a "let's reconsider."
	Suspend everyone. You know, they just, whoever was standing around, just suspend them. . . . Teachers just come and grab a handful of people who you see standing around who look like they were doing something. . . you're all suspended.	There are no exceptions to the policy. There is no exception. Would I change it? I don't know. Should a kid who is caught with a gun in his locker be kicked out or be allowed to come back into this school?. . . You are going to kick him out of here and throw him out in society? Who's going to care for him then?	If you're caught fighting, then you go home and you're suspended. It's either three or five days. If it's a fist fight, they can be suspended to another school.
	I disagree with the administrators. How sometimes like when people are doing good stuff, they may get involved with something bad and they just feel like eliminating them will be the best thing, but they don't look at their good qualities, and stuff like that.	Part of our fear is our knowing that no one gets rid of these kids. They just move from school to school. So, in the middle of the semester when you get a new kid all of a sudden, you know that kid has probably been put out of some other school for carrying a weapon.	If we catch a kid with a weapon. . .we've expelled since I've been the principal here. We've expelled or there has been an expulsion pending on five kids.
	You have to see each individual case and how it affects their lives. You can't just go out and rule for them.	So, in other words, if you're hit in the face and your initial reaction, as a 16-year-old, is to smack this person back, you both will be suspended for 10 days.	Possession of a weapon, using a weapon, you don't get a second chance.

views can be presented on a particular issue—in this case, opinions on the use of suspensions/expulsions to deter violence.

Together, the poster-size map of violent events, the interview data organized by themes, and the information on the potential obstacles can provide very concrete intervention strategies to reduce violence in school communities. Because most unsafe areas usually have few adults, the dialogue between the various school subsystems should include realistic ways to reclaim unowned territory and time. At a minimum, the organized data provides a formal opportunity for various school subsystems to discuss these issues. We believe this assessment process is powerful because the organized information presented back to the school constituents emerged from the setting. It contrasts with other assessment approaches where outside "experts" determine what the problem and intervention should be.

With time, some schools may want to create an ongoing "hot spot" map to track unsafe places and times on a monthly basis. This technique has been used by urban planners, criminologists, and law enforcement agencies to identify and reduce crime in predictable locations. The recent reduction in violent crime across many U.S. cities has been partially attributed to this method on a community level. Interventions designed to increase the safety of housing projects have also relied on similar mapping techniques.

CONCLUSION

The authors of this chapter have argued that entire school settings should be the focus of violence prevention strategies designed for African American male adolescents. We have suggested an alternative school violence procedure that integrates school maps (to locate violent hot spots in the school) and focus groups with students, teachers, school staff, and administrators (to identify social reasons why violence is occurring in certain places and potential solutions). Information obtained through the mapping process could (a) increase the dialogue between students, teachers, and school staff on issues of school violence; (b) serve as an evaluation of school violence interventions already used in a school setting; and/or (c) increase school involvement or participation in school violence interventions. A long research history of failed school violence interventions points to the hard fact that implementation of programs in schools does not work if school staff, teachers, and students are not involved or invested in the intervention. This mapping and interviewing process creates opportunities to generate grassroots interventions to secure the safety of children within the school community.

CHAPTER 11

Getting African American Male Students on Track

DON C. LOCKE

In U.S. society, education is essential to upward mobility. Education is also power. When any group in this society, for whatever reasons, fails to benefit from educational opportunities, a crisis results. It seems reasonable to posit that a crisis exists in the education of African American males. Wright (1991-1992) stated,

> We often read about well-heeled individuals who lead groups of influential citizens on quests to save the manatee, crocodile, bald eagle, the Everglades, Grand Canyon, alligators, whales, the petrified forest, the Sequoia trees, [yet] no visible group seems to be interested in expending any energy to save the African American male. (p. 14)

Regardless of the index used, demographic data indicate that African American males are suffering the most acute reactions from inadequacies in education, employment, income, family support, and health care. Phrases like "endangered," "crisis proportions," "nightmarish," "underserved," and "challenging" are frequently used descriptors for the situation facing African American males.

George (1993) predicted that in 20 years, as many as 70% of the African American males now in the second grade will be unqualified for work, either addicted to drugs or alcohol, incarcerated for criminal acts, on parole violations, unemployable, or dead. These data are magnified by statistics suggesting that African American boys have a 1 in 4 chance of dropping out of school before high school graduation and a 1 in 12 chance of graduating from college. An African American boy has a greater than 1 in 3 chance of being unemployed as a teenager; a 1 in 17 chance of being the victim of a violent crime during his teen years; a 1 in 24 chance of being imprisoned while in his 20s. Finally, when it comes to predictions of success, African American males have a 1 in 372 probability of becoming a lawyer; a 1 in 684 chance of becoming a physician; a 1 in 2,700 chance of becoming a dentist; and a 1 in 94 chance of becoming a teacher (George, 1993).

The problem is brought further into focus by the following staggering statistics specifically related to education of African American males:

- One fifth of all black males drop out of high school, and in some cities, the dropout rate is as high as 50% to 70% (Stewart, 1992).

- Black male students score lower than any other group on standardized tests and are three times more likely to be placed into low-ability or special education classes, from which it is often impossible to escape (U.S. Bureau of the Census, 1993).

- Black children are only half as likely as white children to be placed in gifted learning classes (George, 1993).

- Between 1980 and 1988, black female college enrollment increased by 7% while black male college enrollment decreased by 5% (George, 1993).

- Although black students make up 16% of public school enrollments, only 8% of public school teachers are African American (George, 1993).

- One of seven black male students ages 16 and 17 is two or more grades behind in school (George, 1993).

- Black students are over two times as likely to be suspended from school or to receive corporal punishment (George, 1993).

- African American males are overrepresented in low-track, low-ability classes and programs and underrepresented in high-track college preparatory programs and classes for the gifted and talented (Oakes, 1982, 1992).

- Stress, anxiety, anger, hostility, and frustration levels are higher among African American males than in any other sector of the population (Johnson, 1989).

- The average African American male dropout rate was 15.4% in 1991 (U.S. Bureau of the Census, 1993).

Blacks represent about 3.5% of total enrollment in U.S. colleges and universities; they are disproportionately represented among students forced to withdraw, those with relative lower academic performance, and those who have more negative college experiences (Allen, Epps, & Haniff, 1991).

Wingert (1990) reported that although African American high school graduates are doing better on college entrance exams, fewer are going to college. Specifically, the percentage of low-income African American high school graduates attending college dropped from 40% to 30% between 1976 and 1988; enrollment of African American middle-class high school graduates dropped from 54% in 1976 to 36% in 1988; and enrollment of middle-income African American males dropped from 53% in 1976 to 28% in 1988 (p. 75).

Although there are many perspectives on how African American ethnic group membership affects the education of African American males, most educators express dismay, frustration, and even fear when describing the situation surrounding the education of African American males. Groce (1988) concluded that academic achievement depends on the level of parental involvement, parental support, and parental expectations for their children's educational experience.

Many African American males, especially those in adolescence and older, appear to lack a positive cultural identity derived from their African American experience; a culturally relevant belief system that will promote their survival in a hostile environment; a sense of compassion and respect for other African Americans, especially other males; the willingness to accept the nurturing required to overcome seemingly hopeless situations; and the social competencies needed to carry out their mandated functions and responsibilities. For some, these qualities have been translated into behaviors such as playing the dozens, hustling, gang affiliation, woofing, and so on, primarily as survival strategies. If these beliefs and behaviors are to be attacked, a steadfast commitment on the part of parents, schools, churches, community groups, and state and federal officials will be needed so that African American males may be empowered to affect their world, thus making a future for themselves. African American males must be sensitized to their own biases, perceptions, and assumptions about themselves while they are simultaneously made aware of the biases, perceptions, and assumptions of others toward them.

There are many hypotheses concerning the nature of unique problems faced by African American males. Cummings (1986) attributed the persistent failure of African American males to unchanged relationships between teachers and African American males. McDermott (1987) ascribed the difficulties African American males experience in the educational system to what the school has done to them rather than something they have done to themselves. Two hypotheses that serve as major explanations of African American male school performance are those posited by F. D. Erickson (1982, 1984, 1987) in his cultural difference theory and by John U. Ogbu (1982, 1983, 1987) in his secondary cultural discontinuity theory. Cultural Difference Theory argues that differences in cognitive, linguistic, and interaction styles between teachers and students lead to cultural conflicts that result in mistrust and that interfere with African American male achievement. Remediation for academic difficulties should focus on interactions in the classroom, where a culturally responsive pedagogy is suggested.

Cultural Discontinuity Theory focuses on the political and social structures, both in school and outside school, that lead educators to erroneous conclusions about the schooling of African American males. African American males descended from individuals Ogbu (1982, 1983, 1987) describes as "involuntary minorities." These individuals are frequently skeptical of the American dream and are often cynical about their choices in improving their chances by using the beliefs and strategies of the mainstream.

Although these and other theories on the nature of African American male difficulties in educational settings provide useful insights into the causes of problems, many fall short in providing specific programmatic strategies to remedy the situation.

The process by which African American males, who are different in culture, language, and background, have related to and interacted with the culture of the United States is a major point in understanding African American male ethnic identity and in developing culturally specific education strategies. Ethnic identity comprises four main components: ethnic awareness of one's own group as well as other groups; ethnic self-identification, in which individuals identify with a particular group; ethnic attitudes, which include one's feelings about one's own and other groups; and ethnic behaviors, which are the culturally derived behavior patterns specific to an ethnic group. Specifically, racial identity refers to one's sense of belonging to an ethnic group and the part of one's thinking, perceptions, feelings, and behavior that is due to ethnic group membership.

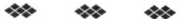

It appears that African American males must learn at least three cultures if they are to be successful. These three cultures are the dominant culture of the United States, the African American culture, and the African American male culture. A number of distinctive characteristics give strong credibility to the uniqueness of an African American culture. Many of the characteristics of African American culture are not characteristic of the dominant culture.

A number of cultural elements have been carryovers from Africa and have survived in the United States. These include dialect, folklore, adult-child relationships, family structure, music, generosity or hospitality, respect for the law, religion, sense of justice, and the work ethic (Asante, 1987).

One specific cultural value is that Africans have a different concept of time than that of the Western world. This difference exists because Africans have no way of expressing a distant future. Another difference is that in traditional African societies, people emphasize that something is being done at the present moment or is done habitually. The Western view of time is linear, with an emphasis on what point on the time line an event occurs, for example, whether it is past, present, or future.

In becoming African Americans, Africans had to develop a new framework capable of holding their beliefs, values, and behavior. What was useful from Africa was retained; what was useless was discarded, and new forms evolved out of the old. This adaptive strategy allowed African American males to carve out a world where they could get on with the business of living, building families, kinship groups, and a way of life capable of sustaining them under the conditions they found in the United States. African American culture is testimony to the process of adaptation and cultural exchange. Although the cultures of West Africa differ in many ways, the traditional worldviews of these cultures are remarkably similar. Among other things, each culture places a great deal of importance on family and kinship relationships, religion, and the care of children.

Hilliard (1976) described the core cultural characteristics of African Americans with the following language. African Americans, he said,

1. Tend to respond to things in terms of the whole picture instead of its parts. The Euro-American tends to believe that anything can be divided and subdivided into pieces and that these pieces add up to a whole. Therefore, art is sometimes taught by numbers, as are dancing and music.

2. Tend to prefer inferential reasoning to deductive or inductive reasoning.

3. Tend to approximate space, numbers, and time rather than stick to accuracy.

4. Tend to prefer to focus on people and their activities rather than on things. This tendency is shown by the fact that so many African American

students choose careers in the helping professions, such as teaching, psychology, and social work.

5. Tend to have a keen sense of justice and are quick to analyze and perceive injustice.

6. Tend to lean toward altruism, a concern for one's fellow man.

7. Tend to prefer novelty, freedom, and personal distinctiveness. This is shown in the development of improvisations in music and styles of clothing.

8. Tend not to be "word" dependent. They tend to be very proficient in nonverbal communications. (pp. 38-39)

A cultural nation is a people with a common past, a common present, and a common future. The society may be that of the United States, but the values are African American. African American values only come through an African American culture. Culture is stressed because it gives identity, purpose, and direction. It tells you who you are, what you must do, and how you can do it. Without a culture, African American values are only a set of reactions to the dominant culture. African American culture is an expression of the desire of African American males to decide their own destiny through control of their own political organizations and the formation and preservation of their cultural, economic, and social institutions.

Those who maintain that African American males must also learn a unique African American male culture suggest that the way to learn culture is with specific manhood training. Among those who have proposed realistic rites-of-passage programs are Brookins and Robinson (1995). They described a formal structured rites-of-passage program that serves to empower adolescents with competencies to face the challenges they will encounter in adulthood. Although this program is designed for all African American adolescents, female and male, its potential for African American male manhood training is obvious. The Adolescent Developmental Pathways Paradigm includes four stages. The preparation stage is designed to "bring closure to the childhood identity and heighten the youth's awareness of the developmental changes that are about to take place" (p. 175). Separation, the second state, includes education on adult responsibilities and an exploration of adult roles and identities. The third stage of transition includes activities that help youth "negotiate the disparities between the suboptimal and optimal values and world views they experience in their expanding social environment" (p. 175). The final stage, reincorporation, signals the establishment of a new identity for the adolescent, one that includes psychological competencies to face the challenges of being an adult and benefit the adolescent's community.

I believe that the most effective programs for African American males are those that actively promote the ideology of multiculturalism. African American males who have developed bicultural competence are likely to be more effective in negotiating the experiences they face in school and in the real world. Rotheram-Borus (1993) found that a substantial proportion of adolescents will choose to identify themselves as bicultural when given the option.

Karenga (1977) described Afrocentrism as a worldview that places Africa and African culture and history at the center of African American efforts to resolve problems. This African worldview emphasizes the following principles: (a) interconnectedness; (b) harmony; (c) balance; (d) affective epistemology; (e) authenticity, spontaneity, and naturalness; and (f) cultural awareness.

The distinguishing characteristics of this Afrocentric paradigm are based on the Nguzo Saba, or the seven principles of nationhood *(umoja, kujichagulia, ujima, ujamaa, nia, kuumba,* and *imani).* These seven principles are traditional precepts in African culture, and they form a coherent value base that guides thoughts, behaviors, and emotional expression (Karenga, 1977; Phillips, 1990). Umoja (unity) reflects the need for harmony and interdependence and the importance of relationships. Kujichagulia (self-determination) reflects empowerment of the community and authenticity. It involves the capacity to choose among alternatives and to determine one's behavior. Ujima (collective work and responsibility) refers to mutual interdependence and balance; active togetherness with family and community; and a collective past, present, and future. Ujamaa (cooperative economics) means financial interdependence and shared resources. There is a belief that the only things one owns are the things that can be given away. Nia (purpose) refers to meaningful contributions that benefit not just the self but the collective. Kuumba (creativity) suggests that there is a creative spirit in everyone that can bring into being a new reality. Creativity is a product of self-determination, and the goal is to build and uplift, not to destroy. Imani (faith) reflects the interconnectedness of the past, the present, and the future. Out of this principle, one derives faith in family, friends, and community.

GETTING ON THE RIGHT TRACK PROJECT

The "Getting on the Right Track" project described in this chapter was developed with the Sedlacek and Brooks (1976) dimensions of success and

Karenga's (1977) principles of the Nguzo Saba as the foundation for specific activities. These dimensions are critical if African American males are to persist in school, and if they are to become successful once they leave school. They are strengths that must be developed or nurtured if African American males are to survive. The following eight dimensions are those that are indicative of successful African American males.

The first is positive self-confidence. African American males who have strong feelings of self-worth, who have strength of character, who have self-determination and independence, have better chances of succeeding than those who do not.

The second is realistic self-appraisal. African American males who have a realistic understanding of their academic strengths and weaknesses have better chances of succeeding than those who do not. When students use their strengths to work on their weaknesses, they seem to be in better positions to persevere academically and to do well in later life.

The third is understanding and ability to deal with racism. African American males who understand and deal with racism effectively succeed more often than those who do not. African American males must learn how to handle prejudice and racism in ways that are not self-destructive or harmful to themselves or others. The school and community must help students identify racism in their personal experiences, to work to eradicate racism in the society, and to respond to racism with effective strategies. By doing this, boys become strong and healthy men who have pride and confidence in who they are as African American males.

The fourth is a preference for long-range goals over more immediate, short-term needs. African American males who accomplish this task will succeed at a greater rate than those who must have their needs met immediately. African American history provides numerous examples of models who had few of their most basic needs met and still made significant contributions to society. These models had a greater than ordinary ability to defer gratification.

The fifth characteristic of successful African American males is the availability of a strong support person. This person may be a family member, teacher, counselor, pastor, or friend. These people help students cope, prioritize, and persevere in the face of great struggle.

Sixth, African American males are more likely to succeed if they have successful leadership experiences. Students who participate in school activities and organizations have a greater likelihood of succeeding than those who only participate in classroom activities.

Seventh, African American males who have demonstrated community service have a greater chance of persevering and doing well than those who do not. Students who are part of organizations and activities in the community that assert African American culture and values have an advantage over students who do not.

Eighth, African American males who have knowledge acquired in a field are more likely to do well than those who do not. If students have culturally related ways of obtaining information and demonstrating knowledge, then they can feel confident about the ways in which they come to new knowledge and understanding.

The Getting on the Right Track project was a pilot program for 160 African American students in two rural high schools in North Carolina (40 students in each high school class). Although the program included both males and females, the strategies employed were of particular relevance for African American males.

The project was initiated as a deliberate psychological educational intervention with three objectives: (a) to make the school an effective social center by cooperative rather than competitive learning, (b) to make the educators involved with the student participants significant adults by addressing the interests of the students and acting as advocates on behalf of the participating students, and (c) to strengthen the ego identity with an Afrocentric perspective to role-taking experiences.

Ninth-grade students were selected for the project; according to middle school personnel, they were academically capable and needed some assistance to be able to pursue a college education after high school. Each student signed a contract that indicated a willingness to participate in all aspects of the program including (a) a commitment to pursue a college preparatory curriculum; (b) permission for the project staff to periodically review school records; (c) adherence to a code of behavior; (d) willingness to meet regularly with a teacher mentor and the project staff; and (e) a promise to maintain regular contact with the teacher mentor, project counselor, or the graduate assistant assigned to the project in case of any educational or personal problem.

Seven teachers volunteered to serve as mentors to students in the project. These teachers made a commitment to meet informally with project participants weekly to monitor their progress. Several mentor teachers took students for lunch on weekends, had breakfast with them at school, or spent time with them in other nonschool settings. Teachers received no compensation for their participation, and they were not relieved of other school duties for serving as mentors. They did receive free conference registration to an annual conference on the education of African American children hosted by a local university.

Parents/guardians of student participants, seen by the project staff as central to the success of the project, were contacted by letter and phone to inform them that their child was selected for the project and to request permission for their child to participate. Parents were invited to a meeting early in the school year where the project was explained to them and where they signed a contract indicating support of the project goals and their commitment to encourage their child to persevere academically. Of special note is that every child in the project was represented in the first parent/guardian meeting. Attendance at all other parent meetings has been 80% or higher.

The primary activity of the freshman year was a 1-hour meeting between the graduate assistant assigned to the project and the student participants every 2 weeks for the entire academic year. Students were taken from their regular classes to participate in the project. Students were taught some African American history and culture; basic communication techniques, for example, importance of eye contact and assertiveness; study techniques; and strategies for successful interracial interactions. The greatest amount of time in these biweekly meetings was devoted to what was called an "Afrocentric Identity-Enhancing Science Project." This deliberate psychological education (Sprinthall & Scott, 1989) aspect of the project, conducted by the graduate assistant, involved developing thinking and research skills and included the following:

1. Identifying student interests and hobbies, which were translated into research questions. For example, one student whose interests included sewing completed a research project on patterns in African fabrics; another whose interests included writing did a comprehensive study of newspaper production.

2. Reflection on naming self *African American,* as opposed to *colored, Afro-American, Negro,* and so on.

3. Exploration of historical evidence of Africa as the cradle of civilization. The primary basis for this evidence was taken from Ivan Van Sertima's (1976) book, *They Came Before Columbus,* a review of evidence of an early African presence in the Americas.

4. Contrasting the Mercator projection with the Peters projection of world maps to see where certain continents are placed on maps and to explore reasons for their placements. Comparisons of map sizes of continents were made between their sizes on maps and their land mass sizes.

5. Writing letters to individuals related in some way to their research project to gain primary information.

6. Writing a research paper on their topic. Topics were often related to students' regular study in science, language, or social studies.

7. Preparation of an oral presentation for a science fair that was held at a local university.

8. A field trip to a local life and science museum. (Locke & Faubert, 1993)

During the second year of the project, sophomores served as peer mentors to new freshmen who entered the program. Sophomores also directed the new freshmen in their Afrocentric Identity-Enhancing Science Project. This mentoring and teaching provided the sophomores an opportunity to participate in a significant role-taking experience (Locke & Zimmerman, 1987). Sophomores also participated in the science fair with their mentored freshmen and took a field trip to a historically black college.

The third year of the project afforded opportunity for the juniors to expand their activities, because the current sophomores assumed the roles of peer mentors for the new freshmen. Junior year activities include researching and writing their family histories, participation in a community service project (e.g., volunteering at a day care center or retirement home) for a minimum of 8 hours, thoroughly investigating a minimum of five colleges/universities, participating in the regular career awareness activities at school, and a field trip to Washington, D.C.

Year 4 of the project involved having the students focus exclusively on college preparation. For those who needed to retake the Scholastic Aptitude Test, help sessions were provided. Students explored financial aid opportunities and narrowed their college choices to two or three institutions. The students took a field trip to the Atlanta University complex of colleges in the spring.

The qualitative results of the project provide evidence that when school is an effective social center where cooperative learning takes place, rural African American students can and will succeed. They are proud of themselves, and significant adults in their schools and communities are pleased with their progress. Of the 40 students who entered the program as freshmen, 32 graduated from high school and all had plans for attending college. Quantitative data revealed that students gained in both abstract thinking and level of ego development (Faubert, Locke, Sprinthall, & Howland, 1996).

TALKING IN THE STREET AND TALKING IN SCHOOL PROGRAM

"Talking in the Street and Talking in School," a speaking skills program, was designed to dispel some misconceptions about black English and offer training for African American high school senior students to understand black English and to learn standard English. Because of the worth our society places on language and "correct speech," black English was described as useful in some settings, and standard English was described as useful in some settings. The most important message communicated to the participants was to learn the appropriate time(s) to use each.

The clear message of the program was that students who wish to move into the mainstream of the dominant culture in the United States must have the ability to speak standard English. It is not racist to encourage African American youth to learn standard English. In fact, it is racist not to encourage these youth to learn standard English. Failure to teach all students standard English, in effect, relegates those who do not to positions of extreme disadvantage.

Prior to the implementation of the program, we assessed the beginning level of communication. Although this does not require the use of a speech therapist, a therapist was used in this program to determine if the youth were speaking black English or poor standard English. Two books were useful in learning about the distinction between standard English and black English: John Baugh's (1983) *Black Street Speech* and Geneva Smitherman's (1977) *Talkin' and Testifyin'*. Students' speech was recorded prior to beginning the program, and progress was monitored during the program and at its conclusion.

The first area to receive attention in the project was self-concept development. African American males need to feel good enough about themselves to be willing to attempt different speaking tasks around their peers and before their teachers and other adults. Self-concept development included discussions about race, ethnicity, prejudice, racism, and discrimination.

The component of the program included a focus on speech skill development in the areas of diction, rate of speech, fluency, general voice characteristics, and vocal inflection. These areas were taught prior to beginning instruction in public speaking, the third major component of the project. Participants were actually taught black English so that they could know themselves when their speech was nonstandard.

The program focused on nonverbal as well as verbal communication. Most writers in communication conclude that the majority of any message communicated is nonverbal (Mehrabian, 1981). Students and teachers jointly developed culturally specific nonverbal behaviors. Students were then shown how their nonverbal messages influence their verbal ones and vice versa. Specific to the area of nonverbal communication is assertiveness and listening skills. Participants were taught how to assert themselves without being either aggressive or passive. Participants were also taught active listening skills.

Once these skills were fairly well developed, students began developing public speaking skills by preparing speeches on topics of their choice. Students were encouraged to write speeches on things about which they were already knowledgeable. Speeches were videotaped, and students were encouraged to analyze their own tapes for examples of good standard English speech as well as nonverbal communication.

Participants explored interracial communication, as well. They were surprised to learn that they speak differently in interracial situations. They also discovered that their nonverbal communication differs in different racial/ethnic situations.

The final component of the project was assessment of change in participants from the initial assessment to the conclusion of the project. The final assessment included communication competence, self-reported attitudinal change, and reports from other educators who had observed the youth in the program. This qualitative evaluation indicated that the program was a success, in that participants significantly changed in their ability to speak standard English.

Strong language development programs are important in the promotion of African American student development, because language is the foundation of all other learning. African American males must understand that it is important to understand black English as well as standard English. Students must see that learning standard English is essential for their future success in the world of work.

OTHER PROGRAMS FOR AFRICAN AMERICAN MALES

Ascher (1992) reported on her study of some 20 alternative school programs designed specifically for African American males. These programs ranged in format from the Martin Luther King African American Immersion Elementary School in Milwaukee and the Ujamaa Institute in New York City to afterschool or Saturday schools like the Save a Star program in Detroit and the Urban League-sponsored Children of the Sun Program in Tampa, Florida. She found that these school and community-based programs for African

American males reflect common characteristics, including (a) appropriate male role modeling and male bonding; (b) identity creation and self-esteem through "transition to manhood" programs; (c) cultural inoculation or protection against the hostile forces of prejudice, poverty, drugs, unemployment, and disease; (d) strengthening parent and community involvement; and (e) a safe haven as a healthy alternative for the streets.

The Holweide School in Germany (Ratzki & Fisher, 1989/1990) is an example of a school with a personalized school environment. The school serves culturally diverse students who previously were classified as noncollege-bound. Teachers work in teams of six or eight with 120 students, who remain as a unit for 6 years. Teachers decide how to group students, who will teach what subjects, how the day will be organized, what curriculum materials will be used, and how much time will be devoted to each subject. The program also has strong community and parent involvement components.

Many programs have been developed at the college/university level for recruitment, retention, graduation, and placement of African American males. One successful program is the Peer Mentor Program at North Carolina State University in Raleigh (Locke & Covington, 1992; Locke & Zimmerman, 1987). The program was initiated to answer the challenges facing African American students in a predominantly white environment. The primary objective of the program is to aid first-year students in their academic, emotional, and sociocultural adjustment to the university. African American juniors and seniors who express a desire to help others and who are themselves academically successful are selected as peer mentors. Each peer mentor is assigned three to five first-year students, and teams are formed of three to five mentors along with those they mentor. The teams are organized to promote program-wide communication, to form a small group of peers for social and personal support, and to provide the peer mentors with support in their helping roles.

Peer mentors participate in a formal and comprehensive training program designed to help them develop effective active listening skills, establish positive relationships with those they mentor, and to learn skills necessary to facility the smooth integration of others into an existing, predominantly white environment. Mentors are then enrolled in a two semester-hour credit course in paraprofessional counseling, with topics such as communication skills, crisis intervention, self-awareness and self-identity, values clarification, developmental needs of first-year students, time management skills, African American awareness, and coping with unique problems of being African American on a predominantly white campus. A unique component of the course is a unit (about one fourth of the course) on African American identity formation, and in particular, the nature and development of African American identity in a predominantly white environment. The rationale for this unit is that students who have accurate information and opportunities to explore racially sensitive issues will develop the skills necessary to succeed in culturally diverse environments. Research results on the program found that peer mentors increased in their level of ego development as a result of participating in the program (Locke & Zimmerman, 1987). Qualitative evaluations of the program indicate satisfaction with the program; graduating students report the program was critical to their retention and graduation.

STRATEGIES TO IMPROVE THE EDUCATION OF AFRICAN AMERICAN MALES

The issue is how schools can educate African American males, perhaps the nation's most disenfranchised group, without substantial macrolevel societal changes. What is the motivation for African American youth who see their place in society as a dead-end experience? Strickland (1989) suggested that if African American males are to survive the educational process, "we must recapture our history for ourselves and our young people, and then, standing on that history, we must develop new strategies of struggle adequate to the challenges that now confront us" (p. 112). Polite (1994) used the elements of chaos theory, borrowed from quantum physics, to examine the social context of schooling for African American males. Chaos theory includes two theoretical assumptions that are relevant to the education of African American males: (a) Minor changes within or outside the system can render profound consequences on it, and (b) the interrelation of components in a system is more important than any one or more of its component parts.

Gibbs (1988) identified a series of recommendations to be implemented at local, state, and national levels to improve conditions in the schools so that the "continuing waste of human potential and the frequent imposition of negative sanctions against students who desperately need to be recognized in positive ways" (p. 88) can be halted. These recommendations identify the role each must play to ensure quality educational opportunity for African American males.

Local/School Level

1. Recruit and select competent, caring, confident, and creative teachers at school sites and district-level administrators.

2. Implement heterogeneous ability grouping (except in cases of severe handicapping conditions).

3. Ensure that teachers, administrators, and school staff are cognizant of the importance of expectations on student achievement.

4. Value school academic performance.

5. Implement early childhood education programs.

6. Use resources from the business community.

7. Develop and use a resource bank of role models.

8. Improve parental involvement in the schools and parents' knowledge of postsecondary educational requirements.

State Level

Items 3, 5, and 8 from the local level-list require state policies and state funding for effective implementation.

National Level

1. Provide student financial assistance for postsecondary educational opportunities.

2. Provide funding for demonstration projects.

3. Provide funding for establishing preschool and early school year programs.

The process strategies that follow (Locke, 1989, 1998) are aimed at providing educators with specific ways to improve competence with African American males. The strategies are:

1. Strive to understand the worldview of African American males and how their views might differ from that of the dominant culture.

2. Be open and honest in relationships with African American males. Leave yourself open to culturally different attitudes and encourage African American males to be open and honest with you about issues related to their cultures. Talk positively with African American males about their physical characteristics and cultural heritage. Make it clear that a person's identity is never an acceptable reason for rejecting him/her.

3. Learn as much as possible about your own culture. One can appreciate another culture much more if there is first an appreciation of one's own culture. Understand, honestly face, and improve the knowledge of yourself, and this will lead to positive interactions with others.

4. Determine the degree to which the client is bicultural (adaptable to the dominant culture and the African American culture) or traditional.

5. Seek to genuinely respect and appreciate culturally different attitudes and behaviors. Demonstrate that you both recognize and value the African American culture.

6. Begin work with African American males by assuming that they may be bringing strengths to education. Strengths might include their religious orientation, a strong family support system, and a high tolerance for environmental stress. Determine how these strengths might be used to resolve the situation that brought them to education.

7. Take advantage of all available opportunities to participate in activities of cultural groups in the African American community. Work to understand and analyze the development of clients' social, home, and community relationships. Try to obtain direct involvement with members of African American groups and/or with organizations working to improve human relationships, including intergroup relations.

8. Use techniques that communicate to African American clients that they are equals in the therapeutic process. Although clients may perceive the counselor as an "authority," clients must be made to feel that they bring a rich supply of resources that might be useful in the resolution of the precipitating situation.

9. Keep in mind that African American males are both unique individuals and members of their cultural group. Strive to keep a reasonable balance between your views of males as unique beings and cultural group members.

10. Eliminate all your behaviors that suggest prejudice, racism, or discrimination against African American males.

11. Have the client help the counselor explore stereotypes held by the counselor that might be inhibiting the education process.

12. Encourage your colleagues to institutionalize practices in each school or agency that acknowledge the contributions of African American males. Strive to work together toward agreed-on solutions and interactions with respect for differences.

13. Hold high expectations of all African American males and encourage all who work with them to do likewise. Initiate activities to build self-identity and teach the value of differences among people.

14. Ask questions about African American males. Learn as much as you can about African American males and share what you learn with your colleagues. Recognize that the cultural heritage of African American males is as much a part of what makes up that client as his physical characteristics.

15. Develop culturally specific programs to foster the psychological development of African American males.

The preceding discussion outlines areas that are appropriate for use with African American males while recognizing the difficulty in translating many of the suggestions into straightforward guidelines. I believe that all efforts to develop programs specific to the needs of African American males must be based on a solid understanding of African American male development, a clear understanding of the view of African American males in the society in general, a clear understanding of the view of African American males in the specific local setting, and the unique interpretation that each African American male makes of his relationship to these factors.

CHAPTER 12

Meeting the Educational Needs of Homeless and Highly Mobile African American Males

WILLIAM R. PENUEL
BERTHA SHERRILL
TIMOTHY DAVEY
ELIZABETH ALLISON

A mong the most difficult youth to reach through school or community-based programs are those who move frequently. These youth are more often than not poor, and their poverty and mobility means that they don't stay in the same school long enough to form meaningful relationships, learn valuable academic skills, or participate in fun social activities. In short, these students seem always to miss out on things that other students experience simply by being in the same school or neighborhood over time.

Mobility is not easy to define. Some studies of mobility measure cumulative moves, whereas others focus on either residential moves or school transfers (Eckenrode, Rowe, Laird, & Brathwaite, 1995). In this chapter, we consider the effect of mobility from the standpoint of school transfers, a challenging problem for many urban schools today. To be sure, most school systems build in regular transfers between elementary, middle, and high school grades, but mobility within the school year often has quite different

AUTHORS' NOTE: This research was made possible through funds from the Tennessee Department of Education to the Metropolitan Nashville Public Schools. All views expressed herein are the sole responsibility of the authors.

effects because all students do not experience the moves at the same time and the schools do not often provide the same kind of support services for the transition. Mobility rates within the school year for many urban schools can range as high as 30% to 40%, suggesting a steady stream of movement of students in and out of school. Understanding how to meet the needs of these mobile students is then important, both from the standpoint of the school, whose climate may reflect this movement and therefore be constantly in flux, and from the standpoint of the students, who must adjust to new schools, develop new relationships with students and peers, and find their way through their new classes and coursework.

Young African American males are among those most at risk for such mobility, and the combined effects of multiple school changes and poverty put healthy self-development, a sense of cultural and community belonging, and student achievement in jeopardy. The fact that they are more likely to grow up in poverty (Johnson, Miranda, Sherman, & Weil, 1992) and to fall behind in school (Resnick, Burt, Newmark, & Reilly, 1992) make the risks of school transfer more pronounced. In addition, many African American males experience the worlds of home and school as disjunctive and opposi- tional (Ogbu, 1978). School-based programs can, however, help to reduce these risks while at the same time building on the strengths of many mobile students. Providing students with a way to belong and feel a part of school communities can help build a strong sense of self. Partnering veteran students with newcomers can give the latter a sense that they have someone to whom they can turn in times of need. Tutoring programs and school social work services can support student achievement and ensure that these students are not lost by schools when they move. Below, we consider in greater detail some of the risks associated with student mobility and the resources that can support student achievement, self- development, and belonging.

A PORTRAIT OF SOCIAL AND EDUCATIONAL RISK: ACHIEVEMENT AND STUDENT MOBILITY

Several educational studies have shown that students who change schools frequently show poorer school performance than their peers who stay in the same school over time (Benson, Haycraft, Steyaert, & Weigel, 1979; Cohen, Johnson, Struening, & Brook, 1989; Eckenrode et al., 1995; Felner, Primavera, & Cause, 1981; Ingersoll, Seamman, & Eckerling, 1989; Levine, 1966; Mundy, Robertson, Greenblatt, & Robertson, 1989; Pedersen &

Sullivan, 1964). Although some studies (e.g., Greene & Daugherty, 1961; Marchant & Medway, 1987) have not shown such an effect, most of these have not included samples of students from backgrounds of low socio-economic status. Other studies have pointed to the critical role poverty plays in making the negative impact of student mobility more apparent. For example, Johnson and Lindblad (1991) found that achievement scores of students who moved within the city (intracity mobility) were lower than for students who moved from city to city. In addition, they found that those who were moving within the city tended to be from lower socioeconomic backgrounds than those moving from city to city. Apparently, city-to-city moves were associated with job advancement, whereas intracity moves were often necessitated by changes in family and housing situations connected to being economically disadvantaged.

Researchers have suggested different reasons for how mobility works against students. For example, Dohrenwend (1966) proposed that students from economically disadvantaged families are exposed to more stressful life events, of which moving from school to school is one among many that contribute to psychological distress. Eckenrode et al. (1995) have suggested that maltreatment figures strongly in the explanation of the effects of student mobility. They found that more maltreatment leads to higher levels of mobility, and higher levels of mobility were related to lower levels of academic achievement. Haour-Knipe (1989) has suggested other factors that might link mobility and achievement: separation and loss associated with friends and familiar places, difficulties in making new friends, changes in curriculum and teacher expectations. Indeed, several researchers have found that mobility can negatively affect peer relations in school (Brockman & Reeves, 1967; Jason et al., 1992) and that mobility for students living in poverty is strongly associated with lower self-concept (Ziesemer, Marcoux, & Marwell, 1994). Whatever the reasons, mobility for students in poverty seems especially detrimental to school success.

Moreover, the risks associated with growing up as an African American male compound the risks of school failure and dropping out associated with mobility. More than half of all African American children are raised in mother-only households, as compared with 17% of European American children and 26.6% of Hispanic children (U.S. Bureau of the Census, 1992). Recent studies show that boys raised in such households are at greater risk for disciplinary problems at school, among other behaviors (Anderson, 1993; Dryfoos, 1990; Sampson, 1991). Young African American males may, more-over, develop a sense of identity and learning that is in opposition to school cultures, which have historically excluded African Americans from opportunities to succeed (Ogbu, 1978, 1991).

One of the factors that mediates school performance of African American males, it has been suggested, has to do with differences between the culture of home and the culture of power, as experienced by students themselves. The culture of home refers to the ways of thinking, acting, and valuing that one learns at home (Delpit, 1988). This culture is one that is learned early, and it is most difficult to hide or change (Gee, 1990). For middle-class white children, the culture of home's norms for thinking and acting closely resemble the norms of schools, but for African American males, these norms may be quite different. Schools foster far more independent, competitive ways of acting and encourage communicative norms that may be experienced as alien by African American students (Collins, 1993).

PROTECTIVE FACTORS AMONG MOBILE AFRICAN AMERICAN MALES

Getting to school is often much more difficult for students who move often. Children who are homeless represent one such group. When they do attend school, however, school serves as an important place for them, an oasis from the chaos of the shelter (Schilit, 1989). In this regard, school attendance for homeless students, like other mobile students, does appear to make a difference in how students perceive themselves within their environments. Timberlake and Sabatino (1994) found that children who attend school regularly had higher levels of self-esteem and lower levels of loneliness. School officials need to remember that attendance is often itself a positive achievement of mobile students and should thus be considered an aspect of resiliency for these students, who get to school each day through their own efforts and choice. Mincy (1994a) points out that in this connection, public schools have a great potential to promote the development of young black males, because they provide opportunities to learn basic skills and an opportunity to interact with people from different cultural and socioeconomic backgrounds.

Besides adopting these progressive strategies to educate African American male students, educators must help support the development of a healthy relationship toward the culture of power. According to Collins (1993), there is a need for educators to support the process of intertwining of students' home culture and the culture of schools, all the while making explicit the possible benefits to students: having the choice to perform competently in both home and school culture, having the choice to synthesize both cultures, and having the choice to legitimize the culture of home. There is a particular need to develop among African American males a sense of cultural belonging and positive group identity, particularly to recognize and reframe the kinds of resistance that Ogbu (1978, 1991) describes in his research. In particular, the historical reasons for opposition or resistance to educational achievement need to be appreciated by school staff. Efforts should be made to recognize the contributions of African Americans to education in the United States, to affirm the identities of people in the classroom, and to provide opportunities to develop a positive sense of belonging *both* to a school community and to one's own cultural group. Belonging is in all likelihood a basic human need (Maslow, 1970), made all the more difficult to meet when students move often and when students' cultural identities are not recognized in the curricula and practices of schools.

SOME DROPOUT PREVENTION STRATEGIES FOR MOBILE AFRICAN AMERICAN MALES

In this section, we present examples of components from programs that share a common measurable objective: reducing the dropout rate among mobile students of low socioeconomic status. Each of these program components has been part of evaluated programs (see in particular, Jason et al., 1992); they are presented together here as possible strategies to use in a variety of settings. We interpret each of these interventions in a different way than they have been previously interpreted, in that we view each intervention as contributing somehow to the goals of introducing students explicitly to school culture and providing students with opportunities to develop a relationship to school culture that prepares them for success.

Orientation Programs

One of the most valuable services for mobile African American male students is an orientation program (see Weine, Kuraski, Jason, Danner, & Johnson, 1993). Placing children in small groups and reviewing school rules, support programs, and clubs in which students can get involved helps students to feel more at home in their school. It's important that such orientation programs take place periodically during the school year, because many students move, not at the beginning of the school year, but in the middle. Research suggests that the negative effects of unscheduled transitions that take place during regular school year as opposed to the summer are greater (Brockman & Reeves, 1967). Often, students who change schools in mid-year miss out on important class events, such as field trips, book fairs, and the orientation program provided at the beginning of the school year. These events are often significant in the life of the school, and mobile students need opportunities to find out about their school's culture and climate and about how they might belong to that school community.

In this connection, schools need to become more like communities of learners, as several advocates and researchers have suggested (Brown & Campione, 1994; Rogoff, 1994). In other words, schools need to have good strategies for making new, diverse students feel welcome and a part of the school. As communities, schools need to inform new members of the community about its characteristic ways of acting, speaking, and being in that school and introduce students to the meaningful events, symbols, and values that help to define the identity of the school. As part of this introduction, norms about how teachers and students communicate, learn, and participate together in group activities should be explicitly named and shared so that young African American male students have the chance to learn what is expected of them to succeed in school. For their part, according to Walling (1990), teachers "need to demonstrate to the new student that he or she is a valued addition—and valued as a person—from the first moments in school" (p. 25). This includes, for Walling, learning about cultural backgrounds of students and discussing school culture with them. Schools, furthermore, need to develop ways to ensure success of mobile students, including the use of multiple teaching modes, cooperative and team-based learning, and authentic assessment of performance. In this way, schools can help develop a greater sense of ownership among mobile students. Cooperative education is especially recommended by researchers for African American male students (Ferguson, 1994) and mobile students (Weine et al., 1993).

Homework Centers

Tutoring is recommended by many educational researchers working with mobile youth. Weine et al. (1993) suggest that tutoring programs include both parents and teachers in learning how to give strategic assistance to students to complete homework and other school tasks. They have found that while academic gains following their program to help transfer students in an urban school have been somewhat limited (mostly to the domain of spelling), participants in their program did improve in the area of social development, possibly through the positive relationships built with adults through the program.

After-school homework centers are one way to organize programs in which adults help young people or peers help each other to complete homework tasks assigned during the school hours. They are designed to meet the needs of students who often do not have a quiet place in which to complete assignments given by teachers at school (Prentiss, 1996). Homework centers may rely on a diversity of teaching methods and strategies. Some rely heavily on peer tutors, whereas others use certified teachers from local school districts. Some take place at school, whereas others may be housed in community-based organizations and faith communities. Although the effects of participation in extracurricular activities for minority males are mixed, those that are school-focused (such as science fairs) have proven to be effective in raising student achievement (Lisella & Serwatka, 1996).

Teachers and tutors at homework centers typically have different roles from school teachers in the classroom, in that instead of selecting tasks for the students, tutors helping with homework must make sense of and work with tasks brought to the center by students (Prentiss, 1996). This means that the relationship between tutor and student is that of two people working to solve a common problem, with one (the tutor) being more expert in solving the types of problems that might come up and the other (the student) being in a better position to define what must be completed. The relationship between tutor and student in homework centers is, moreover, constantly shifting, depending on how many participants are present, the tasks or homework to be completed, and the specific questions of students (Frank, 1996).

Homework centers thus can serve as effective learning environments for children because they can promote the development of a collaborative relationship with an adult or more capable peer that is both personally meaningful and focused on doing well in school. Although homework center activities may look a lot like school activities, to young people, they can seem more accessible than school because adults relate to them more personally and with greater individualized attention.

Cultural Enrichment Programs

Particularly for young African American males, programs that promote the development of cultural awareness, respect for diversity, and positive cultural self-concept based on a sense of competence and values are important to mobile youth. Providing opportunities to participate in a variety of modes of learning that honor the cultural contributions of different groups can provide a context for healthy self-development. Sharing forms of storytelling, healing, dancing, and music is a way to encourage such a context and provide young males with the resources they need to develop a sense of self as capable of doing well in the world.

It is particularly important that schools provide different ways to recognize the diverse identities that make up their student body. Administrators, teachers, and students all need to have opportunities to learn from one another the stories of their families, cultures, and shared practices and to know how others can affirm them. Given mobile youths' specific needs for belonging, it's important that such programs emphasize how members of different cultural groups relate to one another and can form bonds of friendship across difference as well as within one's own group.

School Social Work Services

Mobile students need people within the school system who can act as their advocates and who can keep track of their moves. School social workers are often in a good position to be such advocates. They can engage in a number of activities that help mobile students: case management, provision of school supplies and adequate clothing, advocacy and communication with teachers, and coordination of services for families. Dupper and Halter (1994) suggest that advocates who work closely with parents and schools to coordinate services such as transportation, appropriate clothing, and school supplies can make a differences in the lives of mobile youth. Schools, for their part, can reduce barriers to enrollment, providing adequate transportation and access to special programs, school supplies and a safe place for one's property, and food (free breakfast and lunch).

Johnson and Lindblad (1991) recommend counseling for families and students to help them adjust to school. Such counseling can help young African American males feel a greater sense of connection to the school and to develop a positive self-concept as youths who are able to adapt to new situations and thrive within new environments. Also, working with families in this way can help them to feel more a part of the school community and provide parents with a safe place in which to share their own stresses and frustrations.

Attendance Tracking

One of the ways that many mobile students get "lost" by the school system is a rapid decline in school attendance that goes unnoticed by school officials. Schools can help avert this situation by assigning advocates for mobile youth who track attendance and warn attendance workers when these students miss several days of school. School social workers can make home visits to discover what the reasons for lack of attendance may be. In some cases, a family will have moved again and transferred schools without notifying the school. Sometimes, records take several weeks to transfer, so it appears that a child is missing school when he or she is in fact attending somewhere else. In other cases, the student is having problems getting to school, and having someone tracking attendance can prevent more serious truancy problems and possibly help children stay in school.

Buddy Systems

Jason et al. (1992) advocate the use of buddy systems to help build bonds between new and old students at schools. Having a buddy in a new school can reduce the sense of isolation and alienation for new students and give them a peer to whom they can talk about issues they may be facing in school. Buddies who receive training may be more effective than those who don't, as training can alert buddies to some of the issues the newcomers may be facing and give them some suggestions about how to answer questions and respond to concerns of the new students.

PUTTING IT ALL TOGETHER: BUILDING COMMUNITIES OF LEARNERS

Isolated program components designed to serve students facing particular challenges in their lives are hardly ever effective in themselves. We would do well in our school systems to build cultures of learning within each of our schools, so that they become true communities of learners in partnership with agencies in the larger community (Brown & Campione, 1994; Rogoff, 1994), communities in which students can come to feel quickly a sense of belonging. Measuring the success of programs for mobile African American males in particular requires sensitivity to the issues of inclusion, recognition, and support within these communities. Schools that are inclusive in their instructional practices, recognize the diverse and distinct identities of their students and teachers, and provide support for healthy self-development and academic communities must be built from the ground up, relying on democratic principles for program development, implementation, and evaluation. With these tools, we can make schools a better place for all our children.

CHAPTER 13

The Education of Adolescent Black Males: Connecting Self-Esteem to Human Dignity

GARRETT ALBERT DUNCAN

Over the past decade or so, much attention in the United States has been given to the plight of black men and boys. The statistics are all too familiar: By now, most of us know that the number one killer of young black males is their cohorts; we also know that one in three of these young men, on any given day, is under the supervision of the criminal justice system. The most recent research also reveals that the rates of unemployment, teenage fatherhood, and death for young black males are higher than for any other social group.

We know that, in school, black male children and teenagers are overrepresented in programs for students that are categorized as being mentally retarded as well as for those that are designated as having behavioral problems. Black male students are also underrepresented in college preparatory tracks and classes for gifted and talented youth. Statistics such as these have shaped a public perception that black male children and youth are at risk for failure in American society. Some observers, particularly within black communities, liken the plight of young black males to that of an endangered species (Gibbs, 1988). This metaphor has inspired the publication of books and has led to a number of conferences and workshops across the country; also, one may reasonably argue that concern over the status of black men played a large role in the tremendous success of the Million Man March in October 1995.

It is true that young black men and boys bear disproportionately the brunt of America's social ills, are in the crosshairs of narcotic enforcement agencies and anticrime legislation, and are a sizable part of the labor force that drives the burgeoning prison industry. However, the nearly foregone conclusion that to be young, black, and male is to be doomed to failure and misery glosses over the vast majority of young black males who lead constructive and productive lives. Moreover, metaphors that compare young black males to beasts reinforce beliefs that these young men are a menace to society and fails to consider that society may be, in fact, a menace to them.

This chapter addresses these issues and has the objective of providing strategies to foster the wholesome development of adolescent black males, with an emphasis on interactions within the classroom. As I hint in the subtitle, the broader purpose of this chapter is to move beyond a view of self-esteem that limits our conceptions of the conditions confronting adolescent black males to one that is linked to the affirmation of human dignity. As I shall discuss in greater detail below, the former way of understanding self-esteem often proceeds from the premise that the personal and social problems of young black men originate within them; affirming the humanity of adolescent black males, however, entails acknowledging that we live in a social order that deliberately constructs itself to promote a view of black youth as subhuman, even to the extent of compelling them to accept their lot in life, including the fact of their own inferiority and worthlessness.

WELCOME TO THE TERRORDOME! THE CLASSROOM EXPERIENCES OF ADOLESCENT BLACK MALES[1]

As I suggested above, relationships are critical to fostering the wholesome development of adolescent black males. Understanding the relationships that structure the schooling experiences of adolescent black males is a first step toward creating environments that enhance self-esteem and affirm human dignity. From an instructional standpoint, the placement of relationships as central to pedagogy is consonant with current learning theory. In succinct terms, such a learning theory posits that children and youth learn in settings through their interactions with other people and things. If anything interferes with these dynamics, that is, prevents or disrupts these interactions, the learning process diminishes. In addition, we know that learning not only refers to cognitive development but also is connected to affective (feelings), effective (skills), and intuitive factors, as well. Therefore, teacher practices that disrupt learning in one domain will have an impact in other domains as well.

Certain practices undermine the education of children and youth in general and have particularly disastrous effects on adolescent black males. In the main, these practices include instances where teachers systematically

◆ *Seat black males farther from them than they do other students.* This practice makes it more difficult to monitor the work of these students or to provide them personal feedback. Some studies indicate that black females are used as social translators—or buffers—between teachers, mainly white females or males, and black males.

◆ *Seat black males closer to them than they do other students.* Although this seems to contradict the previous practice, it has a similar outcome—disrupting the relationships between students and the teacher. The practice of seating black males closer to the teacher serves the purpose of surveillance and control of the body as opposed to monitoring work. By seating black males closer to them, teachers are able to record every infraction of class rules, for the express purpose of either generating documentation for referral to special education or for initiating disciplinary procedures. Students readily pick up on this and will generally provide the teacher all the evidence he or she needs.

◆ *Give black males less direct instruction.* This generally contributes to students' confusion and frustration over what is expected of them by way of assignments and/or behavior. In many ways, this practice is related to the culture of power within which teachers are embedded and in which they erroneously assume that their students participate (Delpit, 1995). Here, the lack of direct instruction may have to do with an assumption of a shared system of codes and communication. Thus, less direct instruction occurs when teachers assume that their students already know what is expected of them. In other situations, teachers initiate less direct interaction simply to avoid contact or confrontation with black males.

◆ *Pay less personal attention to black males in academic situations.* This includes smiling less often, maintaining less eye contact, and limiting other nonverbal forms of communication that indicate attention and responsiveness. These behaviors reinforce suspicion and mistrust and the general feeling among black males that they are unwelcome in the classroom.

◆ *Call on black males less often to answer classroom questions or to do demonstrations.* This practice has much to do with unexamined beliefs on the part of teachers that black males do not know the answers or have incomplete or inadequately prepared assignments.

♦ *Interrupt the performances of black males more frequently than they do those of other students.* This often has to do with the unwillingness of teachers to take black males seriously or to show the same patience when working with them that is shown when working with other students.

♦ *Give black males less time to answer questions before moving on.* This also has to do with the unwillingness of teachers to take black males seriously or to show the same patience when working with them that is shown when working with other students.

♦ *Do not stay with black males in failure situations.* This practice, related to the two previous ones, is manifested in the unwillingness of teachers to apply standard instructional strategies, such as prompting, providing clues, or asking follow-up questions.

♦ *Criticize black males more frequently than other students for incorrect public responses.* These responses are more often than not associated with teachers' perceptions of the young men's conduct and less to do with academic performance. In other words, students are given negative criticism about their personal attributes as opposed to constructive responses that critique the actual work in question.

♦ *Praise black males more frequently than other students for incorrect public responses.* While this practice seems to contradict the aforementioned one, praise here may be associated with teachers' lowered expectations for what students are able to do. In these instances, teachers are satisfied to get even an utterance from their resisting black male. This practice is also related to twisted notions of constructivist pedagogy and multiculturalism, which lead teachers to accept whatever students give them for the sake of "affirming the learner" or the "learner's culture."

♦ *Provide black males with less accurate and less detailed feedback than other students.* In many ways, this practice has to do with teachers not wanting to waste their time, energy, and resources doing things that they believe will not make a difference. These practices are also related to deficit theories that posit a genetic basis for the plight of black males; whether one assumes that black males are "part monkey," as 14-year-old Albert believes white people perceive him most of the time (Duncan, 1997), or subscribes to the views advanced in *The Bell Curve* (Herrnstein & Murray, 1994), the tacit belief here is that black males will not benefit from additional attention and resources.

◆ *Fail to give black males feedback about their responses more frequently than other students.* This practice is informed by the same views that inform the preceding practices.

◆ *Demand less work and effort from black males than from other students.* This is another practice that is related to low expectations and the unwillingness of teachers to enter into difficult situations with adolescent black males. The reluctance of teachers to challenge black males to complete demanding work has to with uncritical beliefs that these young men are volatile and may cause physical harm. Unwillingness to call black male students to task for poor academic work has also to do with unfounded concerns that doing so will damage these students' self-esteem.

◆ *Assign lessons to black males that emphasize behavior management and control more often than to other students.* This practice has to do with the punitive character of education that informs the schooling experiences of adolescent black males. It is also related to preconceptions of teachers concerning what preparation is necessary for the economic stations that these students will later occupy in life—whether they are low-paying repetitive jobs, prison, or both—that demand behavioral compliance of their workers.

◆ *Interpret the narrative styles of black males as inarticulate, perceive the speech patterns of black males as inchoate and incomplete, and interpret signifying black males as violent, hostile, and aggressive.* These practices are related to a combination of factors: meanings ascribed to compositional styles that do not conform to topic-centered prescriptions; confusion over the status of black speech; and preconceived notions that connect adolescent black male discourses to hip-hop and rap culture and, by extension, "gang" and urban "street" culture. Also, these views are connected to nonverbal communicative behavior associated with black males, such as "cool" attire, stance, posture, gestures, and facial and visual behaviors (e.g., eye contact, rolling of eyes, gazing, glaring, and staring), as mentioned in an earlier section of this chapter (Majors, 1991; Majors & Billson, 1992).

Many of the above practices are shaped by distorted perceptions that teachers have of black masculinity in general, and young black males in particular. These perceptions are sustained by uncritical habits of mind, or *dysconsciousness* (King, 1991), and by habitually unexamined attitudes, or *habitudes* (Flores, Cousin, & Diaz, 1991). Mental images, here, exist as conceptual cultural artifacts and are buttressed by memories of real and imagined experiences, as well as the emotions, such as fear and anger, associated with them. What is significant about these conceptual cultural artifacts is that they quite readily come to bear in concrete forms (Cole, 1996). As they play out in classrooms, these perceptions create and sustain conditions that disregard the humanity of adolescent black males.

Changing these environments is no easy task. First and foremost, unless a teacher has a proven track record of success with adolescent black males, he or she will be met with institutional resistance to efforts to transform the conditions of these students. Sentiments that young black males are irredeemable and beyond repair are reinforced by a political climate in which black youths are equated with crime and punishment, leaving very little room to discuss anything that has to do with affirming human dignity and promoting the empowerment of adolescent black males—those very issues that are central to responsive education. It is possible to overcome these institutional limitations, but in doing so, teachers will likely have to work through a classroom culture within which black males have been conditioned, often since kindergarten, to accept the fact of their own unworthiness.

A personal experience may help to illustrate this point. Over the course of a year in the early 1990s, I taught both physical science and chemistry in a public high school in the Inland Empire of Southern California. Physical science is a watered-down combination of chemistry, physics, and geology and is placed in the curriculum for the sole purpose of meeting high school graduation requirements. This and like courses in other disciplines (e.g., English, math, and social science) offered at this school have no value in terms of college requirements. This fact was not lost among the students in the course, a number of whom did not want to take a college-prep course in the first place; the school accommodated these students by providing three non-college-prep courses for every single college-prep course in the four major disciplinary areas.

I took it on myself to initiate a shift in the curriculum of the physical science course to one that emphasized chemistry and that shared the same material and equipment to which other students had access. The widespread response to a question posed to students in the physical science class after the completion of their first chemistry laboratory exercise is relevant to the present discussion, illustrating with painful clarity how curriculum and instructional practices work together to shape youth identities. The exercise in question had to do with determining the identities of unknown substances.

When, on a follow-up quiz, I asked what was the purpose of the experiment, students in the chemistry class who, ironically, had to be dragged, screaming, into the exercise, answered, simply and systematically, "to determine the identities of the unknown substances." However, their mostly black and Chicano male peers in the physical science class, who enthusiastically and without hesitation participated in the exercise, just as readily and systematically answered the same question, "to determine if we behave well enough to have future labs." In this instance, the young men in this class had been conditioned to understand the meaning of their schooling in terms of behavioral compliance, whereas their classmates in the college-prep section were taught to view their education in terms of intellectual performance. To paraphrase Madhubuti (1990), the former group of students were being trained to control their bodies from the neck down, while the latter group was learning to work theirs from the neck up.

Indeed, although it was rewarding for both me and my students in the physical science class to engage in a more rigorous and challenging curriculum, the transition did not occur automatically. Moreover, there were minimal attempts to modify behavior directly; it was quite clear that behavior problems had more to do with the lessons prepared in the classroom and how students were treated than anything else. Therefore, emphasis was placed on curriculum development and a constant evaluation of the forces that shaped the class dynamics. Also, there were setbacks (I expelled a student from class who purposely placed a white-hot metal spatula in another student's hand, to name the most severe case). However, the greatest reward was in the increased enthusiasm for learning (for instance, one student confided that science was the only reason he showed up for school), shifts in attitudes, and the development of skills on the part of the majority in the class. In addition, we were able to convince the principal and department chair to support the opening of additional chemistry (college preparatory) courses for the following school year.

WORK IS LOVE MADE VISIBLE: TRANSFORMING EDUCATIONAL SETTINGS FOR ADOLESCENT BLACK MALES

In the context of my practices as a classroom teacher, as sketched above, as well as current research in education, I offer the following suggestions to both enhance self-esteem and promote the wholesome development of adolescent black males. I divide these suggestions into three areas: curriculum, instructional practices, and teacher behaviors.

Curriculum

◆ *Involve students with issues they regard as vital concerns and place them ahead of the curriculum.* This includes making explicit issues that relate to race, class, gender, and sexuality. In the physical science class, for instance, we explored the scientific and social ramifications of environmental racism and medical sexism. Both issues were initiated by published news reports. The first article, published 400 miles north of our city in a San Francisco Bay Area daily newspaper, reported on the concentration of hazardous waste materials in East and South Central Los Angeles—figuratively in our own back yards and literally in the backyards of a number of our relatives. The second article was published in a local newspaper and reported on the failure of medical science to develop technology able to synthesize Taxol, a substance that is vital to women's health and, at that time, obtained primarily from the bark of an ever diminishing natural resource.

Responsive pedagogy does not need to be restricted to science. The involvement of students with issues they regard as vital may be accomplished across the curriculum. As it relates to the traditional curriculum, the most basic way of transforming cultural dynamics in the classroom is through the inclusion of literature that speaks to the reality of adolescent black masculinities. There are the familiar works, such as *The Autobiography of Malcolm X* (Haley, 1965/1992), *Manchild in the Promised Land* (Brown, 1965), *Invisible Man* (Ellison, 1947/1989), and *Black Boy* (Wright, 1945) as well as more recent works, such as *Makes Me Wanna Holler* (McCall, 1994), *Monster* (Shakur, 1994), *Living to Tell About It* (Dawsey, 1996), *Parallel Time* (Staples, 1994), and *Brotherman* (Boyd & Allen, 1996). The inclusion of literature that connects to the lives of adolescent black males is more than simply an issue of promoting ethnic boosterism, racial pride, or surface-level self-esteem. As research indicates (Ball, 1995; Lee, 1991), such literature provides an interface that promotes cognitive scaffolding or, in other words, lasting and transformative learning, in schools.

◆ *Make explicit relations of power at work in the classroom, school, community, and society with respect to the students' lives.* For the most part, adolescent black males have some level of awareness of the relations of power that shape their realities. However, articulating the actual mechanisms is a process of making the political pedagogical (Giroux, 1985), or making explicit in concrete terms the forces that shape social reality. Only when adolescent black males are able to visualize and articulate the circumstances that bind them will they be able to transform them. Self-destructive behavior is the product of invisibility and silence.

◆ *Engage students in the use of technologies that access information.* This task promotes not only self-development and economic participation, it is also related to transforming the broader U.S. culture as it relates to dominant constructions of black masculinities. With respect to the economy, schools where black youth are concentrated are slow in coming to terms with the reality that society is no longer based on an industrial economy organized simply around capital and labor. Rather, the United States is swiftly becoming a society where access to and manipulation of symbols and information define the economy. The Bureau of Labor Statistics anticipates that between 1995 and 2010 over 90% of the jobs to be created in the United States will be related to information and service (Anderson, 1994). Two major considerations become evident here as it relates to the present discussion.

First, U.S. industries in the immediate future will produce jobs that will be divided between a disproportionately high number of opportunities in low-paying, low-status, unstable positions and a small number of high-paying, high-status, more secure ones. Black males are generally confined to the former category and often are left out of the latter altogether, putting them at risk of contributing to the economy as workers in prison, "America's newest growth industry" (Bloomer, 1997, p. 14). Thus, responsive curricula attend to the economic realities that face black males and provide them opportunities to master the technologies that will play large roles in shaping the quality of their adult lives.

Second, any economy based on the flow of symbols and information necessarily involves the production and reproduction of culture and the formation of identities. These symbols have everything to do with the construction of perceptions of black males in the wider society, including how black males come to perceive themselves. Thus, access to informational technologies is a means to obtain both control over the material forces and the flow of information that shape the lives of black men and boys.

◆ *Involve students in re-doing, polishing, or perfecting their work.* In terms of curriculum, this is perhaps the most difficult but most critical task in fostering the wholesome development of adolescent black males. In addition to promoting the values of perseverance, self-discipline, and tenacity, it provides the opportunity to reinforce the fact that individuals are not merely passive objects but are, in fact, active agents in the social construction of reality. It fosters a disposition of vibrant participation, a disposition that is necessary for adolescent black males to become *the* major force in their lives. Madhubuti (1990) says that this practice in the classroom distinguishes the development of those who are trained to depend on and work for others and those who are educated to take charge of and control their destiny. Research bears this out: In its annual report, the Education Trust (1996) lists rigorous curriculum as one of the defining characteristics of high-achieving schools in poor neighborhoods.

Instructional Practices

◆ *Communicate the objectives of the lesson.* Although this strategy may seem obvious, the fact that teachers systematically avoid adolescent black males in the classroom makes it one that bears highlighting. Students need to be told what they will learn, how they will learn it, the behavior needed for the mastery, and how the new learning is related to prior knowledge. Also, objectives are concrete, as opposed to the ambiguity associated with *purposes, aims,* and *goals.*

◆ *The teacher understands the relationship between theory and practice.* This strategy is related directly to the preceding one. Indeed, teachers must have a vision—that includes purposes, aims, and goals—of what they want for their students. This vision, or theoretical foundation, however, must be linked to well-defined and concrete practices in the classroom. Peter McLaren (1989) describes these distinctions in terms of larger macro-objectives and discrete micro-objectives; Paulo Freire (1970/1990) describes the critical union of these two pedagogical dimensions as *praxis.*

There is also a political dimension involved in this strategy, apparent in the manner in which teachers perceive their roles, such as in the distinction between being agents of change or control; how they relate to black males, their parents, and their community; how they define expectations for their students and work to bring these expectations into fruition through the creation and establishment of new curriculum; and whether they acknowledge their personal limitations.

◆ *Plan activities so that students have a high rate of success.* This strategy is often misunderstood to mean to water-down the curriculum or to promote self-esteem without demanding academic achievement.

On the contrary, as I have indicated throughout this chapter, students generally excel in classrooms with rigorous curricula because they offer more interesting as well as more purposeful and stimulating lessons. In this vein, by orienting presentations toward active involvement and using a variety of approaches (for example, discussion, inquiry, concept development, peer tutoring) and entry points (which is common in project-based curriculum), teachers adjust for individual differences in the way students learn. Also, within these learning experiences, teachers should establish routines and structures in the classroom. Doing so enables teachers to foster the conditions that support cognitive scaffolding, as described earlier, and that assist students in transforming scholastic knowledge organized in schools into the intuitive knowledge that leads to empowerment (see Gardner, 1991, for a discussion on learning processes and the organization of knowledge in schools).

Teacher Behaviors

◆ *Foster a supportive socioemotional climate.* As I indicated in the beginning of this section, the learning process is fundamentally a social process and is informed by cognitive, effective, affective, and intuitive factors. Emphasis thus far in this chapter has been placed on strategies that involve primarily the first two factors. The latter two factors are closely related and are often downplayed as being unimportant in the learning process. For instance, some teachers are known to say that students do not have to "like" them in order to learn from them. On some levels, this position may be true. Yet, in a society that is stratified by relations of power, such sentiments overlook the fact that many teachers not only dislike black males but in fact despise and are fearful of them.

Elsewhere, I (Duncan, 1993) described how children detect negative teacher perceptions and respond to these teachers in adverse ways. More recently, a 6-year-old black boy, a participant in an afterschool computer club, indicated to an adult white participant that he and his mother, who happened to visit the club that day, were "different" from black people and, at the same time, from other white people. These distinctions were made spontaneously and to affirm the relationship between the child and the adults. Moreover, the child's remarks were responses to the respect and dignity with which the young man, a first-year college student, treated the young boy over the course of several weeks in the computer club. If a boy of 6 years old can make distinctions such as these, it goes without saying that adolescents can, too.

In concrete terms, then, a supportive socioemotional climate is characterized by more smiles, head nods, forward body leaning, eye contact, friendliness, and demonstrated empathy for students' expressions of feelings, which may include an occasional outburst. Also, there is an absence of the use of shame and humiliation, screaming and haranguing in these settings. Defuse, sidestep, and redirect all challenges to authority. Do not try to control students by knowingly putting them on the spot or attempting to embarrass them; the latter is done, often inadvertently, by asking for private information publicly.

Along these lines, Martin Haberman (1994) argues that "teachers who start out intending to dominate poor children or youth are doomed to failure" (p. 133) and suggests providing the conditions for their empowerment as the only alternative. This does not mean that teachers should allow disrespectful behavior from adolescent black males. The aim here is for teachers to assist young men to overcome limiting and debilitating forms of resistance and, at the same time, to understand and support their resistance to subordination and injustice (Darder, 1995).

◆ *Provide more verbal input.* This is another suggestion that appears self-evident but, because of existing classroom conditions for black males, is being made explicit here. Specifically, when teachers fear, dislike, or do not understand their students, they avoid talking to them and thus limit the opportunities for these students to engage new and rigorous curricula. Even when such curricula are provided, the absence of dialogue may lead to confusion and frustration, resulting in students being penalized for their behavior and beliefs being reinforced concerning their motivation or intellectual capability. Also, as is true in any learning situation, students should also be provided with increased verbal outputs, such as clue giving and rephrasing, as well as being given additional opportunities to respond to tasks. Along these lines, teachers also will do well to give more effective feedback to adolescent black males, which means more praise for achievement and less criticism that, in many situations, is driven more by animus and less by concern for the students' development.

◆ *Model cooperation with all other adults in the school and demonstrate respect for parents in the presence of their children.* As I indicated earlier, my focus on the role of teachers in promoting the wholesome development of adolescent black males does not ignore the fact of the broader institution of schooling and the relations of power that are intrinsic to shaping classroom environments. Also, differences in style and approaches among teachers and administrators are natural to any school setting. It is important that teachers work through differences, not only to model these processes for students, but to form the alliances that are necessary for the success of adolescent black males.

In addition, it is not inconceivable for teachers who demonstrate respect for black males to be the target of suspicion by their colleagues. In some instances, adult coworkers may even openly express their disdain for or disapproval of the work of that teacher, even in the presence of students. Teachers who are the objects of such politics cannot afford to react to this kind of treatment in an uncritical fashion. This does not mean that poor treatment is to be accepted or tolerated. It does mean, however, that teachers run a tremendous risk of undermining their good work by entering into what are often petty battles. In addition, students have expectations about the way teachers are to conduct themselves in such instances, even if these expectations are at variance with their own behavior. Furthermore, students often lose respect for teachers who take on the characteristics of those teachers who disrespect them. The rationale for students is simple: If a teacher can be harassed into speaking ill of colleagues, including administrators—and especially behind their backs–a teacher can also be driven to do the same with students.

In a related vein, many of the paraprofessionals, custodians, office workers, and cafeteria personnel in the schools where adolescent males are concentrated come from and reside in the school community. It is not impossible for the school's custodian to be the popular and well-respected pastor of a neighborhood church or the office manager to have a prominent role in the civic life of the community. In other words, these individuals may be a teacher's greatest ally at the school, assisting her or him to marshal resources or to mobilize the community on behalf of students or possibly even a teacher.

Finally, it goes without saying that teachers must show respect for students' parents and/or family members. Respect, here, also means understanding the boundaries and limitations of the authority that a teacher has. Even teachers with the best intentions may undermine their work by presenting themselves as a savior or by presuming to know more than the parents about what is best for their child. Indeed, teachers have critical knowledge and are in fact invaluable, even essential, to the livelihood and wholesome development of adolescent black males. However, it is up to the families, however defined, to determine the terms of a teacher's participation in their lives.

CONCLUSION

Although this chapter highlights issues incident to the education of adolescent black males, I hope to impress on readers the larger issue of how identities are constructed not only within the institution of schooling but also within the context of the broader society. To reiterate a major premise that guides my thinking along these lines, the construction and experience of adolescent black masculinities is a dynamic relationship that, in the United States, is under constant negotiation within an often hostile context. When we speak of individuals and groups in terms of their relationships, we begin to develop a greater understanding of the circumstances that shape their lives. By viewing black males in relational terms, we begin to comprehend that young black men and boys live in a society that deliberately and systematically conveys and reinforces images of them as violent, unintelligent, irresponsible, and irredeemable.

Also, by rethinking some of our most basic beliefs about schooling, we begin to see that the entire educational enterprise is about changing lives—of both students and teachers. For the most part, schools have not sought to change adolescent black males in ways that foster self-esteem or affirm human dignity. Indeed, to respond to adolescent black males in schools in ways that acknowledge their humanity and promote their empowerment is not without its difficulties. In some instances, this entails going into uncharted areas where we, to paraphrase Cornel West (hooks & West, 1990), jump out on nothing and hope to land on something. As West suggests, the greatest limitations may be those that we impose on ourselves. The fact that most secondary classrooms are relatively autonomous arenas of learning should be grounds for optimism, however. Furthermore, given the bureaucracy of schooling in urban districts, where most adolescent black males attend schools, teachers may largely dictate what goes on in their classrooms on a day-to-day basis.

Such freedom runs counter to teacher perceptions of what they can do in their classrooms and points to possibilities for teachers to forge spaces for new sets of assumptions and practices that affirm the dignity and worthiness of young black males and, furthermore, promote self-esteem that is based on empowerment and a heightened sense of one's humanity. Such freedom also keeps alive both the possibility that teachers will continue to take risks with their adolescent black males and the promise that they will be rewarded with the success of their students and the support of the communities within which they teach.

NOTE

1. In the next two sections, I draw on the work of Darder (1995), Haberman (1991, 1994), Moody and Moody (1989), and the Education Trust (1996), and on my own practices and work as an educator, teacher-educator, and educational researcher.

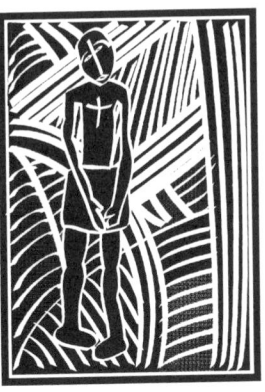

PART IV

Familial
Relations

Familial relations are more important to African American males than most of us realize. Families serve to make men more civil, if not indeed more civilized. It has been suggested that family life for men has a number of benefits for them and society: It controls and focuses their sexual energy, children make them aware of themselves as role models, and the material needs of their families promote regular work and self-sacrifice (Courtwright, 1996; Durkheim, 1951). Indeed violent crimes are largely committed by unattached males (Courtwright, 1996). Family men have better mental and physical health, live longer, make more money, and have a greater sense of personal self-worth. Moreover, the positive involvement of African American males in family life affects both fathers and their children. It serves to increase the probability that fathers will spend more of their energy "doing the right thing" and that their sons and daughters will have a greater probability of "seeing what the right thing looks like."

However, the past 20 years have seen a dramatic decline in rates of father-present African American families (Tucker & Mitchell-Kernan, 1995). Major structural changes in our society have negatively influenced the quality and types of familial involvements for many African American males (Bowman, 1989; Wilson, 1987). It remains imperative for those who practice, at either individual or programmatic levels, to encourage and promote positive, nurturing, nonviolent, and supportive familial relations for all African American males. We must act in contrast to many social welfare efforts, which have consistently attempted to assist African American families while largely ignoring African American males. Although some may attempt to minimize the importance of father presence, asserting that others will step in to fill their shoes, reality suggests that too few others do so. As is true for mothers, there is no real substitute for fathers (McLanahan & Sandefur, 1994; Vosler & Robertson, 1998). In addition to their breadwinner roles, males provide social-emotional support as well as a much needed male perspective to family life. All this is not to suggest that organizations such as Big Brothers and 100 Black Men do not provide valuable services to the rearing of African American children. Still, it should remain our foremost goal, as practitioners, to enhance the functioning of as many original family units as possible. This goal will require those who practice with African American males to work to sustain their existing familial relationships, reunite those that have fallen into dissolution, and improve those that have become problematic or dysfunctional for any of their members.

African American males have too frequently been invisible components of African American families. And although it is true that about 58% of African American families are headed by females, it is also true that African American males are sole parent to 4.3% of all African American families (U.S. Bureau of the Census, 1996). Most will agree that there are still far too few fathers in African American families. But by the same token, this figure is higher than many might imagine, given the numbers of African American males lost yearly to unemployment, prisons, drugs, and homicides.

The foremost goal of this section is to promote healthy relationships between African American males and their families. These efforts serve to enhance all African American males including those who reside with their partners and those who do not. It must be remembered that to improve the familial relations of African American males is to improve the quality of life for the entire African American community.

CHAPTER 14

Family Practice With African American Males

RUTH G. McROY
SADYE M. L. LOGAN
EDITH M. FREEMAN

African American families are often portrayed in the literature and the media as primarily single-parent families in which the African American male figure is either absent, marginally present, or dysfunctional. However, recent statistics show that in 1990 there were 3.8 million African American married couple families and 3.7 million African American single-parent families. About 39% of African American families with children were headed by married couples in 1990, 57% of African American families with children were headed by females, and 4% by males (U.S. Bureau of the Census, 1991a). Attention must be given to the daily stresses faced by African American families and in particular the roles of African American men in those varying family structures (Daly, Jennings, Beckett, & Leashore, 1995). This chapter focuses on unique economic, social, and cultural issues associated with African American males and their families. It presents theories guiding practice, obstacles to treatment, and guidelines for practice with African American males and their families.

ECONOMIC PROBLEMS AND MARITAL RELATIONSHIPS

Studies on economic status and marital satisfaction among African Americans (Belle, 1982; Gray-Little, 1982) have reported a direct relationship between satisfaction with marriage and income and education. Marital satisfaction decreases as income and education decrease, probably due to the stress associated with poverty, unemployment, and bleak outlook for the future.

For dual-earner African American families, median incomes were about $39,601 in 1990, whereas in families where only the husband was employed, the median income was $25,037; it was $21,400 when only the wife was employed. When both spouses were not working and living primarily on retirement income, the couples received an average of $13,789 (U.S. Bureau of the Census, 1991a).

As black women are often hired instead of African American men for the same positions, there will be increasingly more African American women who may be earning more than African American men. In 30% of African American families, women earn more than their husbands (Davis, 1993). For African American men who desire to be the main breadwinner, an inability to fulfill this goal can sometimes lead to marital distress (Whetstone, 1996). Moreover, when African American marital partners judge each other by the size of the partner's paycheck, problems may develop in the marriage.

The prevalence of marital instability and divorce among African American families is increasing. For example, in 1990, there were 28.2 divorces per 100 African American marriages and 13 divorces per 100 white marriages (U.S. Bureau of the Census, 1991a). The disparity between couples' earnings and the low earnings of many African American men may lead to higher rates of marital dissolution and may make some men and women less likely to remarry. Moreover, increasing rates of joblessness, as well as declining incomes, have been found to be associated with the trend of African American men to never marry, to delay marriage, and to be less likely to remarry, especially those who are poor (Chadiha, 1992).

Some couples have been successful in finding ways to withstand the tensions resulting from job instability. For example, Chadiha (1992) reported the findings of her study of 64 urban African American couples in which husbands' economic problems were viewed as "a dysfunction in the transaction between people and their environments" (p. 545), rather than dysfunctions within the family. These couples reported that they generally had to delay marriage plans due to husbands' job layoffs, unemployment, or lack of money. They found strength in one another throughout these difficult times and tended to adapt through mutual decision making, to postpone marriage, to save money for marriage, to accept help from family; in some cases, both partners work, and if needed, work more than one job. Mutual interdependence, communication, flexibility in family roles, and an understanding that the problems did not stem from family dysfunction led the couples in this study to survive and adapt to difficult economic times.

Employed husbands may also experience anxiety associated with the possibility of job loss. For example, Staples (1985) noted that one in three African American employed males will experience unemployment in a given year. Referring to males in precarious employment situations as "the working worried," Lawson and Thompson (1995) noted that African American males often work several jobs at one time to buffer the effects of periodic employment. However, their long work hours often limit the amount of time for a spouse and may lead to marital dissolution (Booth, Johnson, White, & Edwards, 1986). Research has shown that both husband and wife must work in most African American families in order to have incomes equivalent to one white spouse working. If the wife becomes unemployed, additional financial stress may occur, which may lead to more marital dissatisfaction. Moreover, issues such as financial strain due to periodic unemployment, differences in spending practices, incompatible personalities, differences in religious practices, and failure to negotiate conflict were found to be causes of divorce among working- and middle-class African American men (Lawson & Thompson, 1995).

LIFE COURSE ISSUES: STRENGTH AND RESILIENCE IN AFRICAN AMERICAN FAMILIES

Despite negative experiences with such life course issues as racism and economic insecurities, most African American families have proven to be resilient and have found ways to successfully cope and survive. The African American community remains a source of strength, recognition, and support for building self-esteem and improving overall life satisfaction of African American males over time (Daly et al., 1995). Although the majority of African American males feel that they are providing well for their families, younger African American males, due to the lack of available jobs, are less likely to perceive themselves as being good providers than males 65 and older (Taylor, Leashore, & Tolliver, 1988). Older males' positive self-perceptions may be derived over time by receiving positive feedback and recognition from the community as being good providers to their families and having taken responsibility to give back to the community.

Life course issues, for African American males, are shaped within a bicultural, often racially oppressive, hostile environment. Within this context, predominant life course issues include or are influenced by (a) the level of nurturance within the home and family, (b) availability of educational opportunities, and (c) level of stress in the world of work. The interplay of these factors underscores the complex nature of African American family life as well as the need to study and understand the deeper layers of African American growth and development.

THEORIES GUIDING PRACTICE WITH AFRICAN AMERICAN MALES

Given the complex nature of family practice and the unique concerns of African American males and their families, it is imperative that appropriate theoretical lenses be used when viewing this population. We propose that a developmental perspective coupled with ecological and family systems theory within an African-centered context provides the necessary framework for understanding and working with African American males. Ecological systems theory offers a conceptual framework that supports a vision of people, places, and things as an interrelated, interconnected whole (Germain & Gitterman, 1995). Systems ideas further reinforce the notion of wholeness, as well as openness or growth and development (Compton & Galaway, 1994). This view shifts attention from placing blame to searching for solutions. Family systems concepts suggest that we are inextricably linked to our family of origin and all of the generations preceding, that everything that happens in life is affected by past life experiences (Bowen, 1978).

McAdoo (1993) noted that ecological theory allows one to consider the varied roles of African American men and allows for understanding these men individually and collectively. Furthermore, these conceptualizations focus our attention on the interface between the transaction of African American men and the different levels of their environment, particularly the physical or natural world, which includes ancestors, deceased and living (the spirit world), and the cultural world, which includes values, beliefs, attitudes, artifacts, rituals, myths, and the overlapping social world, which includes neighbors, self-help and support groups, and organizations.

In general, the helping professions have focused most, if not all, their attention on the third level of the environment, which includes elements broadly shared across families and organizations. But to fully exploit the implicit promise of ecological and family systems conceptualizations in providing a culturally appropriate assessment of and treatment to African American men and their families, it is necessary to use an African-centered paradigm. This paradigm provides a functional, cultural framework that reflects the cultural and political reality of African Americans men. It is useful for understanding and talking about approaches to reaching African American males in treatment.

GETTING MEN INTO TREATMENT

Often, African American men display distrust of social service agencies and may be very reluctant to participate in family or individual therapy (A. J. Franklin, 1992). Some, feeling that they have not been effective providers for their families, may be reluctant to begin a therapeutic relationship and may discourage their wives from sharing the private details of their lives with a therapist. Having often developed a "healthy cultural paranoia," as a result of historical experiences with racism and possibly personal experiences of betrayal in their lives, many African American men will find it hard to overcome their distrust and concerns about getting involved with yet another white institution. Practitioners must not only have historical and contemporary knowledge of the experiences of African American men, they must also be aware of African American men's developmental and life cycle issues and how they have coped with these issues over the years. It has been our experience that along with a strong knowledge base, a strong therapeutic alliance is not only critical to getting African American men into treatment but also to supporting them so they stay with the process. Factors that should be considered are the sex and ethnicity of the therapist, gender role issues, power issues, and self-disclosure.

Sex of the Therapist. Due to the historical and contemporary, perceived and real, power and privilege issues between African Americans and whites, as well as ongoing stereotypical images of African American males as being often hostile, aggressive, and sexualized, the gender and ethnicity of the therapist can become overlapping issues influencing family practice with African American males. Some African American men may be uncomfortable with a female therapist of any ethnicity due to their reluctance to reveal personal vulnerabilities. Some may see females as a threat to their own employability, as many affirmative action programs have benefited white females at the expense of minority males. Others may be reluctant to work with a white female due to the historical stigma and vulnerability associated with interracial relationships. Some may also be reluctant to enter therapy with a white male therapist if they see economic opportunities being controlled by white men. Others may express a preference for a male therapist due to fears that a female therapist might be less likely to see problems from the husband's perspective. Still others may prefer to enter therapy with an African American male with whom the client may feel greater self-identification and rapport. Others may express no gender preference. This is a complex matter and must be individualized based on the male's masculine identification regarding dependency, level of acculturation, previous experiences in therapy, and emotional expressiveness, as well as feelings of support and trust toward the therapist.

An initial evaluation should be conducted at intake to determine if the African American male expresses a specific desire for a therapist of a particular gender. Questions can be asked about the client's relationships with both men and women and how comfortable he feels in discussing issues with a male or female therapist. Such an evaluation may suggest the need for a male or female therapist or a male-female co-therapist team. The primary issue in relationship building between an African American male client and the therapist is trust. Trust building is often related to such qualities as ethnicity, empathy, warmth, genuineness and true respect for the family in treatment.

Ethnicity of the Therapist. Some African American men may prefer to see an African American therapist because they feel that they can more readily connect and trust another African American. As mentioned earlier, they may feel anger toward white males and females, whom they may perceive to be responsible in part for job scarcity and the ongoing legacy of race relations in this country. However, other African American men may actually express a desire to see a white therapist, primarily due to their assumption that a non-African American therapist is less likely to know the client or to know others who may know him. Again, the key to therapeutic relationship development with African American men is trust. They must be able to feel comfortable with sharing personal information. If this is in doubt, the African American male is likely not to continue in therapy (A. J. Franklin, 1992). These issues must be discussed with the client and his family early in the therapeutic encounter.

Gender Role Issues. Men and women are taking a new look at sex role stereotypes and their impact on their overall relationships. These explorations are also forcing clinicians to examine their own stereotypical notions and to be more constructive in supporting and encouraging greater self-actualization. Available literature and experience supports the notion that African American men, like men of other ethnic groups, are becoming more sensitized to gender issues (Moore Campbell, 1986). Effective helping not only allows men to explore femininity within themselves but also lets women achieve feelings of self-worth and personal power. The practitioner can encourage the African American male client to compare the roles played by women and men in his parents' generation to the roles now being played by men and women, given today's changing family structures. The positive benefits of role flexibility and expansion in adapting to difficult economic times and problems in the marital and other interpersonal relationships should be addressed. Male and female co-therapists in family practice can model ways to address gender issues, mutual interdependence, and dyadic communication about changing gender expectations and nontraditional roles in families.

Power Issues. The discourse about African American men and oppression focuses on the stripping away of their manhood. They are almost always depicted in all facets of life as powerless and lacking in dignity and self-respect. This image has taken its toll on the overall psyche of African American men and many feel invisible (A. J. Franklin, 1992, p. 353). Therefore, when they come into treatment, they may feel the need to prove to their therapist that they are strong, competent, and "in charge." The therapist who is genuine and accepting would be able to demonstrate by example that the aim of therapy is to foster an honest, empowering relationship, not a competitive struggle.

Self-Disclosure. In therapeutic encounters where the focus includes racial and gender role issues, the therapist must be more active and prepared to share personal experiences to express genuine emotions and to relate in a natural caring manner. In this regard, the therapist becomes a powerful role model for the client. The therapist enhances the client's change process, not only by self-disclosing appropriate personal experiences but also by encouraging and affirming nontraditional masculine attitudes and roles (expressing feelings, doing housework, cooking, or caring for children).

CASE EXAMPLE

The following family situation involving Roger serves to illustrate some of these issues faced by African American males, as well as the process of treatment.

Roger is 56 years old and the father of a 14-year-old son and a 10-year-old daughter. His wife, Karen, is 43 years old. Roger has a graduate degree in business but is currently unemployed due to a recession. This situation has produced tremendous stress in this family, but especially in Roger, who defines family roles and responsibilities in fairly traditional terms.

Roger grew up in a two-parent family in the segregated rural South, the fifth of 12 siblings. The family's overall income was below the poverty level and created situations where many dreams were deferred. Roger is a sensitive individual who grew up in a religion-oriented family and perhaps was most affected by the context of his upbringing: extremely modest financial means, a segregated social and educational environment, a strict father, a gentle loving mother, and overcrowded housing conditions. Roger always felt somewhat ashamed of his background. Furthermore, he not only saw on a daily basis but experienced that life for African Americans in the South was separate and not equal.

In Roger's terms, he wanted to be somebody, to achieve something and do something with his life. He felt constrained by the inadequate southern educational system for African Americans. Although Roger struggled to obtain an education, he felt constrained by his ethnicity in finding and maintaining employment in the white corporate world. The pain and disappointment that accompanied Roger's upbringing in a mostly hostile, racist world tends to resurface unconsciously in stressful work- or life-related concerns. Generally, these emotions are expressed as feelings of inadequacy or that someone is out to get him.

At present, Roger's son has begun speaking to him in what Roger describes as a disrespectful manner, and there is a great deal of stress in Roger's relationship with his wife. At one point, she moved out of their bedroom.

Life course issues, as illustrated in Roger's story, create a unique context for development and socialization and must be considered in working with this family. Role strain is a significant outgrowth of this unique context. It manifests across the life cycle from the pre-adult stage to old age. In the pre-adult stage, the role strain may result from educational preparation; in early adulthood, from career considerations; in middle adulthood, from fulfilling familial obligations; and in old age, from the aging process itself (Bowman, 1989).

Roger clearly has felt the constraints of societal racism while growing up as well as in his adult life. He is feeling a sense of failure, anger, and helplessness as he slowly loses his primary sources of self-respect and self-esteem. The loss of his job, the means of providing for his family, the respect of his son, and his relationship with his wife have led him to seek help. He may exhibit a great deal of defensiveness and skepticism initially in the therapeutic encounter. It will be important to demonstrate respect; acknowledge his negative experiences as a child, in the corporate world, and in his family; and simultaneously find ways to begin to empower Roger. He will need to realistically focus on the external causes of the job loss and to identify the disempowering statements that Roger may be using to explain his job loss. Roger must become aware of how his own demeanor may be affecting others at home as well as in his interactions in previous job settings, and how he can draw on his strengths to rebuild his career.

GUIDELINES FOR PRACTICE

It is clear that biased descriptions of African American males and families in the professional literature and mass media have contributed to and exacerbated the problems confronting this population. New, more positive perspectives are needed that reflect the realities and marginalized voices of these men and their families. As noted earlier, family practice with African American males is complex. Therefore, it is critically important that practitioners adopt not only the kind of multicontextual framework described above but also a working set of practice guidelines. The following principles based on the theoretical discussion presented earlier are designed to enhance the process of treatment:

1. Regardless of the presenting problems that bring African American males into family practice settings for services, their strengths and common environmental barriers (e.g., institutional racism) to achieving their goals should be identified and addressed. For example, with Roger, it is important to do a complete social assessment, which includes the extended and augmented family system as well as the nuclear family system and social networks. The therapist should review Roger's wife's expectations of his instrumental role in the family and her perception of her role. If she is not currently working, she might consider trying to get a job to help out the family during this time of economic crisis.

2. Afrocentric values and traditions offer a positive, strengths-focused framework for understanding and implementing solutions to the problems that bring clients in for services. The strengths, in Roger's case, include achievement of a graduate degree, despite his family's modest means; his commitment to being successful; his commitment to his family; and his overall accomplishments throughout his 56 years. His family of origin's strong bonds, flexibility, strong achievement, and work orientation against the odds should be highlighted.

3. Culture-related family and community supports, often ignored in traditional services, can be enhanced to provide an ongoing self- and mutual-help system of care. Roger may be encouraged to connect with community resources through the church or other community programs. He may begin to offer low-cost business consulting services within the community to begin

establishing credibility while helping others in need. This may lead to positive references that may aid his job search. In so doing, he "gives back" something to the community while continuing to build his own knowledge and skills in the business arena. If successful, he may decide to begin his own consulting business or at least earn enough money to assist his family while he continues his job search.

Roger may also get his son and daughter involved in his business to begin to teach them job skills. This is also another opportunity to involve the entire family in building money management skills. It may be necessary for Roger to explore job possibilities in other locations, if it is unlikely that he can find a job in his current locale. Role playing with Roger can be effective in assessing how he presents himself during a job interview and to determine if there are changes Roger needs to make that may increase the likelihood of getting a job.

4. Recognize the importance of effective joining with the family. Given the challenges connected with getting African American men into family treatment, therapists need to not only acknowledge this difficulty but also use active action-oriented strategies such as homework, contracts, role playing, genograms, and ecomaps to allow the male client to experience a sense of empowerment and active involvement in the process. It is also critical that the presenting concerns be universalized. In this way, any guilt and shame connected to the concerns can be diffused. It will be important to acknowledge Roger's expertise and experience and to get Roger and his family involved in activities that will help them see positive growth and outcomes early in the counseling experience. Giving Roger's son an opportunity to role-play his father will help him to develop empathy for his current situation and may lead to improved relationships. The family should regularly be given homework assignments, which may involve activities that all four participate in together to improve communication and relationships.

5. Identify and promote strengths within the family and in each member. Through this process the family gains a broader view of each other and their overall capabilities for growth and change. In Roger's case, the therapist should involve the entire family in identifying strengths of each individual member as well as the family unit. In the past, Roger had been very involved in the church, and there may be ways that Roger can become reinvolved at this time. Life course issues for each member of the family should be explored. For example, Roger's wife is 13 years younger than her husband is. She may have very different goals and expectations at this stage of her life than her husband has.

6. Identify the meaning of manhood for the men in the family. Through this process, the therapist is able to evolve an approach that integrates both the male and female voices in the helping encounter. Roger and his son may have different understandings of manhood, given the generation gap. Moreover, as Roger defines family roles in traditional terms, it is important for the therapist to explore the similarities and differences in his situation to help him recognize the external factors that may influence his current employment situation. His son should be helped to explore how he views manhood and his perception of his own manhood and his own outlook for the future.

7. Discuss the ways gender-related behaviors affect each family member. Roger and each member of his family should be asked to explore how they perceive the influence of gender and ethnicity on their life course as a family and as individuals. The therapist might explore how each family member interprets the job loss. If blame is being placed, this should be addressed.

8. Promote the positive ways in which African American partners have supported each other and teach ways to replace manipulative nonnurturing uses of power in the relationship. Roger and his wife have been married for over 14 years. They should take time to recall challenging situations in which they have found ways to support each other. The therapist should point out ways in which their current interactions have led to a power clash. Finding ways for Roger and his wife to feel positive about each other and to empower one another is essential.

9. Recognize and promote the need for intimacy in the family. Roger's family seems very disconnected at this time. It is essential, as the therapist joins the family, that he or she is able to identify the disconnections and facilitate positive interactions. The therapist might suggest ways that the family can have "fun times," despite the bleak job situation.

10. Emphasize the need to be in touch with and clearly express feelings in the family. Communication is a key to improving marital relationships, and the therapist should introduce and model active listening techniques to facilitate communication. Roger's wife has moved out of the bedroom, presumably to passively demonstrate her dislike of their current relationship. The therapist should explore how feelings are shown in the family and assumptions that each may have about the other. Focus should be on the identification of new more effective and active ways of expressing feelings in the family.

Assessment and intervention must, therefore, focus on developing or enhancing existing supports as the process of family practice unfolds. This positive "perspective allows us to predict alternative outcomes to the racial barriers to employment, experiences of social isolation on the job and in the mainstream community, and the development of roles that African American men may play in their families" (McAdoo, 1996, p. 289) as essential and valued members.

Supports may include social networks, support groups, leadership development and mentoring, natural healing, entrepreneurial resources, and other factors. Mutual help and responsibility for the clan are part of the African philosophy and value system (Crawley & Freeman, 1993). Helping to strengthen clients' participation in these supports as well as their role in developing and maintaining them should be a goal of family practice in this area (Freeman, 1990). The implications of such supports are that family and community rebuilding will increase as self-sufficiency improves and a sense of empowerment and mutual competence occur (Freeman & O'Dell, 1993).

It is also important to examine issues of economic and social development with African American males. This element involves reaching the business and economic leaders whose policies and practices affect the social and economic development of African American communities. Some aspects of development will need to involve collaboration with these leaders, African American women, members of other ethnic groups of color, the media, and others with social influence who are willing to join and facilitate, rather than to lead, the process of change. Empowerment at the political level is a critical element for addressing the problems and building on the strengths of African American males, and therefore, for family practice with this population. Two major sources of political empowerment are a shift in some decision making from large institutions to the communities where the population lives (power sharing) and increased cultural sensitivity about these clients' needs by policy makers in other areas.

In characterizing the plight of African American men, Allen-Meares and Burman (1995) pose the question "What happens to an individual who perceives the larger society as hostile, intolerant, and uncaring; opportunities for survival and advancement as limited; and little hope of rising above the status quo" (p. 270)? In response, these authors propose a model for activism, which includes advocacy, empowerment, and class action social work. The focus is on micro and macro issues that affect these clients' goals and aspirations as well as on the consequences of those issues, including racism, discrimination, and poverty (Devore & Schlesinger, 1991).

A single voice appears to be emerging from scholars of African American family life regarding the need for public policy relevant to African American males (Allen-Meares & Burman, 1995; Leashore, 1991; Staples & Bowlin-

Johnson, 1993). Given that many African American males are often unable to secure full-time employment, have a variety of health and educational problems, and experience life as hopeless, the call is for a national effort to provide job training, full employment, health care, and equitable and fair practices under the legal system. Staples and Bowlin-Johnson (1993), among others, believe that for change to occur it will be necessary to advance a public policy to reverse the trend toward an upward redistribution of wealth.

SUMMARY AND CONCLUSIONS

This chapter has presented both conceptual and practical perspectives for practitioners who are engaged in family practice with African American males. African American men and their families are influenced by a variety of social, economic, and political forces that must be understood in order to provide effective services. Societal and familial expectations of the male provider role and economic vulnerability may limit the African American's ability to perform this role, which may lead to personal and familial distress. The African American male's experiences and relationships in his own family of origin, in the community, and during his education may influence his family relationships. Often, due to the negative experiences many African American men have had, they may approach the therapeutic encounter with some distrust and misgivings. Practitioners must convey respect, sensitivity, and genuineness in the therapeutic interaction and must work toward the development of trust. Rather than moving quickly toward a diagnosis, workers must acknowledge economic vulnerability, feelings of anger and despair, and reactions to societal racism. Negative portrayals of African American men and feelings of invisibility may be a part of the problem the African American male client is experiencing. Exploring these issues with the client through appropriate cultural lenses, and identifying the strengths of the male and his family, will make it possible to begin working toward an empowering intervention with African American males.

Activism and systems change are also needed to help develop public policies that reflect the needs, priorities, and social realities of African American men and families. Key policies should aim to improve opportunities for employment, education, recreation, health and safety, housing, and other needs, while helping to achieve individual and family goals identified in family treatment. The African value of *kujichaguilia* or self-determination is consistent with this perspective about the need for African American men

204   FAMILIAL RELATIONS

to advocate for and secure power over their lives and communities. This value requires them "to define ourselves, name ourselves, create for ourselves, and speak for ourselves instead of being defined, named, created for, and spoken for by others" (Gordon, 1993, p. 83). Thus political action becomes an avenue for ethnic and individual self-determination.

CHAPTER 15

Culturally Sensitive Interventions With African American Teenage Fathers

MARK S. KISELICA

In late August 1993, as I strolled through an airport to catch a plane bound for Indianapolis after attending the annual convention of the American Psychological Association in Toronto, I was stopped dead in my tracks by the alarming cover of the August 30, 1993 issue of *Newsweek* magazine, which was displayed on a rack at an airport newsstand. The cover depicted a color photograph of the face of a 7-year-old African American boy named George Martin. George gazed at the camera with a solemn expression that seemed to convey the tone of the cover title, which read, "A World Without Fathers: The Struggle to Save the Black Family."

I remember experiencing an array of ambivalent feelings after I purchased the magazine and read its contents during my flight to Indianapolis. On the one hand, I was relieved that a national magazine was calling attention to the many difficulties faced by a substantial number of African American families, particularly those headed by single mothers who first became parents as teenagers. Also, I was glad that the articles corresponding to the cover title provided an in-depth and accurate analysis of the historical and economic events that have assaulted the institution of marriage among African American couples, especially those from the lower socioeconomic echelons of our society. On the other hand, I was deeply disturbed that this issue of *Newsweek* failed to portray the complexity of the roles that African American men play in the lives of their families. Moreover, I feared that the casual passerby, who happened to spy the cover page of this issue but did not read the articles inside it, would be hit by yet another destructive stereotype that has been transmitted by the media in this country in recent years: that young black men callously exploit black adolescent women and then coldly discard their partners and their children to fend for themselves in this world.

Moving beyond such simplistic images is not only the starting point but also the most essential feature in helping adolescent African American fathers. The primary purpose of this chapter is to provide the reader with a complex understanding of the joys, hardships, and challenges experienced by African American males who become fathers during their teenage years and to offer culturally sensitive recommendations for clinical practice. This chapter begins with an overview of adolescent pregnancy and parenthood among African Americans, including a discussion of the life circumstances that propel many young African Americans to early parenthood. Next, the experiences of African American teenage fathers are described. Strategies for engaging African American teenage fathers in counseling and assisting them with the transition to parenthood are discussed.

ADOLESCENT PREGNANCY AND PARENTHOOD IN THE AFRICAN AMERICAN COMMUNITY

Although teenage pregnancy and parenthood are phenomena that cut across race, ethnic, and socioeconomic lines, national statistics reveal that a disproportionate number of African American adolescents are becoming parents. In 1991, the birth rate among African American adolescent females was more than twice that among white teenagers, and the vast majority of births among this population occurred to females who were unmarried (see Children's Defense Fund, 1994).

What accounts for the higher birth rate among African American teenagers? According to Moore, Simms, and Betsey (1986), many of the factors that independently predict early childbearing—that is, inadequate information about human sexuality and contraception, poorly educated parents, school dropout, poor employment prospects, single-parent families—are found to be concentrated in those neighborhoods where African American children are particularly likely to be growing up. The authors surmised that the aggregate influence of these separate factors may be greater than the simple sum of the separate effects, thereby placing African American youth at greater risk than other ethnic groups to engage in high-risk sexual behaviors, such as unprotected sexual intercourse, and consequently to become teenage parents. Similarly, the Children's Defense Fund (1994) has argued that the far higher poverty rates and weaker basic academic skills among African American teenagers are key reasons why their teen birth rate is much higher than that of whites. Finally, several scholars (e.g., Abrahamse,

Morrison, & Waite, 1988; Battle, 1988/1989; Butts, 1989; Scott-Jones, Roland, & White, 1989; Smith, 1988, 1989; Sullivan, 1985) have proposed that the historical restriction of opportunities and the bleak future of a substantial number of African American adolescents play a major role in the high pregnancy and birth rates among African American teenagers. According to these scholars, impoverished African American youth may see less opportunity in their own futures and hence less to lose by becoming teenage parents. Because African American males perceive so many of the adult roles valued by American society as being closed to them, they may view parenthood as a way to display maturity and a sense of achievement (Gabriel & McAnarney, 1983; Smith, 1988, 1989).

Limited economic prospects and life opportunities have also made the prospect of marriage tenuous for many young African American fathers. Because African American youth tend to reside in communities struggling with high rates of unemployment, they are likely to be either unemployed or earning insufficient income to support a family and marry (Furstenberg, 1976; Hardy & Zabin, 1991; Salguero, 1984; Sullivan, 1985; Williams, 1991). Moreover, welfare policies historically have discouraged marriage among young, impoverished African American couples, because a family's support payments were reduced, or even eliminated, if a male lived in the household (Erickson & Gecas, 1991; Moore & Burt, 1982). Thus, although marriage is still a strong value among African Americans (see Hatchett, 1991; Moore et al., 1986; Williams, 1990), the majority of African American teenage parents do not marry (Children's Defense Fund, 1994). Instead, the teenage mother tends to live with her family, rely on their economic and emotional support, and delay marriage until the child's father or another male can prove his worth as an adequate provider (Furstenberg, 1976; Hardy & Zabin, 1991; Marsiglio, 1987; Salguero, 1984; Sullivan, 1985; Williams, 1991).

What, then, are the perspectives and experiences of African American males who become fathers as teenagers within the context of poverty, limited opportunities, and noncustodial parenthood? An answer to this question is provided through the following overview of research that has been conducted with African American teenage fathers.

ADOLESCENT FATHERHOOD: THE AFRICAN AMERICAN EXPERIENCE

Among African American teenage fathers, issues of paternity, child support, and visitation tend to be negotiated in large part by folk rather than legal norms, although legal sanctions are often brought into play when folk negotiations break down (Sullivan, 1985). An examination of these folk traditions furnishes insights about how adolescent fathers, their partners, and their respective families adapt to the arrival of the baby, typically within the context of the difficult life circumstances described earlier. In spite of these adaptive patterns, however, the transition to parenthood for African American teenage fathers is complicated by the stressors associated with adolescent paternity.

Folk Customs for Establishing and Demonstrating Paternity

Sullivan (1985) observed that folk traditions dictate that the father experience genuine concern for his child and that he express this concern in the form of some type of concrete assistance to his new family. If these steps are taken, then the paternity of the father will likely be recognized, even if he does not fulfill the legally defined responsibilities of a father, such as providing court-defined levels of child support (Sullivan, 1985).

Data from several studies suggest that most African American teenage fathers meet these folk criteria, at least during the early stages of their children's lives. The vast majority of African American unwed adolescent fathers have reported feeling love for their partners during and after the pregnancy and concern for their children's future (Hendricks, 1981, 1988; Hendricks & Solomon, 1987). Data from other studies suggest that most maintain an ongoing relationship with the mother and contribute their financial and emotional support to the mother and the baby during the early years of the child's life (Sullivan, 1985; Vaz, Smolen, & Miller, 1983; Williams, 1991). Several investigators (Achatz & MacAllum, 1994; Rivara, Sweeney, & Henderson, 1986; Sullivan, 1985) have documented that African American teenage fathers tend to support their partners and children in ways that might not be accounted for by official records of child support. Although most young fathers have minimal economic resources to contribute to the support of their children, they tend to compensate in a number for ways for what they cannot contribute monetarily. For example, most of the fathers interviewed by Sullivan (1985) described playing with their children and assisting with such tasks as providing part-time child care, feeding their children, changing diapers, providing diapers and clothes, and taking their children on recreational outings.

These forms of providing support to the adolescent mother and interacting with the child are a source of great joy and pride for young African American fathers (Achatz & MacAllum, 1994; Sullivan, 1985). They commonly express affection for their children and sincere hopes that their children will have better lives than they had (Achatz & MacAllum, 1994; Hendricks, 1981, 1988; Robinson, 1988; Sullivan, 1985). For many, fatherhood prompts them to behave more responsibly and provides them with a greater sense of meaning (Achatz & MacAllum, 1994). In spite of these positive aspects, however, adolescent fatherhood has a number of complications.

Complications Associated With Adolescent Paternity

Although African American teenage fathers appear to support their partners throughout the pregnancy and during the first year of the child's life, the interaction of a complex host of factors tends to contribute to a deterioration of the relationship between the young fathers and their partners and children. Data reported in several studies indicate that the frequency of contact between the couple and between the father and his child gradually declines over time (Hardy & Zabin, 1991; Rivara et al., 1986; Salguero, 1984). If the father and his family also reduce concrete forms of support for the child, then the recognition of his paternity and his right to visit may be jeopardized (Sullivan, 1985). Hostilities between the two families can follow, contributing to rifts between the young father and the mother of his child and her family (Hendricks, 1981, 1988; Hendricks & Solomon, 1987). In a climate of such tensions and stressors related to other hardships, contact between the father and his partner and child can wane even further (Furstenberg, Brooks-Gunn, & Morgan, 1987; Hardy & Zabin, 1991).

These troubled relationships are just some of the many complications associated with adolescent paternity. In addition, African American teenage fathers report experiencing the following problems: difficulty completing school, getting a job, and fulfilling the financial responsibilities of fatherhood; a lack of knowledge about parenting skills and contraceptives; restricted freedom imposed by parenting duties; and not being able to see their children as often as they would like (Hendricks, 1981, 1988; Hendricks & Solomon, 1987).

The employment difficulties of African American adolescent father may be related, in part, to their truncated educational experiences. The educational achievement level of African American adolescent fathers is not as high as their non-father classmates (Card & Wise, 1978; Hendricks, Montgomery, & Fullilove, 1984; Marsiglio, 1986).

It is unclear whether early fatherhood precedes or follows school dropout. Some young men who have dropped out of school may drift into parenthood in an attempt to add a meaningful purpose to their lives. Adolescent males enrolled in school at the time of conception tend to be poor achievers or disconnected from the school environment. It seems that these youth are at risk to drop out, and the pregnancy is the precipitating event to leave school (Brindis, 1993). In the latter case, early fatherhood may limit the number of years adolescent fathers might otherwise spend in school and, consequently, curtail their occupational opportunities.

Racism and stereotypes about black males compound the many hardships encountered by African American adolescent fathers by discouraging their interest in seeking professional assistance. Wyatt (1982) observed that African American males are the victims of societal stereotypes depicting black men as super studs with savage sexual appetites. Kiselica (1995) warned that unquestioned adherence to such stereotypes may cause Caucasian service providers to treat African American teenage fathers in a pejorative manner. Smith (1989) reported that many of the African American service providers and community leaders who had participated in her research project also appeared to have internalized negative societal attitudes about black adolescent fathers, as evidenced by their strong opposition to providing outreach programs for this population, whom they viewed as being irresponsible and "no good" (p. 217). As a consequence of such attitudes, many African American teenage fathers believe that society could care less about their perspectives and circumstances (Achatz & MacAllum, 1994) and that they will be treated judgmentally by service providers (Hendricks, 1988).

IMPLICATIONS FOR SERVICE PROVISION

Service providers must carefully clarify their attitudes and divest themselves of stereotypes regarding African American teenage fathers before they attempt to work with this population (Kiselica, 1995). Those practitioners who are unable to do so have an ethical obligation to refer African American adolescent fathers to colleagues who are committed to helping these young men with the transition to parenthood.

Ideally, teenage parenting programs offered in African American communities should be staffed by personnel who understand the complex context in which adolescent pregnancy and parenthood occurs. Clinicians must communicate this understanding through the practice of culturally sensitive outreach, rapport building, and intervention strategies. An overview of these strategies, gleaned from recommendations by Kiselica (1995), follows.

Outreach and Rapport-Building Strategies

Many service programs targeting African American fathers have been unsuccessful in recruiting participants. Typically, in these instances, well-intentioned professionals have developed a fatherhood training service, identified potential clients for this service, and then invited those clients to participate in a program that will help them "to become responsible parents." To the dismay of the outreach workers, most of the young fathers either don't avail themselves of the services or do so on a very sporadic basis. In response, the outreach staff become frustrated, erroneously conclude that adolescent fathers are irresponsible parents who don't want help, and terminate the program.

The primary flaw of this approach to outreach is the failure of the program developers to anticipate the many hardships experienced by African American teenage fathers and their understandable wariness of service providers. In contrast, successful programs with this population have been designed to address the multifaceted needs of African American youth, not just those issues specifically related to paternity. Particular components of young father programs found to be valued by African American teenage fathers include the following: comprehensive case management (Achatz & MacAllum, 1994), recreational services (Barber & Munn, 1993), vocational counseling and job training (Achatz & MacAllum, 1994; Brindis, Barth, & Loomis, 1987; Brown, 1990; Hendricks, 1988; Klinman & Sander, 1985; Sander & Rosen, 1987), high school diploma equivalency classes (Achatz & MacAllum, 1994), free medical service such as physical examinations and diagnosis and treatment of sexually transmitted diseases (Hendricks, 1988), legal advice regarding paternity establishment, child support enforcement, child custody, and visitation rights (Achatz & MacAllum, 1994; Barth, Claycomb, & Loomis, 1988; Hendricks, 1988), free transportation to and from the service site (Barth et al., 1988), specific information about how to become involved in the pregnancy and delivery (Achatz & MacAllum, 1994; Barth et al., 1988; Brindis et al., 1987; Hendricks, 1988; Klinman & Sander, 1985), parenting skills training (Achatz & MacAllum, 1994; Barth et al., 1988; Brindis et al., 1987; Hendricks, 1988; Klinman & Sander, 1985), and assistance with other concrete needs, such as help in obtaining a driver's license or protection from violent gangs (Barber & Munn, 1993).

In addition to providing holistic services, successful programs have employed a variety of rapport-building strategies designed to allay the young fathers' apprehensions about being judged by program employees. Training the staff to understand the customs of, and slang expressions used in, the local community will facilitate staff-client contact throughout all of their interactions together (Barth et al., 1988; Smith, 1989). Because African American teenage boys are accustomed to building friendships through group recreational activities, Barber and Munn (1993) recommended that program staff spend a considerable amount of time joining program participants in athletic events, such as playing basketball games or practicing karate skills, so that the staff can establish a comfortable rapport with the fathers before formal program activities are initiated. Practitioners are cautioned to avoid confronting the youths about issues of male responsibility during these early contacts; it is more fruitful to allow the clients to take the lead regarding what topics they wish to discuss (Hendricks, 1988). Although the program staff may have an agenda of topics (e.g., vocational counseling, followed by legal counseling and then parenting skills training) they wish to cover in the service program, they must be willing to adjust the agenda to respond to the participants' most pressing needs (Hendricks, 1988). For example, Barber and Munn (1993) reported that they have periodically postponed planned activities in favor of assisting young men with urgent social and practical matters, such as visiting a friend in the hospital or driving several young men to a driver's license center. Hendricks (1988) added that it is crucial to have flexible program hours so that young men can juggle their visits to the program site with their other responsibilities. In addition, case management offices in which individual or group counseling or skills training classes are held should be "male-friendly" environments, furnished with magazines that are likely to be of interest to teenage boys (e.g., *Sports Illustrated*) and posters of positive male role models (Kiselica, 1995). Taking these measures is likely to help African American teenage fathers feel comfortable at the program site and believe that staff are truly dedicated to helping them.

The staff who serve African American teenage fathers should not be discouraged if the early stages of program development are sparsely attended or if participants attend inconsistently over time. Many young fathers are understandably reluctant to invest themselves in programs until they have had a chance to "check them out" thoroughly. After a handful of the participants begin to trust program employees, the positive reputation of the program gradually spreads throughout the community, and then more and more adolescent males join the program. Although a core cadre of fathers will become regular participants in program activities, others will attend irregularly, drifting to the program site at critical times when they need help, drifting out when they are preoccupied with concerns that, in their minds, take priority over what is being offered by the service program. By being patient, persistently reaching out to the program participants, and remaining sensitive to their concerns, practitioners will develop ties with the fathers that transcend periods of absence from the program. In addition, ongoing outreach will have the effect of boosting the cumulative participation of young men in the program over time (Kiselica, 1995).

Intervention Strategies

These outreach and rapport-building strategies create an atmosphere of trust in which African American teenage fathers are willing to participate in formal activities, such as individual and family counseling, preparation for fatherhood, and educational and career counseling.

Individual Counseling. For individual counseling to be most effective, it must be tailored toward the life experiences and perspectives of African Americans. Cheatham (1990b) has argued that counseling approaches over-emphasizing client responsibility and introspection are ill-suited for African American clients, whose sociocultural experience is infused with themes of powerlessness. Cheatham added that unless the realistic, extrapsychic problems of African Americans are addressed, counseling is likely to be ineffective. In light of these recommendations, Kiselica (1995) warned that beginning the counseling process with an African American teenage father by abruptly confronting his lack of sexual responsibility or by exploring his hidden motivations in becoming a father is likely to alienate the youth. Instead, Kiselica advised mental health professionals to help the father immediately to resolve his urgent, concrete concerns, such as finding a job or medical services for his partner and their child. After such practical assistance is rendered, many young African American fathers trust that the counselor will sensitively handle their intrapsychic issues, such as the unresolved pain and anger harbored by those boys who were abandoned by their own fathers (Kiselica, 1995).

Throughout the course of individual counseling, the helper must be prepared to respond to several race-related issues that commonly arise with African American clients. For example, many African American clients are mistrustful of professional counselors due to the historical maltreatment of blacks by the mental health system in the United States. This is particularly true when an African American client who carries resentment toward the dominant white culture encounters a white counselor. In such circumstances, the counselor must avoid reacting defensively, empathize with the perspective of the client, and demonstrate his or her sincere concern for the client by taking rapid, concrete action to address the client's most urgent concern (Kiselica, 1995). In addition, both black and white counselors are advised to carefully monitor countertransference issues pertaining to race, which sometimes surface during work with African American clients (Jones, 1985). For example, white counselors might avoid racial issues by referring the client to another counselor, whereas black counselors might overidentify with the client's racial issues and overlook other concerns of the client (Smith, 1981). Keeping attuned to these potential issues will help the counselor maintain objectivity with the client.

Family Counseling. If possible, family counseling should be conducted concurrently with individual counseling for two reasons. First, traditionally, African Americans have relied extensively on the extended kinship network as a mechanism to cope with the many hardships they have faced living in an oppressive society (Boyd-Franklin, 1989). As evidence of this tradition, African American families have provided varied forms of support to their adolescents facing parenthood during their teenage years (Furstenburg et al., 1987; Hendricks, 1988; Sullivan, 1985; Williams, 1991). Tapping into this natural support system is likely to enhance any efforts to help African American teenage fathers. Second, the occurrence of an unplanned adolescent pregnancy and the subsequent birth of the child poses hardships and often prompts a number of intra- and interfamilial conflicts (Furstenburg et al., 1987; Hendricks, 1988; Sullivan, 1985; Williams, 1991). Family counseling can help the families of the young mother and father resolve these problems.

Before any family counseling is initiated, several preliminary steps should be taken. As a sign of respect for the young father's autonomy, the counselor should obtain his permission to contact his family, and, if need be, his partner's family to solicit their help or to mediate problems between the youth and either family (Hendricks, 1988). Through individual counseling sessions, the counselor can process the client's feelings about working with family members and clarify which family members to contact first. Once the counselor calls or visits these family members, it is important to convey to these individuals a sincere interest in helping both the teenage father and the other members of the family with their respective concerns, even those that may not pertain to the crisis pregnancy (Kiselica, 1995). Authentic gestures of this kind help to establish rapport with African Americans, who are often suspicious of the motivations of mental health professionals due to the discriminatory and culturally insensitive historical treatment of African Americans by the mental health system (Smith, 1981; Sue, McKinney, Allen, & Hall, 1974). Several contacts with family members may be necessary before the counselor is trusted and accepted by the family (Kiselica, 1995).

Once key family members agree to participate in counseling, it is recommended that the counselor ask the family to identify relatives who have a special relationship with the teenage father. These relatives may include friends of the family who are not blood relatives but are nevertheless considered by the family to be kin. As Boyd-Franklin (1989) has noted, acknowledging and using this network communicates respect to the family and increases the likelihood of conducting a successful intervention. Once family counseling has started, the practitioner should be willing to address whatever concerns the family brings up. Although some of these will pertain directly to the young man's adjustment to fatherhood, such as identifying family support for the father and negotiating roles within and between families pertaining to the raising of the child, other problems, such as long-standing conflicts between family members, may emerge and take precedence over fatherhood issues from time to time. This point was illustrated by Kiselica (1995) in a case study regarding his work with an African American teenage father named Maurice. Although Kiselica conducted several family interventions designed to address Maurice's parenting skills deficits, employment difficulties, and problems coping with racist behavior, he also assisted Maurice's family to cope with the death of his grandmother and to address long-standing tensions between Maurice's mother and her sister.

Preparation for Fatherhood. Adolescent males facing fatherhood need to clarify their conceptions of masculinity and fatherhood, learn effective parenting skills, and develop skills for preventing additional unplanned pregnancies (Kiselica, 1995, 1996; Kiselica, Rotzien & Doms, 1994). These tasks can be completed in fatherhood training programs specifically geared to the needs of the fathers.

Due to their cultural preference for communal relations and group educational activities (Franklin, 1989; Lee, 1989), African American adolescent males are likely to respond well to parenting skills training conducted through group psychoeducational classes. Ideally, such training should be conducted by adult African American men, who can teach young fathers Afrocentric perspectives on masculinity and paternity (Kiselica, 1995).

Parenting skills trainers can employ a number of resources that have been effective in preparing African American adolescent males for adulthood and the responsibilities of parenthood. A three-module course on fatherhood training, replete with a variety of pertinent educational videos and readings, is described in detail in *Multicultural Counseling With Teenage Fathers: A Practical Guide* (Kiselica, 1995). Other notable resources include the following: Wynn's (1992) *Empowering African-American Males to Succeed,* a 10-step approach to teaching an understanding of the African culture to black males; *The Black Teenage Parenting and Early Childhood Education Curriculum* (Nobles, Goddard, & Cavil, 1985), a six-module curriculum that prepares adolescents for parenthood from an African American cultural perspective; and Lee's (1989) *Blackness: A State of Mind, A State of Being,* a six-session model that incorporates Afrocentric education into a self-enhancement program for black adolescents.

Educational and Career Counseling. Educational and career counseling with adolescent fathers typically occurs in two phases that are related to the course of the pregnancy. During the prenatal phase of counseling, counseling is crisis oriented and focused on helping the expectant father to make important decisions regarding school and work. For example, the counselor provides decision-making counseling designed to help the youth decide whether or not he should drop out of school and how he will support his partner during the pregnancy. During the postnatal phase of counseling, long-term educational and career plans are formulated, and job-training services are provided with the hope of maximizing the young father's chances of realizing a fulfilling career and a life of economic self-sufficiency (Kiselica & Murphy, 1994; Kiselica & Pfaller, 1993).

Practitioners can gear educational and career counseling to the needs of African American teenage fathers by incorporating an Afrocentric orientation to the counseling process (Kiselica, 1995). According to Baly (1989), Cheatham (1990a), and Parham and Austin (1994), Afrocentric career counseling addresses the following culturally salient issues of African Americans: the individual's perception of certain factors in the environment (e.g., one's view of the opportunity structure) and locus of control; the influence of significant others; the effects of racial identity attitudes on values, perceptions of opportunities, occupational stereotyping, career decision making, and workforce diversity; and experiences of racism, disenfranchisement, economic hardship, and structural discrimination and their effects on the self-concept.

A career development program developed by D'Andrea and Daniels (1992) is a good example of an Afrocentric approach to helping African American youth. Implemented by a collaborative team of school, community, and business leaders, the program combined traditional career counseling strategies with an Afrocentric cooperative group approach. Career development activities were focused on addressing racial identity issues as they related to career concerns and on facilitating racial identity and career development.

A noteworthy feature of the D'Andrea and Daniels (1992) program is the cooperative venture that had been forged between schools and their communities in an effort to expand the experiences and opportunities available to African American adolescent males. Such collaborative efforts are required to help African American youngsters overcome the limited opportunity structure of many African American communities (Carrera, 1992; Hendricks, 1988; Lee, 1989; Smith, 1988). On a related note, Carrera (1992) proposed that institutions of higher education work with high schools to enhance the life chances of poor and alienated youth. Youth who complete such a program could be guaranteed admission to college. Such a commitment can serve as an incentive to young people interested in furthering their education, and it will affirm the fact that college is part of their future.

CONCLUSION

The practice suggestions offered here are likely to enhance the work of helping professionals assisting young African American fathers with the transition to fatherhood; to maximize the efficacy of the strategies described in this chapter, however, they must be supported by major policy initiatives designed to improve the status of African American families. Since 1980, the response of governmental policy to the needs of African American families has been insufficient to improve the quality of life and opportunities of this population. Consequently, the status of African American families has been sliding backward, and large segments of the African American community are in danger of becoming trapped in a permanent underclass (Children's Defense Fund, 1994; Gibbs, 1988). Until this sociological crisis is resolved, mental health professionals will, to a great extent, be handcuffed while they attempt to address the many problems associated with adolescent pregnancy and parenthood. For this reason, the leaders of the professional organizations representing psychologists, counselors, social workers, physicians, nurses, educators, and other professionals are urged to (a) learn about proposed policy changes that have been designed "to address the circumstances that make it so difficult for low-income, young fathers to achieve economic self-sufficiency, and discourage them from fulfilling their personal and legal obligations to their dependent children" (Achatz & MacAllum, 1994, p. 99; see Lawson & Rhode, 1993; Lerman & Ooms, 1993; for pertinent discussions); and (b) consolidate their respective lobbying forces to fight for government-sponsored services that will help African American children to delay childbearing and assist African American youth who already are parents with their adjustments as young mothers and fathers.

CHAPTER 16

Working With Incarcerated African American Males and Their Families

ANTHONY E. O. KING

A s the number of African American males incarcerated in state and federal prisons sets new records each year, there is a need to provide these men and their families with a variety of prison- and community-based family-centered services and programs that address the multifaceted and unique problems they experience. This chapter describes the impact of incarceration on African American males and their families. Moreover, it describes several types of programs and services that could improve the lives of incarcerated African American males and their families.

THE IMPACT OF INCARCERATION ON AFRICAN AMERICAN MALES

In general, imprisonment exacts a terrible toll on inmates in part because it separates them from their families, friends, and communities. The stress and anxiety triggered by this separation are similar to what individuals experience when a loved one dies or when a divorce occurs. Moreover, it can lead to depression and suicide among African Americans (Houston, 1990; Moore, 1989). Furthermore, the rigid and authoritarian environment of prisons creates and enhances dependency in inmates. Prison administrators encourage and reward conformity. As a result, the prison experience undermines African American males' capacity and willingness to think and act independently of coercive authority (Lichtenstein & Kroll, 1990). Studies have suggested that, on release, men who were once characterized as "model prisoners" typically have a more difficult time adjusting to the outside world, where independent thought and effective autonomous behavior are essential (Lichtenstein & Kroll, 1990). Prisons also pose a major health threat to inmates.

The average American prison is more violent than the worst inner-city neighborhood, and the HIV infection rate is more than seven times the rate in the civilian population (U.S. Department of Justice, Bureau of Justice Statistics, 1996). These conditions add to the emotional stress inmates experience.

THE IMPACT OF INCARCERATION ON MALES' FAMILY LIFE AND RELATIONSHIPS

The high incarceration rate of African American males has contributed to an alarming growth in the number and percentage of poor female-headed households and children in African American communities (U.S. Bureau of the Census, 1995b). Few inmates are able to contribute to the financial support of their families and children while incarcerated (Fishman, 1988; Jorgensen, Hernandez, & Warren, 1986; King, 1993c; Shaw, 1987; Swan, 1981). Moreover, a prison record makes it extremely difficult for a former inmate to secure employment and/or find a good-paying job upon his release from prison. Without jobs, formerly incarcerated men cannot support their families.

In addition to financial difficulties, family life in general, and family relationships in particular, suffer and are strained when a man goes to prison (Adalist Estrin, 1995; Finney Hairston, 1991; King, 1993a, 1993c; Lanier, 1991). Family members are forced to pull together and replace the incarcerated male's income as well as any emotional support he contributed to the family. All of this must be done while each member of the family struggles to cope with the anxiety and fears associated with having a loved one in prison.

On the other hand, the inmate must cope with his concerns about the fate of his family and loved ones. I have worked with hundreds of incarcerated African American males. Most of the men I encountered expressed tremendous guilt over the hardships their families faced as a result of their imprisonment. The guilt many men experience frequently leads to behavior that only makes their family situation worse (Adalist Estrin, 1994, 1995; King, 1993c).

THE IMPACT OF INCARCERATION ON INMATES' CHILDREN, YOUNGER SIBLINGS, AND COMMUNITIES

Children suffer the most when their fathers go to prison (Lloyd, 1993; Rainey Ranson, 1994). Many develop serious emotional and behavioral problems during their father's imprisonment (Jorgensen et al., 1986; Lloyd, 1993; Sack, 1977; Schneller, 1976; Shaw, 1987). The social stigma associated with having a father or brother in prison is an additional burden that children must bear. Studies have found that the psychosocial development of children, especially boys, is adversely affected when their father is imprisoned (Sack, 1977; Shaw, 1987). The incarceration of an older brother also has a tremendous impact on younger male siblings. Younger males who idolized or looked up to their older brothers can lose faith in them because they feel abandoned by them. Some younger male siblings maintain their allegiance and begin to emulate their incarcerated brothers' criminal behavior. This is a way of strengthening the bond that has been strained by the older brother's incarceration. Predictably, the behavior of the younger siblings places them on the same road that led their brother to a life of crime and imprisonment.

Lastly, the incarceration of so many African American males has a negative impact on the communities to which they return (Swan, 1981). After serving time in prison, many African American males return to their communities angry, frustrated, poor, and stigmatized for the rest of their lives. The emotional problems they bring back to their families and communities simply compound the poverty, violence, family instability, and overall misery and cynicism that may already exist.

Recently, there has been a significant increase in the number of prison- and community-based family-centered programs and services for incarcerated inmates (Adalist Estrin, 1995; Bloom & Steinhart, 1993). Most of these programs have had a positive impact on inmates and their families. In spite of the success of these programs, they suffer from three important limitations: (a) Most target women inmates and their children, who represent less than 7% of the state and federal inmate populations (Bloom & Steinhart, 1993; U.S. Department of Justice, 1995b); (b) there are not enough programs and services available to serve the majority of needy individuals and families, regardless of gender; and (c) few programs meet the unique needs of African American male inmates and their families. If these men and their families are to survive the trauma of incarceration and begin to address the myriad of problems that contribute to their high incarceration rate, community- and prison-based individual and family-oriented programs and services must be made available to them.

INTERVENING WITH INCARCERATED
AFRICAN AMERICAN MALES AND THEIR FAMILIES

The five types of programs and services that incarcerated African American men and their families need are (a) culture awareness and socialization programs, (b) Afrocentric clinical services, (c) community-based family support programs, (d) prison-based family life education programs, and (e) community-based inmate reentry programs.

Culture Awareness Groups and Programs

During the past decade, culture awareness groups and programs have emerged as one of the most popular and important interventions for working with African American males in their communities. Recently, human service professionals and community volunteers have begun to offer these groups and programs in prisons. However, I found only one article in the social service and/or prison rehabilitation literature that described such a program (King, 1994). As a result, the model described here is offered only as an example and not as a definitive model. Before starting a cultural awareness group, practitioners should check with the warden in their prison to ensure that the group's activities do not violate the institution's administrative rules and regulations.

Prison-based cultural awareness programs/groups are usually designed to accomplish one or more of the following goals: (a) enhance African American males' social and cultural identity; (b) teach them about their African and African American culture and history; (c) encourage and help inmates' development of a sense of social, historical, and spiritual connection between themselves and their African and African American foremothers and forefathers; (d) develop a sense of responsibility for their families and communities; and (e) generate a sense of respect and appreciation for African American males.

The size of a cultural awareness group typically varies from as few as 10 to as many as 30 or 40 men. Group members participate in a variety of culturally relevant celebrations and activities such as Kwanzaa and Black History Month. Group members also attend lectures on African and African American history and culture presented by local and national experts. Some programs develop special libraries, which contain books, monographs, scholarly articles, and video- and audiotapes about African Americans. These materials are discussed in group sessions (which last anywhere from 1 to 4 hours). Inmates are allowed to check out all of these materials for their personal use except the videotapes.

Another important aspect of cultural awareness groups is the ongoing intellectual discussions that take place during the sessions. Spirited but respectful debates and discussions teach inmates how to respect and interact with other African American males in a candid but nonaggressive manner. Inmates who participate in cultural awareness groups develop a greater appreciation for their history and culture and a strong desire to rehabilitate themselves while in prison so that they can contribute to their families and communities once they are released. Cultural awareness groups and programs are easy to organize, inexpensive, and require very little time to facilitate. Moreover, they are appropriate for all age groups. Thus, practitioners can develop cultural awareness groups for younger males in both short- and long-term youth correctional facilities.

Rites-of-Passage Programs

Traditionally, rites-of-passage programs have been used to help children and adolescents develop character and integrity and learn about their cultural heritage (Coppock Warfield, 1990, 1992; Hill, 1992; Kunjufu, 1986; Nobles, 1988; Perkins, 1986). They also have been used to help children develop a strong sense of personal responsibility and respect for their communities (Coppock Warfield, 1992; Hill, 1992; Nobles, 1988). Participating in a rites-of-passage program also can reduce the probability that a child will engage in antisocial and self-destructive behavior (Hill, 1992; Oliver, 1989; Trotter, 1991).

Incarcerated African American males need such programs for several reasons. Most of these men are the products of some of the worst social, economic, family, and environmental conditions in America (Irwin & Austin, 1994). For many incarcerated males, childhood was shaped by poverty, drug abuse, violence, and family disruption. Thus, hundreds of thousands of incarcerated African American males have some of the same needs as the children who participate in youth-oriented rites-of-passage programs. It is imperative, therefore, that these programs be made available to incarcerated African American males.

The basic goals or program objectives of adult rites-of-passage programs are to (a) enhance adult personal development, (b) help adults bond and develop a sense of community, (c) teach adults the virtues of selflessness and community service, and (d) help adults develop the capacity and skills required to serve youth effectively and efficiently (P. Hill, Jr., personal communication, February 10, 1997).

Personal Development

Rites-of-passage programs provide African American inmates with a culture-specific ethos and value system by teaching them the Nguzo Saba, or the seven principles of nationhood: unity, self-determination, collective work and responsibility, cooperative economics, purpose, creativity, and faith (Karenga, 1977). Participants' self-awareness and cultural identities are enhanced by studying African and African American history and culture. In addition, inmates are taught the importance of maintaining optimal well-being and spirituality. These activities and experiences help incarcerated African American males rehabilitate themselves by helping change their attitudes and beliefs about themselves and their relationships with others.

Bonding and Developing a Sense of Community

When inmates are involved in rites-of-passage programs they participate in a variety of activities that help them bond as a community. The development of an authentic community helps inmates recapture or develop an appreciation and respect for others.

Moreover, it provides them with a support network that can help them address personal problems and concerns that might contribute to antisocial behavior or general distress and anxiety.

Extolling the Virtues of Selflessness and Community Service

In rites-of-passage programs, inmates can be taught the virtues of becoming a servant leader. A servant leader is a person who leads by joining with others to participate in activities that strengthen or support their community.

One of the ways inmates are encouraged to express their servant leadership is by developing and implementing community services. Incarcerated African American males can satisfy their community service responsibilities by serving as tutors in the prison literacy program and peer counselors in their units or by helping to develop or expand the prison library. Through their participation in these types of activities, incarcerated males develop a strong sense of responsibility for others.

Develop the Capacity and Skills Required to Serve Youth

Rites-of-passage programs for adults teach participants the knowledge and skills necessary to nurture and support children and adolescents in a variety of roles and contexts. Many incarcerated males have children; therefore, increasing their knowledge about child and adolescent development increases their ability to function more effectively as fathers. Furthermore, armed with this knowledge, a commitment to servant leadership, and a greater sense of community service, formerly incarcerated African American males can return to their communities and serve as role models and mentors for youth who are at risk of engaging in criminal activities.

Afrocentric Clinical Services

African American men and their families need clinical services that address the unique social and intrapersonal problems that undermine their individual and family functioning. The need to provide African Americans these types of clinical services has been well documented (Acosta, Yamamoto, & Evans, 1982; Akbar, 1981; Boyd-Franklin, 1989; Crawley, 1996; Harvey, 1995; Jones, 1979; Poitier, Niliwaambieni, & Lamar-Rowe, 1997; Schele, 1996; Taylor, Neighbors, & Broman, 1989).

For instance, clinical services in prisons and community-based mental health agencies need to help African American males and their families cope more effectively with institutional racism and discrimination. These men and their families need help developing healthy cultural identities and raising their children in a racist society. Both of these problems are particularly relevant to African American males (Boyd-Franklin, 1989; Gilbert, 1974; Gochros, 1966; Grier & Cobbs, 1971; Houston, 1990). Repressed anger and frustration generated by personal experiences with actual or perceived racial discrimination frequently contribute to African American males' antisocial behavior (Grier & Cobbs, 1968; Wilson, 1990).

Through my clinical work with incarcerated African American males, I have found that most exhibit a tremendous desire to discuss their experiences as black men in this society. Practitioners should encourage inmates to discuss their experiences as black men with them. If they are handled sensitively and skillfully, such discussions and interactions can help inmates grow, and reduce the defensiveness and mistrust that traditionally characterize the relationship between clinicians and African American males. As the men increase their self-awareness, many become more willing and able to confront their personal weaknesses and shortcomings. This confrontation, in turn, facilitates the habilitation and rehabilitation processes.

Lastly, during the past 10 years, practitioners have developed numerous Afrocentric therapeutic models and approaches (Akbar, 1991b; Azibo, 1989; Myers, 1988; Phillips, 1990; Poitier et al., 1997). Therefore, practitioners can now choose from a range of culture-specific models and approaches to address the problems cited above.

Community-Based Family Services

The previous discussion has documented the problems incarcerated African American males and their families experience. It also documents the need for community-based family services that target these men and their families. Community-based family counseling, group work, and case management services, specifically designed for families of incarcerated men, can help them cope with the problems associated with incarceration. In addition, community-based family services can help inmates' families examine their strengths and weaknesses in the light of present and past problems and crises. Community-based family services can also help the custodial parent or guardian to help the inmates' children and siblings cope more effectively with their fathers' or brothers' absence.

Finally, community-based family services can provide immeasurable practical support to the wives, mothers, and grandmothers of incarcerated African American males. These women frequently need help applying for public assistance, locating child care providers, or finding a second job. In addition, many mothers, grandmothers, and female companions need help negotiating the myriad of confusing rules and regulations concerning prison visits and mail.

Prison-Based Family Life and Education Services

Incarcerated African American males and their families need prison-based family-oriented programs and services. These programs provide inmates and their families opportunities to interact with one another, as well as to address a wide range of family issues and concerns while the inmate is still in prison. Prison-based family-oriented programs and services also provide special activities and programs for the children of inmates, which can help these children cope with the difficulties associated with their fathers' incarceration.

Inmates also need short-term family education and relationship groups (King, 1993b). I have facilitated numerous short-term family relationship groups with incarcerated African American men and women. Participants stated that these group experiences helped them reevaluate their family relationships, improve their communication within their families, and understand the developmental needs of their family members. In addition to these benefits, family education and relationship groups provide inmates with many opportunities to discuss male-female relationship concerns, parenting problems, and other family issues within the context of a supportive group.

I have observed older African American males helping younger and less experienced men cope with their personal anxieties and the family problems they may have been experiencing. This is a very positive and important experience for African American males, given the degree and amount of intragender conflict and hostility many have experienced in their families and communities.

Reentry Programs and Services

Finally, once they are released from prison, African American males need assistance reestablishing themselves in their communities. Imprisonment isolates and stigmatizes an individual and his family. It also forces an individual to think and behave in a manner that is not necessarily consistent with thriving outside of prison. Moreover, former offenders are often poor and unemployed before they go to prison. Consequently, to avoid engaging in criminal activities to support themselves and their families, they will need a great deal of assistance upon release. Minimally, reentry programs should provide the following: (a) employment and job training assistance, (b) individual and group counseling services, (c) opportunities to engage in community service activities, (d) mentors, and (e) referral services to other human services and programs. With the assistance of an effective and well-managed reentry program, the chances that a formerly incarcerated African American male will return to prison diminishes significantly.

CONCLUSIONS

In this chapter, I have discussed the impact of incarceration on African American males and their families. I have also described five types of programs and services that incarcerated African American males and their families need to survive the trauma of imprisonment and improve their individual and family functioning. If one of the important roles of imprisonment is to help offenders rehabilitate and/or habilitate themselves, then offenders and their families need access to these programs. If practitioners continue to overlook the very important social service needs of incarcerated African American men and their families, we will condemn these men and their families to a life of misery, frustration, and unnecessary pain and suffering. When this happens the entire society suffers. Thus, meeting the needs of these men and their families improves their lives and enhances the safety and well-being of all citizens.

CHAPTER 17

Working in Groups With African American Men Who Batter

OLIVER J. WILLIAMS

More effective group treatment methods must be developed to transform men who batter, hold them accountable for their behavior, and reduce the victimization of abused women. But what is the most effective group treatment method to use with these men? Many African American men who batter have a different experience in batterers' treatment groups than their white counterparts. African American men reportedly drop out of treatment sooner and complete at lower rates than whites. Most batterers' treatment programs employ a one-size-fits-all model of treatment that characteristically focuses on the violent behavior, the gender of the perpetrator, and cognitive approaches to inducing behavioral change. In a national survey of batterers' programs, Williams and Becker (1994) found that most of the programs they surveyed do not consider race or culture in service delivery or design of treatment groups. As a group, all men who batter are resistant to treatment. But clinicians who lack cultural competence create an additional barrier to treatment that can increase resistance (Williams, 1995). Group treatment methods will be more effective with African American men who batter if it is delivered by group workers who are familiar with the population and incorporate such knowledge into group practice skills and group treatment design. This chapter examines how to blend traditional batterer's intervention treatment methods with culturally competent group treatment strategies for African American men who batter.

TRADITIONAL FOCUS OF BATTERERS' GROUPS

Historically, a feminist perspective has influenced the group treatment design and the issues that are addressed in treatment with men who batter (National Research Council, 1996). We have learned from the battered women's movement that sexism and male privilege have historically contributed to the abuse of women. From this perspective, abuse is not just a random act; rather, it is a behavior focused on the selection of the victim, a female partner. In group, men who batter learn that they are predisposed to violence due to societal and familial exposure to violence toward women. From this perspective, batterers' treatment has historically focused on the following issues: developing alternatives to male violence, increasing perpetrators' awareness of their need for power and control over their partner, and restructuring their sexist attitudes and behaviors.

EXPANDING THE FOCUS OF GROUP TREATMENT

Often, these men discuss long-standing or current unresolved issues that seem indirectly related to their violence. Treatment groups can contribute to the resocialization and education of the client even though not all of the material discussed seems directly associated with partner violence. But the extent to which these secondary issues get addressed depends on how comfortable the group worker is in addressing the content clients present in treatment. For example, a client wants to discuss issues such as work conflicts with fellow employees or supervisors. Some group workers may feel that this gets men off track and avoids focusing on the abuse of women. This type of worker would redirect clients to address their relationship with their partner. In contrast, other group workers may find such content important. First, they may ask the client to assess the situation and their behavior with employees or their supervisor. Did he handle the situation appropriately? If not, what could he have done differently? Is such conflict a pattern? Group workers and members can help the client gain additional insight into the problem, develop appropriate responses, and rehearse how to address these types of problems in the future. Second, this group worker could require the client to examine how conflict on the job influences what occurs with his partner. Was he verbally abusive or physically abusive to her after the conflict at work? Did he blame her for his frustration? When these types of stresses occur, is the partner at high risk for physical or emotional abuse? What should be done to handle his problem and not make his partner a scapegoat? How should he inform her about his predisposition? In this case, the group worker facilitates insight by assisting the client in linking the content at work and his abusive or violent behavior toward his partner. Group workers must develop the capacity to hear the content and help the client to make connections between his feelings, experiences, and behavior.

DEVELOP THE CAPACITY TO ADDRESS CONTENT OF AFRICAN AMERICAN MALE CLIENTS

Group workers leading treatment groups that include African Americans must be especially cognizant of the types of content that they may presented in treatment. African American men may discuss material associated with their social realities and experiences. Among the themes that could emerge with some of these men are their experiences with racism—both personal and institutional—and themes associated with stressful or violent living environments. Experiences either with racial oppression and/or violent community and social environments can result in maladaptive responses among some African American men.

Racial Oppression

Although African American men abuse women for many of the same reasons that all men do (sexism, power and control issues, etc.) in some instances, African American male violence toward women may be a result of displaced anger due to oppression (Gibbs, 1988; Staples, 1982; Williams, 1998; Wilson, 1991). It is imperative that group workers assist clients to make the connection regarding oppression and violent behavior. For example, in one treatment group, an African American client explained how he was oppressed on his job. He described how he was a target of ridicule by a group of white coworkers. He explained that the leader of this group was a good friend of his supervisor. In the past when he complained, his supervisor was not responsive. In the most recent episode, his coworkers took the keys out of his pocket and moved his car without his permission. Then a truck came along and smashed his car. The client felt that this behavior was directed toward him due to racism. He was very angry and stated he wanted to "go off on somebody."

How should that problem be addressed? Certain workers would feel as though this situation was not relevant to the group. Other workers might feel the situation has merit but deny any racial discrimination or association. A culturally competent worker and group members would know when to acknowledge the racism, when to confront what is not racism, and when to confront violent/abusive behavior. Even if the situation at hand dealt with less extreme and more subtle forms of racism or oppression, the group workers and members would have the capacity to address the issues with the client. In this case, the workers and fellow clients acknowledged the racism and helped the client to consider appropriate strategies to negotiate and confront his problem on the job. But such a group would go much further. The group could explore what the client did after the incident. What were his interactions with his partner? Did he displace his anger about the racism to his partner? If so, in what ways? If not, how did he manage to avoid it? If he did direct his anger at her, what other feelings did he have? Did he feel a sense of powerlessness, frustration, and so on? How did he behave toward her? Was he short with her, did he yell? To what extent did his feelings compare to his states of abusiveness? Was he aware of escalating? Did he hit her? The group members could explore appropriate nonviolent and non-abusive methods of interacting with his partner when he feels powerless or frustrated. They could also contribute to improving clients' insight into teachable moments. That is, the group worker or members could compare the client's feelings of powerlessness, helplessness, and frustration due to oppression on the job with how his partner feels when she is the target of his abuse.

Practitioners who incorporate this content into treatment acknowledge clients' experiences with racism in society. They support and explore strategies to assist the client to negotiate the conflict. They link client experiences to their behavior. They also help clients make the connection between the oppression they experiences and the oppression they are responsible for.

Overwhelmed Community Environments

African American men are uniquely affected by overwhelmed community environments, where they tend to be at high risk for physical harm (Blake & Darling, 1994). Homicide is the leading cause of death among African American men ages 15 to 34 (Rich & Stone, 1996). African American young men have higher rates of acquaintance violence and suicide compared to whites. What is important to recognize here is that most people in that environment are operating on the same set of cognitive and behavioral imperatives. Violence toward women may be one maladaptive behavior that results (Gibbs, 1988).

Accordingly, when such themes are discussed in treatment, group workers must be prepared to address the content and make connections to clients' behavior toward their partner. For example, a client describes living in a neighborhood and being "fronted-off" by some male acquaintances. He lived in a violent community environment. These young male acquaintances were trying to force him to join them in harming people in the community. If he did not, they would use violence toward him. He was trying to find a way out of this situation and struggling with the choices: Do I join with them in violence against others? Do I use violence against them in defense of myself? Do I run away? Can I run away? What about my manhood? Am I really a man if I don't confront them? In this situation, the men in the group explained that violence was not the best choice. One member noted the comment of a policeman who said, "Sometimes people are caught in a circumstance with two bad choices—both can get you into trouble." The group encouraged the man not to use violence because either choice could land him in jail. They acknowledged his reality and helped him to examine his options. One message that the man came away with was that it was not unmanly to move away from danger. In this situation, too, the important action, guided by the group worker, was to acknowledge the reality and to confront negative behaviors and choices.

In strictly focused batterers' groups, such content would likely be ignored because it is not directly related to partner violence. Another group worker may acknowledge the situation but merely view it as another example of male socialization and not an example of social context for some African American men. A culturally competent group worker would acknowledge that this situation is qualitatively different. Furthermore, lack of skill in negotiating the situation could result in violence. Group workers and members would support the client and explore strategies to assist him to negotiate the conflict in nonviolent ways. They would also explore the client's feelings and actions toward his partner. Did he displace his frustration, fear, and anger toward her? When he is faced with situations (caused by high stress and stressful choices), how does he relate to his partner? Finally, the group would assist the client to make the connection between the oppression he experiences and the oppression he inflicts on his partner.

SIXTEEN-WEEK INSIGHT-ORIENTED TREATMENT GROUP CYCLE WITH AFRICAN AMERICAN MEN WHO BATTER

I recommend that groups be conducted in seven phases: pre-group preparation; beginning, middle, and end phase; post-group aftercare; and follow-up.

Pre-Group Phase

In the pre-group phase, the group worker should individually meet with each client prior to his admission to the group. Each client should be oriented to the group treatment process: number of weeks, how groups function, the purpose of the group, the rules, and the goals. Group workers should also contract with the client around informed consent. For example, acknowledgment of the worker's responsibility to report to his partner or authorities if the client appears to be a threat to himself or others, and to report to his probation officer, if applicable, regarding his participation in the group. Batterers' treatment programs should also conduct evaluations of their treatment effectiveness in pre- and post-treatment phases. In the pre-group phase, clients should be evaluated regarding areas that may include the following: their knowledge of domestic abuse, levels of abuse toward a partner, and substance use. If possible and if the partner is in no danger, it would be useful to obtain the partner's or key informant's evaluation of the client in these areas. Post-treatment evaluations must also occur to determine the clients' gains in treatment. Again, such information should be obtained from the client and key informants.

Beginning Phase

In the beginning phase, the following areas should be addressed: group orientation, group rules, purposes of the group, rituals, check-in, and dyadic presentations. During the first group session, the group worker should provide an orientation about the group process and what is expected of a member.

Group Rules

Group rules should be recited during every session. Rules should address attendance, time, drug or alcohol sobriety during groups, appropriate client conduct in groups, and confidentiality and its limits (a limit to confidentiality would be if the man who batterers is a threat to himself or his partner).

Purposes of the Group

The group should recite the purpose of the group every week: (a) to end the violent and abusive behavior, (b) to help them address other issues of concern associated with their violence, (c) to address issues they experience as African American men that they perceive affect their violent and abusive behavior, and (d) to take responsibility for ending their abusive behaviors.

Rituals

Rituals can be effective tools to increase mutual aid or support in treatment groups with African American men who batter. Some programs emphasize community and cultural responsibility to change. In some racially homogeneous groups, codes of conduct and standards of behavior frame group rules and are drawn from African principles. History of the culture is studied, and men learn about the legacy of their people, which demands respect for others. In my work with African American men, I have been surprised to see how many have low self-esteem. It is also surprising to see how many devalue other African Americans, in what hooks (1994) describes as internalized oppression. One consequence of cultural low self-esteem is the devaluation and dehumanizing of others from that culture. Often, such perceptions are based on incomplete information about the culture. For example, one man in the group stated that "niggas ain't shit." He noted that, as a group, African Americans must have done something very horrible historically as a people to deserve slavery and the type of oppression they experience as a people. To increase self-esteem and to provide accurate cultural information, some African American male group leaders—including myself, James Bransford, and Kamal Kambui—use themes that challenge the African American historical representation that has resulted in internalized oppression among many African Americans. The exercise is also used to explore how African American men who batter use internalized oppression to destroy and oppress their female victims and reduce their self-esteem.

Antonia Drew, from ASHA Family Services in Milwaukee, and Raven Mason, from Harriet Tubman Battered Women program in Minneapolis, have used lybations with African American treatment groups to help these men get in touch with the history of their people. Lybations is a ritual where African Americans reflect on important people (usually relatives), either past or present, who have been a support and inspiration for clients. The men are asked to reflect on the history of African Americans in the United States; despite efforts to exterminate and hinder the progress of African Americans, they continue to survive. This ritual helps men get in touch with the fact that they stand on the shoulders of others who have come before them. It is because they lived that he lives. Men who batter are told that they have a responsibility to keep the culture and community strong. They must not behave in ways to destroy it. Leo Hayden, of the TASC program in Chicago,

Illinois, uses a method to get each group member to reflect on the people who have come before him, but he also expects each man to identify a person who is alive today who will build a more peaceful world. Another ritual, used by an African American men's group at the Wilder CAP program in St. Paul, Minnesota, is the whipping ritual, developed by Dion Crushson. In this exercise, at the beginning of each group, men in the group pass a whip around the room. One purpose is to remind men of the pain associated with violence perpetrated on their ancestors. The second purpose is to remind the men of the violence they do to their partners through partner abuse. Finally, another example of a ritual comes from Jim Smith's prison group of African American men in Wisconsin, called The Circle. Each week, members recite a poem focused on the purpose of the group, the types of behavioral changes they must achieve through participation in the group, and the responsibility of African American men to behave in adaptive ways and stay strong for each other and their community. Such rituals and activities can inspire men to change.

Check-In

Each week men should do check-in. This is done when each man in the group briefly shares the positives and the negatives of his week. Such information may produce content for attitudinal and behavioral restructuring among group members.

Dyadic Presentations

During the first phase of treatment, group workers should conduct dyadic presentations regarding the following: the problem of domestic violence; the cycle of violence; identifying differences between physical, emotional, verbal, and sexual abuse; exploring the relevance of the violence to the victim, the man who batters, and the African American community and culture; discussing contributors to violence: social learning, male socialization, sexism, displacement due to oppression, and environmental codes; learning nonviolence; discussing parenthood and intergenerational violence; and teaching and modeling nonviolence. Group leaders also discuss learning techniques to prevent violence, which include taking time out; leaving positively and returning positively; identifying healthy places to go and people to contact; increasing awareness of physical and emotional cues that lead to abuse; encouraging clients to take responsibility for violent behavior—for example, identify most violent incident, admit their level and frequency of abuse to partner; reframing thoughts and feelings; challenging irrational thoughts and feelings; and learning nonviolent approaches to handle conflict. In this phase, some programs give clients readings and homework to increase their knowledge about the problem of domestic violence. By the end of this phase, clients must identify four goals for self-transformation, as well as new methods to handle problems. One goal must include to end violent and abusive behavior, but the other goals can be the client's choice.

Middle Phase

In the middle phase of treatment, the focus of the group should shift to identifying client problem patterns, situations, and behavior. Then, the group members work on restructuring attitudes, thinking, and behaviors, as well as learning new ways of handling conflict. Role playing, rehearsal, and coaching can be used in this phase. For example, in the earlier situations, we explored client conflict at work due to racism. In this case, two clients could role-play the particular circumstances surrounding the event. Group members could give feedback concerning the situation and nonviolent ways to respond. The particular client who is confronted with this problem can rehearse or practice his nonviolent responses. Fellow group members could provide their insights about the appropriateness of the response.

Once this has been accomplished, the group could then also identify proactive, assertive actions that would confront the racism of coworkers and nonresponsiveness of the employer. The group would then turn its attention to the client's behavior with his partner. He and another group member may be asked to role-play his interactions and behavior with his partner. Again, group members can offer feedback about his interactions. They confront his negative attitudes and behaviors. They discuss how his partner must feel during these encounters. Often, she may feel helpless, powerless, vulnerable, and victimized. Members may make comparisons to the client's feelings during his oppressive experiences. The group discusses appropriate non-abusive approaches to employ with his partner. The client rehearses and the group offers feedback and comments, coaching the man who batters through the process. In this phase, clients must ask themselves the question: Why do they resort to abuse rather than alternative approaches? Also, how is their behavior different than when they are nonabusive?

End Phase

In the end phase, group workers should focus on assisting clients to integrate knowledge and skills obtained through group with problems, situations, old patterns, and conflicts outside of group. In other words, the focus should be on new techniques and how to use them in daily situations. Also, clients must begin to identify support systems that will encourage and sustain new behaviors (e.g., other men in the group, churches, sober bars, aftercare groups, community involvement, resources and programs for self-development, new friends, sobriety). Last, the men should identify some way they can contribute to reducing the problem of domestic violence individually.

Post-Treatment Phase

Three evaluations should occur during the end phase of the group: posttest evaluations during the last day of group and 3-month and 6-month follow-up. Among the issues that should be examined during follow-up are the reduction in the levels of client physical abuse and emotional abuse, their knowledge of domestic abuse, and substance use. Furthermore, although it is important to obtain his self-report, when appropriate or possible, it is important to also obtain his partner's report.

Aftercare services must be another consideration of batterers' programs. In my practice experience, I have found that many men want to continue coming to group after the group has ended. These are men who have learned new ways of behaving and see group as a resource to support change. These also tend to be men who have few other supports of this kind in their life.

ADDITIONAL GROUP TREATMENT CONSIDERATIONS

Client Recruitment

From a cultural perspective, the method of recruiting clients and the type of treatment group—voluntary, court-mandated, or some combination—are important considerations for providers of domestic abuse counseling. The choice may affect levels of client involvement when African American men are concerned.

As court-mandated programs emerged, men of color started to show up in batterers' treatment in greater numbers. Because of historical experiences with oppression, certain segments of the African American community view the police and legal systems with distrust. As a result, African American clients referred to court-mandated treatment perceive the programs with distrust. In some localities, batterers' treatment programs only accept court-referred clients, which exacerbates the problem. There must be a way to address this dilemma. Police and court intervention are necessary to protect women from abuse and hold men accountable for their behavior. But court-mandated treatment should not be the only method used to get men who batter into treatment. Batterers' treatment programs should not be only voluntary or court-mandated. Both approaches are important methods of getting African American men into treatment. Voluntary options may be seen more favorably, but men must be encouraged by family, friends, community leaders, and the community at large to participate in treatment. As a result, domestic violence service providers must direct more primary and secondary prevention and educational efforts in the African American community. In addition, these communities must be informed about and directed to available treatment services, and they must create access points for service within the community.

Poverty, Other Stressors, and Resources

Very often, African American clients who live in stressful and violent community environments also live in poverty. In fact, several urban court-mandated programs anecdotally report that a disproportionately high number of poor African American men are referred to treatment.

In addition to violence, poverty is also associated with problems such as substance abuse, unemployment, homelessness, inadequate nutrition and education, child abuse, and neglect. Certainly, these other issues are influenced by a lack of resources, information, and service delivery. Group workers should consider bringing other types of information and resources to groups to respond to the needs of these men and to increase the perception that group is a resource. Connecting men to treatment services for substance abuse is important. Providing information on a group bulletin board concerning access to food, housing, employment, training, and educational opportunities is also useful.

Fee for Service and Poverty

Another important issue is how group treatment services are paid for. Due to poverty, many men are not able to pay for services. For that reason, some programs reportedly drop men from treatment, even when there is a sliding scale. In those cases, programs must determine whether fees for some clients are a barrier to service delivery. If the inability to pay for group treatment is because of poverty, programs and funders must work creatively and collaboratively to offer treatment under different circumstances.

Abuse, Partner Loyalty, and Women's Safety

Many abused women choose to remain in an abusive situation because of love, children, lack of alternatives, loyalty, and/or their understanding of African American men's experiences with oppression. This should not be the reason for women to stay in a dangerous relationship. Although the male's experience may be real, this does not excuse his abusive behavior. Furthermore, change from abuse to recovery takes time. Women who remain in such relationships, waiting for change, risk further injury and harm. Battered women should be informed about the limits of treatment; it is not a guarantee of change. If a woman choose to remain in their relationships, it is the group worker's responsibility to promote her safety. This must be a consideration of treatment. Group workers must determine if the battered woman has a safety plan, that is, a course of action in the event she needs to leave the relationship due to his abuse. Among the things included in this plan should be the following: places to go, people to inform, clothing, and financial resources. She should be connected to a battered women's shelter. If she does not have a safety plan, someone in the agency should collaborate with battered women's services programs and help her to develop one. Programs must also put into policy the responsibility to inform. That is, the woman must be informed if her partner is ever determined to be a threat to her or himself.

GENERAL OVERVIEW OF DOMESTIC VIOLENCE GROUP TREATMENT CHARACTERISTICS

Number of Sessions

- Insight-oriented voluntary groups or court-mandated groups—between 16 and 26 weeks

- Information only educational groups—between 4 and 6 weeks

Treatment cycles vary. Some programs may have much longer treatment cycles. It depends on the program's treatment philosophy. On average, programs tend to last up to 26 weeks (National Research Council, 1996).

Length of Each Session

- Voluntary groups or court-mandated groups—2.5 hours
- Educational groups—2.5 to 3 hours

Open or Closed Format

- Voluntary groups or court-mandated groups—although most tend to be closed ended, there are open-ended models
- Educational groups—tend to be closed ended

Number of Men in the Group

- Voluntary groups—8 to 10
- Court mandated groups—12 to 16
- Educational groups—16 to 25

SUMMARY

Scholars who research maladaptive behaviors of African American men attempt to discern the social realities and antecedents that produce such behavior among these men without excusing the negative behavior. Group workers who work with African American men who batter must incorporate these realities with the conventional wisdom in the field of domestic violence. Traditional treatment groups may only focus on a partial reality and not other important experiences. Cultural competence on the part of group workers will increase the capacity of treatment groups to address the authentic social and cultural experiences of African American men who batter, which influences his abusive behaviors toward women.

Developing effective approaches that confront the behavior of men who batter are imperative to save women's lives, Just as the use of group treatment, cognitive behavioral approaches, and court mandates have helped to enhance the participation of batterers in treatment, culturally competent approaches must be considered within such a context. For many African American men who batter, the use of culturally competent approaches is essential to increase their involvement in treatment and the likelihood of a successful outcome. The information presented above is designed to assist group workers seeking to be more effective with this population. Moreover, it may have implications for the successful involvement and treatment of men from other ethnic and cultural groups, as well. In any case, it is important to recognize that ethnocultural factors should not be permitted to obscure the uniqueness of each client or to allow the worker to neglect each client's individuality. At the same time, the use of culturally competent group treatment approaches is a crucial element in reducing partner abuse among African American men who batter.

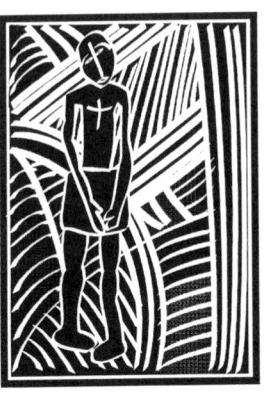

PART V

Gangs, Risky Behavior, and Delinquency

Given the carnage and mayhem taking place among young African American males, few efforts deserve more serious attention than those to reduce gang involvement, risky behaviors, and delinquency. So common has the association between crime and African American males become that for many, the mention of one invokes the image of the other. A simple literature search on African American males will quickly lead to citations on crime, delinquency, drugs, and violence. And although crime and violence committed by African American males continues to remain a central political issue at local, state, and national levels, few with the power to "make a difference" bother to ask why so many African American males are in trouble.

A variety of psychological and sociological explanations have emerged to explain "black crime." Even genetic arguments have been put forth as reasons. However, those who put forth genetic explanations must consider the fact that the level of gang violence and other forms of deviant behavior has risen much faster than any possible concomitant genetic or biological changes. Causes for the growth in gang activity, delinquency, and violence among African American males are not to be found in genetic causes but rather in larger, more encompassing societal forces. However, for African American males who are involved in gangs or other risky behaviors, it has become out of vogue to argue for interpersonal or psychological interventions to assist them, and quite in vogue to lobby instead solely for their punishment.

Hence, it is the state penitentiary, not Penn State, and the "Big House," not Morehouse, that are the destination of increasing numbers of African American males. Without a doubt, prisons have become the method of choice for intervening with this young male population. Although African Americans make up only 12% of all males in America, over 48% of all males confined in prison are African American (U.S. Department of Justice, 1995b; see King, 1993a). Many have been shocked by reports that one in four African American males between the ages of 20 and 29 is incarcerated, on parole, or on probation, or that there are more African males in prison than in college (Mauer, 1994). Indications are that on any given day, 480,000 African American males are enrolled in college, whereas over 525,000 are in jail or prison (King, 1993a). Some in the African American community have wondered aloud that if one in four young white males were experiencing such difficulties, would there not be calls for something akin to a Marshall Youth Plan to correct the situation.

Actually, African American youth are more likely to see a policeman than a doctor or mental health worker. It has been suggested that police are the front line of social service for African American youth (Stark, 1993). This reality only lends credence to the fact that we as a society have become increasingly unforgiving of young African American males. Offenses committed by them are unlikely to be viewed as youthful mistakes made by confused and immature young men. Instead, these youths are more likely to be perceived as hardened criminals. They are often not diverted from, but directed into the criminal justice system (Walker, Spohn, & Delone, 1996). The system now seems frequently only too eager to get their records started, while failing to realize that African American youths are themselves often the victims. Indeed, they are 50% of all homicide victims, making their rate nearly eight times higher than that for white males (Walker et al., 1996). And they are exposed to and witness crime and violence at astronomical rates (Fitpatrick & Boldizar, 1993; Williams, Stiffman, & O'Neal, 1998).

Risky behaviors such as gang violence and drug use are also public health issues, as they contribute to the death and morbidity of African American males. Hence, many of the concerns expressed in this section might well have been placed in the section on health. The same might be said for the economic considerations addressed in this volume, as difficult life conditions, loss of earning power for workers, and the flight of manufacturing from inner cities have led to harsh lives for many African Americans and their children (Staub, 1996). In short, the causes of social anomie for African American males are many and could have easily been addressed by any of the topic areas identified in this book. We encourage practitioners at all levels of intervention to borrow from the insights offered in this section, as well as others, to reduce the numbers of African American youths whose lives are being traumatized and ruined by delinquency, gangs, drugs, violence, and crime.

Chapter 18

Gang Prevention and Intervention With African American Males

Scott H. Decker
G. David Curry

What motivates young men (and women) to join gangs? And more important, what can be done to intervene and prevent gang involvement by African American youth? This chapter examines these and several related issues. We begin with an examination of many of the background issues regarding gangs, then attempt to isolate the distinctively African American elements of contemporary urban street gangs, emphasizing how homes, schools, and communities can affect the lives of gang members, fringe members, and non-gang members. Three levels are identified for explanation and action in dealing with gangs, the motivations of individuals to join gangs, and the persistence of membership even in the face of violence and potential death. We focus on (a) individual level factors; (b) social factors, such as family issues and the social needs of adolescents to belong to groups; and (c) environmental causes, such as the impact of neighborhoods, social structure, and culture. These three levels frame our curative hypotheses and our recommendations for mobilizing the resources, in terms of human, social, and physical capital, that are required if community-based strategies are to succeed in reducing the costs of gang-related violence.

STATEMENT OF THE PROBLEM

One dilemma in responding to gangs is the difficulty in finding consistent definitions of what constitutes a gang, a gang member, and a gang incident. The differences in definition are many and have significant consequences for crafting intervention programs. This issue is crucial in responding to African American gangs because of the stereotyping black males generally face. All definitions of a gang include the group character of membership, but consensus breaks down at that point. A variety of definitions of *gang* require that symbols—clothes, signs, or other forms of nonverbal communication— be a part of the definition. Community activists, as well as scholars of contemporary African American social life, express concern that "any" collective activity by minority youth that is not connected to some mainstream institution such as a social service agency or school may be labeled as a gang. It is this concern that makes it so crucial that any definition of a gang include collective involvement in criminal activity. For our purposes, we define a gang as a group of individuals who have symbols of membership, permanence, and criminal involvement. In a similar vein, a gang member is a person who acknowledges membership in the gang and is regarded as a gang member by other members.

It is critical to have estimates of the number of gangs, gang members, and gang incidents for the nation. Curry, Ball, and Fox (1994) estimated that in 1992 there were 249,324 gang members, 4,881 gangs, 46,359 gang crimes, and slightly more than 1,000 gang homicides. The 1994 estimates found growth in each of these numbers, particularly for gangs, which had nearly doubled to 8,652, and gang members, which had grown to just under 380,000. In addition, gang-related crimes increased dramatically to 437,066. The 1992 survey results also document the ethnicity of gang membership. Nearly half (48%) of gang members in the national survey were African American. Just under 43% of gang members were Hispanic. These data are consistent with the results of the Maxson, Woods, and Klein (1996) study of gang migration, which found that 60% of gang migrants were black. Although these data may be subject to some measurement error, it is difficult to argue that prevention efforts for African American gang involvement are not needed.

A number of observers of and participants in the current gang scene have observed that gangs are related to features of life in the African American community. Shakur (1993), a Los Angeles gang member, argued that gangs were a form of neighborhood protection, a position endorsed by Sanchez-Jankowski (1991). Useni Perkins (1987), a former street gang worker, argues that gangs are the key to the regeneration of the black community. Perkins contends that gangs have the potential for political action that can lead the black community to a position of social, economic, and political power. Brown (1978) studied gangs in Philadelphia and concluded that black gangs were an extension of the African American family. His argument centered on the fact that a large number of young black men grow up in homes without a father figure, and as a consequence, they seek the gang as a surrogate family. Similarly, Taylor (1993, p. 9), in his study of African American gangs in Detroit, included *ethnic families* as one type of group that fit his operational definition of a gang. The dilemma for each of these findings is that the conclusions are drawn from one-shot case studies or more expansive studies where the nature of the underlying sample is difficult to determine. In 1965, Short and Strodtbeck concluded that the black street gangs of Chicago had little political ideology or agenda. The majority of current research has reached a similar conclusion.

The role of gangs in violence has been well documented. In some cities (Los Angeles, Chicago, St. Louis), gangs are responsible for one third of all homicides. And surveys of juvenile detainees indicate that gang members are far more likely to possess and use firearms than their non-gang counterparts. Gang violence has a reciprocal character. That is, the violence of one gang leads to violence from another gang. As Decker (1996) observed, gang violence resembles contagion, in that it can lead to increased involvement from one to the other. Decker and Van Winkle (1996) had 99 subjects in their study; 11 were dead within 2 years of the conclusion of their study. Hutson, Anglin, Kyriacou, Hart, and Spears (1995) documented a phenomenal growth in violence and mortality among African American gang members.

THEORETICAL EXPLANATION

Although individual-level theories of gang involvement are not as common as other kinds of explanations, two 1995 books by senior gang researchers, Irving Spergel and Malcolm Klein, included theoretical perspectives that placed some emphasis on individual-level characteristics. For Spergel (1995), central elements of a theoretical explanation of gang behavior are poverty, social disorganization, and racism. Still, he argued, there has to be some explanation for why only some of the youths who live in at-risk communities where gang involvement is high become gang members and why some youth who become involved in gangs do not become involved in crime. Spergel (p. 163) proposed a collection of social and psychological— but not biological—traits in what he termed personal disorganization theory. These traits included lower intelligence (or at least limited ability to perform academically), estrangement from family and/or school, and a tendency to respond aggressively and physically to adversity. Malcolm Klein (1995, p. 76), who over his career has placed a greater emphasis on group and social dynamic influences on gang involvement, identified a set of personal characteristics that he felt distinguished "gang joiners and heavy participators" from other youth. These characteristics included difficulty in school, low self-esteem, lower impulse control, defiance, aggressiveness, and pride in physical prowess.

For studies specifically attentive to African American gang involvement, individual-level factors have been de-emphasized. In a study of at-risk minority youth in Chicago, Curry and Spergel (1992) found community factors such as the influence and prevalence of gangs and gang members in community, school, and family to be more significant predictors of gang involvement than individual-level factors. African American youths have not been the only populations for which community-level factors have been given greater emphasis in explaining gang involvement. Community-level theories have been *the* explanation of gangs for most of this century. Thrasher (1927) described the gang as an *interstitial* phenomenon, developing and flourishing in the gaps left void by other institutions, such as the family, the school, and the labor force in the turbulent immigrant communities of turn-of-the-century Chicago. Clifford Shaw and Henry McKay (1942) used their studies of delinquent gang members in the 1930s and 1940s to develop the theory of social disorganization. Under classic social disorganization theory, weak ties among community residents result in limited social control of youth. Gangs, serving as collective purveyors of delinquent subculture, develop and become strong in those communities where personal ties between community members are weak. However, the communities that served as the model for these classic theories of social disorganization were communities composed predominantly of European immigrants.

Studies of African American communities led to a general rejection of classic social disorganization theory. Unlike immigrant communities, where population movements and residential instability can be perceived as weakening personal ties among residents, many African American communities, although characterized by poverty, are residentially stable and characterized by strong personal ties among community residents. The persistence of high levels of crime, delinquency, and gang activity in such communities cannot be easily attributed to traditional forms of social disorganization theory. Alternative theoretical perspectives are required.

One of the most important social theories to attempt to explain life conditions among African Americans dwelling in poor neighborhoods in inner cities was offered by William Julius Wilson (1987). He opens the first page of his first chapter with a compelling observation:

Blacks in Harlem and in other ghetto neighborhoods did not hesitate to sleep in parks, on fire escapes, and on rooftops during hot summer nights in the 1940s and 1950s, and whites frequently visited inner-city taverns and nightclubs. There was crime, to be sure, but it had not reached the point where people were fearful of walking the streets at night, despite the overwhelming poverty of the area. (p. 3)

For Wilson, the change between those comparatively peaceful streets and the more violent streets of today's inner cities can be attributed to two types of social dislocations. The first was the de-industrialization of the U.S. economy and an associated decline in blue-collar jobs. The second was the movement of the African American middle and working class out of the neighborhoods where they had been forced to live under the discrimination of prior decades. The results were communities composed of women and their children and a declining pool of marriageable males. Marriageability of African American males has been diminished by persistent joblessness and involvement in the criminal justice system. According to Wilson (1987), "the most dramatic indicator of the extent to which social dislocations have afflicted urban blacks is crime, especially violent crime" (p. 21).

Bursik and Grasmick (1993) have expanded classic social disorganization theory in a way that can incorporate Wilson's theory of the underclass and account for consistently high rates of gang-related crime in stable African American neighborhoods with strong interpersonal ties among residents. Social control, they suggest, operates at three different levels: private, parochial, and public. Private levels of social control are ties at the personal level, which can often exist alongside chronic levels of criminal activity. Parochial levels of social control represent ties between people and people's control over community-level agencies and businesses in their communities. Finally, the public level of social control is concerned with community members' control of public resources, such as law enforcement and social services. Under Bursik and Grasmick's approach, members of Wilson's underclass may share strong interpersonal ties but lack parochial and public social control.

Curry and Spergel (1988) examined community-level variations in gang violence and delinquency using data on the city of Chicago. The authors began with the observation that violent delinquency rates and gang-related violence were not distributed in the same patterns in the city. From 1978 to 1985, the gang homicide rate in Chicago's Latino communities was more than twice the homicide rate in African American communities. Non-gang violence over the same period was much higher in Chicago's African American communities. An analysis of the correlates of gang homicide and delinquency across communities revealed that gang homicide was related to the distribution of the city's Latino population and poverty whereas general delinquency was only related to variations in poverty rates. Poverty was measured as a composite of three indicators: housing values, proportion of families living below the poverty level, and unemployment rate. Once poverty was controlled, the distribution of neither gang homicides nor delinquency rates were statistically related to the distribution of African Americans across communities.

Examining changes in gang homicide rates over the two periods 1978 to 1981 and 1982 to 1985, Curry and Spergel (1988) found that the only significant predictor of increases in gang homicide rates was the distribution of poverty. Over the time period from 1978 to 1985, the gap in the level of gang homicides between African American and Latino communities had narrowed. From their analysis, Curry and Spergel predicted that if trends in their data continued, gang homicide rates in African American communities where poverty was greatest would be subject to the greatest increases over time. A 1996 analysis (Block et al.) of gang-related crimes in Chicago showed that the risk of being an offender in a gang-related homicide had increased for both African American and Latino males when the two periods, 1980 to 1984 and 1990 to 1994, were compared. The rate for Latinos increased from 16.3 to 26.5 per 100,000. The rate for African Americans increased from 10.6 to 32.0 per 100,000, underscoring the risk of violence posed by gang membership, especially for African Americans.

Models that approach the problem of gang involvement from multiple levels perhaps offer the most complete theoretical model of gang involvement. Decker and Van Winkle (1996), in analyzing gangs in St. Louis, proposed a model that incorporated variations in perspective at the individual level, group process variables at the gang level, and community-level influences. St. Louis is a city that has undergone profound social change as a result of the restructuring of the U.S. economy and the growth of the urban underclass. As well as the impact of these changes, the structure of African American gangs and processes in St. Louis reflects a unique combination of local neighborhood dynamics and what Klein (1995, p. 230) has identified as the national level diffusion of gang cultures. In the late 1980s, St. Louis's neighborhood rivalries (dating back for decades) and contemporary friendship networks were transfigured into a system of conflict structures that bear the names and symbols of California's long-standing conflict between the Bloods and the Crips (Covey, Menard, & Franzere, 1992; Jackson & McBride,

1986), with occasional symbolic manifestations of Chicago gang culture. Gang violence has become a disproportionate part of a larger violence problem in the African American communities of St. Louis.

Central to the theoretical model of Decker and Van Winkle is the concept of threat. Perception of the threat of violence at collective and personal levels drives gang involvement and conflict in St. Louis. Above all, gang life in St. Louis was ubiquitously integrated into a socially organized and culturally grounded pattern of violence. It is a violence that determines the community-level emergence and development of gangs and a violence that defines the day-to-day substance and meaning of gang activity.

Families, schools, and communities are weakened by the social disruptions associated with economic restructuring. In the face of this weakness, the importance of gang social organization takes on an exaggerated significance. Youths drawn to gangs as a response to threat actually become at greater risk for violence. Hence, their membership poses a threat to family members, schools, neighbors, and other social institutions. The violence and the reaction of those not involved in gangs to this violence increase gang member marginalization. Therefore, efforts to reduce gang violence have important policy consequences for reintegrating gang youth into mainstream social institutions.

CURATIVE HYPOTHESES

In a search for promising gang intervention programs, Spergel and Curry (1993) interviewed 254 representatives of community agencies across the nation. We propose a pattern of responses that are congruent with the hypothesized causes of the gang problem in the African American community as reviewed above.

In a study of why violent crime rates in the United States are so much greater than those in other comparable nations, Messner and Rosenfeld (1994) concluded that cultural as well as structural changes are required if the national level of violence is to be reduced. Central to U.S. culture, they argue, is the American Dream. Messner and Rosenfeld found that the structural arrangements of U.S. society "are conducive to and presuppose" the cultural orientations that make "the most important feature of the economy of the United States . . . its capitalist nature" (p. 76) and economic institutions dominant over all other institutions. The structure and strength of noneconomic institutions, such as the community, school, and family, suffer from this arrangement. The functions and roles of noneconomic institutions are devalued. Economic norms penetrate community, school, and family functions, and these institutions and their participants make accommodations to the economy. The cost of this accommodation is weakened communities, schools, and families, the very institutions for which strength is required for social control. It takes both the cultural valuation of succeeding and acquiring at any cost and the absence of strong institutions of social control to result in the levels of violent crime that currently exist in the United States. Messner and Rosenfeld call for a cultural regeneration that is associated with strengthening and valuing noneconomic institutions. Such changes are linked to the fundamental causes of gang violence and associated problems in the African American community.

In the short run, strategies for responding to gang violence that move toward these long-term goals should be given preference. Strategies that strengthen families and schools can enhance the personal and parochial levels of social control identified by Bursik and Grasmick (1993) as being required to allow communities to control crime. Community organization strategies that move toward community access to public levels of social control will also be required. Provision of opportunities for legitimate livelihood will be essential, but the continued allocation on the basis of noneconomic criteria of the benefits required to take advantage of those opportunities is just as essential.

A number of proximate interventions are also greatly needed. Research (Decker & Van Winkle, 1994; Klein & Maxson, 1994; Klein, Maxson, & Cunningham, 1991) has shown that whereas gang members frequently use drugs and individual gang members frequently engage in drug sales, particularly at the street level, drug selling organized by the gang is relatively uncommon. A study of gang-related homicides between 1987 and 1990 in Chicago (Block & Block, 1993) revealed that gang homicides were more often turf-related than drug-related. Where specialization in drug crime did occur among Chicago gangs, the practice was found to be more common for African American gangs (Block et al., 1996, pp. 13-14). At least half and perhaps more of the offenses attributed to each of the major African American gangs in Chicago between 1987 and 1994 were drug offenses. (The comparable statistic for Latino gangs was under 25%, and for white gangs, 13%.) Controlling drug markets may prove to be an essential short-term approach to reducing gang-related violence for African American gangs.

Another major factor in contemporary levels of gang-related violence is the availability of guns. From his study of Milwaukee gangs, Hagedorn (1988, pp. 143-144) concluded that guns were a major factor in increases in gang homicides. Nearly half of the African American males interviewed by

Hagedorn reported owning more than one gun. Block and Block (1993) found that guns were the lethal weapons in practically all Chicago gang-related homicides between 1987 and 1990. Sanders (1995, p. 56) suggested that the availability of guns was key to the transition from gang fighting to drive-by shootings and armed robberies. Among African American gang members in St. Louis, Decker and Van Winkle (1996, pp. 175-176) found guns to be "the overwhelming weapon of choice for gang-motivated and gang-related violence." For gang members interviewed in the St. Louis study, the average number of reported guns owned was 4.5. From an analysis of interviews with those arrested in 11 cities where the National Institute of Justice's Drug Use Forecasting Program was being conducted, Decker and Pennell (1996) discovered a strong association between carrying a gun and gang membership. Of those interviewed who identified themselves as gang members, 36% reported carrying a gun all or most of the time. A majority of the total sample reported that obtaining a gun illegally was easy. A third said that they could get a gun in less than a week. Reducing access to firearms is a very promising proximate step in reducing gang-related violence.

PROGRAMS AND THE STRENGTHS OF THE AFRICAN AMERICAN COMMUNITY

A multiyear research and development project funded by the Office of Juvenile Justice and Delinquency Prevention attempted to identify promising community-based responses to youth gang problems across the United States. The major product of this project was a set of prototypes integrated into the Comprehensive Communitywide Approach to Gangs. Usually, it is identified by policymakers and program practitioners simply as the Spergel model. The Spergel model is an extremely flexible format for responding to gang problems at the community level. Its central tenet is community mobilization. Crime control and gang intervention through community mobilization form a formidable national and local challenge.

To underestimate the magnitude of the problem would be a mistake. The incarceration rates of inner-city African American youth as a response to the growing level of violence have been characterized by a former president of the American Society of Criminology as a major assault on the black community (Blumstein, 1993). The level of violence against people and the punitive criminal justice response produce a torrent of disruption that afflicts struggles to rear African American children (Kotlowitz, 1991; Wilson, 1987). Mitchell Duneier (1992), in *Slim's Table: Race, Respectability, and*

Masculinity, produced a compelling portrait of African American men who collectively draw on their inner strength to deal with the problems of day-to-day life in the inner city. In an interview in *The New Yorker* (Remnick, 1996), William Julius Wilson noted "the tragedy that there are so few [Slims]" (p. 106). Wilson argues that an even more massive effort to provide meaningful work at livable wages will be required to supplement existing programs.

The current policy emphasis on community mobilization promises solutions to gang problems that take advantage of the resilience, creativity, and adaptability of members of the African American community. African Americans have developed and maintained their culture and sense of identity in the face of overwhelming adversity, from slavery to service in the Civil War to Jim Crow and segregation. Repeatedly, African Americans have overcome adversity by acts of individual heroism by ordinary men and women integrated into the strength of community organization (Branch, 1988). Local political structures must be used to ensure that federal and state efforts are accessible to community residents and lead to the creation of social capital in the African American community.

An example of the strength that must be incorporated into the effort to control gang-related violence in the African American community has been the efforts Dr. Booker Yelder and other African American professionals. Using volunteer efforts and limited funding, they have brought a continuing array of services to the residents of the Shaw community in the District of Columbia. From 1990 to 1993, Yelder, a former school teacher, supervised a street worker program funded by the Family Youth Services Bureau of the U.S. Department of Health and Human Services, which operated out of an office in one of the District's most crime-ridden housing projects. There are many more projects like this one in many other cities. The task is to unite the efforts of scattered collectivities of African American men and women into a truly comprehensive effort to reduce gang-related violence.

RESOURCES

Despite the many strengths of the target group, progress in dealing with African American gangs is not likely without marshaling resources. These resources must include financial resources, although they are by no means the most important. A variety of other resources—most notably social capital—will be necessary to ameliorate the gang problem in the African American community. And finally, institutional resources must be brought to bear in finding solutions to the violence, family disruption, and imprisonment that has been wrought by the growing problem of gangs in the African American community.

At the center of any effective response to African American gangs, we see the creation of social capital, mutual obligations between members of a community, expectations for appropriate behavior, and sanctions to meet violations of those expectations. Such obligations create links between gang members and the legitimate world of social institutions, tying gang members to the social and institutional fabric of their communities. Much of the gang research and programmatic interventions has identified the marginalization of gang members as a key element in the decision to join a gang and remain a member even in the face of high levels of violence. This marginalization is appropriately countered by efforts to increase social capital. Relationships between gang members and their families, gang members and the institutional world of work, and gang members and their community are cited by many ex-members as the reasons they left their gangs (Decker & Lauritsen, 1996). Strengthening these relationships is a way to make it easier for current gang members to leave their gang and to prevent prospective members from joining.

The role of institutional resources is an important one. Institutions such as the family, school, recreation, and labor market play an important role in preventing gang membership initially and reducing it for those who have joined the gang. Family ties, even for hard-core gang members, remain strong and have consequences for the choices made by gang members (Decker & Van Winkle, 1996). Policies and programs that strengthen the family by building on its innate resiliency are desperately needed. Schools are a natural resource because they touch so many lives and are physically positioned to have maximum impact. Too often, recreation programs have been substituted for more meaningful interventions. A youth worker we have worked with often comments that the struggles of the black community will not be solved by "rolling a thousand basketballs down ghetto streets." To this we say "Amen." However, recreation can be used as a hook to attract at-risk youth to programs with more meaningful goals, such as literacy, high school completion programs, computer skill building, and preparation for trades.

This brings us to the role of the labor market. The creation of new jobs, jobs with a living wage and prospects for a future, is a cornerstone of any gang intervention program. Jobs provide a variety of important benefits in addition to their monetary return. Employment provides a way to fill the day with activities away from the street and nonworking peers. Such diversions have important consequences for reducing the opportunities to become involved in gangs and gang activities. In addition, a job helps to build social capital through the development of networks that extend well beyond neighborhood peers and age-graded peer activities. Finally, a job represents a tangible commitment to and belief in the future. Work is an essential element of American culture, and participation in the labor force provides meaning as well as money.

Among the greatest challenges in responding to gangs in the African American community is the challenge to do so in a depoliticized way that does not reinforce stereotypical images or make the problem worse. Many aspects of the contemporary gang scene in American make this a difficult task. In many communities, there is a great tendency to overidentify the number of gangs and gang members, in large part as a response to the involvement of African Americans in gangs (Huff, 1991). The identification of African American males as gang members because of their clothes or color is a real and damaging correlate of today's gang problem. Such behavior adversely affects the very population that faces the greatest challenges for acceptance in American society, in many cases further marginalizing young men and moving them toward gang membership. Another problem to confront is the tendency among some to glorify gangs or excuse their behavior because of its causes. Neither of these approaches is likely to be productive, as each ignores much of the reality of contemporary African American gangs. Intervention must take great pains to avoid making the gang organization stronger by providing it with resources or status it might otherwise not have access to. Prior research has repeatedly shown the dangers of strengthening the gang.

Amid the current generation of street gangs, many of which are composed of African Americans, it is important to be mindful that three generations of gangs have come and gone in the United States over the past century. As their Irish, Italian, and Polish counterparts did 100 years ago, African Americans must become better integrated into the social and economic fabric of the country, like the European immigrants, whose ancestors, in most cases, came to this country after the ancestors of African Americans.

CHAPTER 19

Preventing Delinquency Among African American Males

JANICE JOSEPH

Official data consistently find that blacks are more delinquent than whites. Black youths are overrepresented in the arrest statistics. Whereas black youths made up 15% of the general population in 1995, they constituted 28% of all juvenile arrests. Also in 1995, 49% of all juveniles arrested for violent crimes, and 27% of those arrested for property crimes were black (Federal Bureau of Investigation, 1996). Official data indicate that black youths are overrepresented in homicide, illegal drugs, and gang activities.

In 1994, 59% of all juveniles arrested for murder and nonnegligent manslaughter were black, compared to 39% who were white and 2% other ethnic groups (U.S. Department of Justice, 1995a). The homicide offense rate for black males between age 14 and 17 in 1993 was 147.3 per 100,000 people compared to 14.0 per 100,000 for whites. The rate for black females in the same age group was 6.6 per 100,000 people, compared to 0.9 per 100,000 for white females (Fox, 1995).

The arrest data for 1994 indicated that 39% of those arrested for drug violations under the age of 18 were black. Black youths under the age of 18 had an arrest rate for drug violations in 1994 of 483.9 per 100,000 people, compared to 88.5 per 100,000 for white youths (Federal Bureau of Investigation, 1995). The Drug Use Forecasting (DUF) data for 1994 also indicated that 50% of black juvenile arrestees, compared with 40% of white arrestees

259

and 46% of Hispanic arrestees, in Cleveland tested positive for drug use. In San Antonio, Texas, the numbers were 33% for black and 16% for white; in Washington, D.C., the numbers were 65% for blacks and 29% for whites (National Institute of Justice, 1995).

Black youths are also involved in gang activities. One of the major illegal acts of black youth gangs is drug trafficking, which is an important source of income, wealth, and power. Black gangs are often linked to the sale of cocaine and crack and operate "rock houses" or "stash houses" that yield thousands of dollars a week for these businesses. Black youth gangs also engage in a great deal of violence (McBride & Jackson, 1989). The Jamaican Posses are extremely violent and would kill anyone they feel is in their way. They are also antipolice and are particularly ruthless in disposing of their enemies (Albrecht, 1992). Of the street gang-motivated offenses recorded during 1987 and 1990 in Chicago, 28% were committed by the Black Gangster Disciples Nation, 18% by the Vice Lords, and the remainder by other types of gangs (Block & Block, 1993). In such cities as New York, Chicago, Los Angeles, Miami, and Washington, D.C., gang-related homicides reach several hundreds annually (Reynolds, 1993).

Self-report studies are alternatives to official data. Many of these studies find relatively smaller differences between black and white youths, compared to official data on delinquency. Several studies (Elliott & Voss, 1974; Gold, 1970) found no difference in delinquency between black and white youths. Hirschi (1969) found slight differences by race, with the rates for blacks higher than those for whites. In addition, many researchers have found that blacks tend to be overrepresented in specific types of offenses (Elliott, Ageton, & Canter, 1980; Hindelang, Hirschi, & Weis, 1981; Huizinga & Elliott, 1987; William & Gold, 1972).

EXPLANATIONS OF DELINQUENCY AMONG BLACK YOUTHS

Biological Explanations

Genetics have been used to explain delinquency among black youths, especially males. Wilson and Herrnstein (1985) implicitly suggest that the higher incidence of crime and delinquency among blacks in the United States may be evidence of biologically inherited propensities. They argue that there is a causal link between physical or biological characteristics and crime. Their argument suggests that because people with black skin make up a disproportionate number of people involved in crime and delinquency, then the black skin, which is genetically determined, must be the cause of crime and delinquency.

Low intelligence has also been linked to black delinquency; it is an association that has been embroiled in controversy. Blacks, on average, score 15 points lower than whites on intelligence tests. Some scholars have used this difference in intelligence test scores to explain the difference in delinquency rates among black and white youths. Some researchers have contended that intelligence is inherited and, when blacks score lower than whites on intelligence tests, it is solely the result of genetic differences between the two races (Gordon, 1976; Hirschi & Hindelang, 1977; Jensen, 1969).

Additional support for the association between intelligence and delinquency has been presented by Herrnstein and Murray (1994), who recently reignited the debate regarding intelligence and race. More important, they argue that intelligence levels differ among ethnic groups and that a range of social problems, such as crime, unemployment, and poverty, are related to low intelligence. They state that blacks score lower than whites on every known standardized test of cognitive ability, but they dismiss cultural factors or socioeconomic status as contributing to these differences. Instead, they conclude that differences in test scores between blacks and whites are largely related to genetic differences in intelligence between the two groups, with blacks having lower intelligence.

The use of intelligence tests to attempt to demonstrate the genetic inferiority of blacks is very dangerous. To link the delinquency of blacks with low intelligence can have serious ramifications for young blacks in the way the criminal justice system and society at large treat them.

Sociological Explanations

Subculture of Violence Perspective

The subculture of violence theory was proposed by Wolfgang and Ferracuti (1967), who maintained that young lower-class black males possess a distinct subculture that emphasizes the use of violence and accounts for their relatively high rates of violence. According to these researchers, although the members of this subculture share dominant values, they use violence to solve disputes and conflicts. Violence is condoned, legitimized, and considered appropriate for members of this subculture.

Curtis (1975) also claimed that the emphasis on manliness in the black community encourages the use of force and violence: Instead of backing down and looking for alternative solutions for problems, black males typically resort to force for settling disputes. Other research, however, questions the racially based subculture of violence by reporting that on attitudinal measures of approval/disapproval of violence, minority groups were no different than the general population (Ball-Rokeach, 1973; Erlanger, 1974).

Environmental Factors

Urban ecologists (Shaw & McKay, 1942; Thrasher, 1927) maintain that the physical and social environments can promote deviant behavior, such as crime and delinquency. Several researchers have found that there are delinquency-producing areas in large cities. Such areas are characterized by high mobility, high population density, substandard housing, family dysfunction, and slumlike conditions. The residents are transient and have low incomes with minimal occupational skills (Bursik, 1988; Heitgerd & Bursik, 1997; Shannon, 1982).

About 56% of the black population lives in such areas, and these neighborhoods are socially toxic, characterized by high unemployment, poverty, overcrowding, public housing, and physical decay (Pace, 1993). Drug addiction, welfare dependency, female-based households, and other pathologies are prevalent in these neighborhoods. Residents are often excluded from the mainstream and are increasingly trapped in poor neighborhoods from one generation to the other (Bartollas & Miller, 1994). Rose (1990) and Farley (1980) suggest that the ghetto environments are pathogenic for black youth. Overcrowding, social isolation, and social disorganization contribute to feelings of powerlessness, despair, social alienation, crime, and delinquency.

Sociohistorical Perspective

Joseph (1995) proposed a sociohistorical perspective: The historical past and structural factors of poverty, inadequate education, disorganized and deprived environments, unemployment, and other social ills interact to weaken the bonds that some black youths have to society. The underlying factor appears to be the degree of social integration of black youths in American society. Given their weakened bonds and lack of integration into the society, the gang becomes very significant to many black males, providing status, acceptance, respect, and prestige they might otherwise not receive.

In fact, the gang in the inner city is believed to have taken over the socialization of many black males by replacing the family, the school, the church, and government agencies (Voight, Thornton, Barrile, & Seaman, 1994). As the saliency of gangs increases, so too does the probability of delinquency. This perspective views the underlying causes of delinquency as the historical and structural factors that predispose black youths to delinquency, with bonding to delinquent peers serving as an important inducement to delinquency.

DELINQUENCY PREVENTION

Common sense indicates that it is better to prevent a problem than to react to it once it arises. This is true of delinquency. In 1993, Attorney General Janet Reno stated, "America would rather build prisons than invest in a child and we've got to change that. Unless we invest in children, we will never have enough dollars to build all the prisons necessary to house people 15 to 20 years from now" ("Reno Calls," p. 1A). If society wants to prevent black males' involvement in delinquency, especially violence, it has to go beyond treating the symptoms to examining the causes.

There are three levels of delinquency prevention: primary, secondary, and tertiary. Primary prevention of delinquency among black males is directed at modifying and changing conditions that lead to delinquency. Prevention strategies are aimed at reducing risk factors and providing protective factors that are now nonexistent in black male environments. Secondary prevention seeks early identification and intervention into the lives of black males who are found to be in delinquency-producing circumstances. Secondary prevention focuses on changing the behaviors of black males likely to become delinquent. Strategies would include deterrence, strengthening of social bonds with institutions, and goal attainment. Tertiary prevention is aimed at reducing recidivism by focusing on preventing further delinquent acts by black males already identified as delinquent. This would involve treatment and rehabilitation techniques or strategies.

Most juvenile delinquency efforts have been unsuccessful because of their negative approach—attempting to keep juveniles from misbehaving. Positive approaches that emphasize opportunities for healthy social, physical, and mental development have a much greater likelihood of success. Another weakness of past delinquency prevention efforts is their narrow scope, focusing on only one or two of society's institutions that have responsibility for the social development of children. Most programs have targeted the schools or the family and ignored the community (Brewer, Hawkins, Catalano, & Neckerman, 1995).

When possible, practitioners should engage in prevention. Prevention strategies need to start early in the lives of black males, before the onset of delinquency. Intervention programs beginning as early as elementary school years will be most effective in the long run. Strategies need to be comprehensive in terms of multiple and interrelated causes associated with delinquency. They should be designed for the long term because risk factors usually have a long-term effect on black males' behavior.

Prevention strategies seek to reduce existing risk factors and provide protective factors that are missing from a youth's environment. In many ways, preventive strategies attempt to provide for at-risk youths what effective parents, schools, and communities provide in the natural course of youth development. Successful delinquency prevention strategies must be positive in their orientation and comprehensive in their scope. Comprehensive strategy is based on a risk-focused approach; it states that to prevent a problem from occurring, the factors contributing to the development of the problem must be identified, and then ways must be found to address and ameliorate these factors.

INTERVENTION STRATEGIES

This chapter identifies four critical avenues of intervention and some of the strategies used.

Family

The family is the most important influence in the lives of children and the first line of defense against delinquency. Programs that strengthen the family and foster healthy growth and development of children, from prenatal care through adolescence, should be widely available. These programs could encourage bonding between parent and child, and they should provide support for families in crisis. Black families should be provided with the following:

Child-Rearing Education. Seminars, conferences, and workshops on parenting techniques and skills for teenagers who may not be parents. The purpose of this is to provide them with the skills necessary to become good parents.

Parental Training. Educating black parents in child management skills. Such techniques include teaching parents positive reinforcement, problem-solving techniques, ways to reduce family conflict and improve communications skills, the importance of networking with other parents, and identification of early antisocial behavior. This training should be conducted by a therapist from the black community who can bring an Afrocentric approach to this training.

Teen-Parent Education. Special parenting education and services for pregnant teenagers, including counseling, child-rearing techniques, and birth control.

Family Volunteers. Recruits from the community to work with families and at risk males. This would include surrogate parents and Big Brothers. One of the problems of the black family is that there is often no father or father figure in the home.

The School

Outside the family, the school has the greatest impact on the lives of children. The school profoundly influences the hopes and dreams of black males. Many black males bring one or more risk factors to school with them, and these factors may hinder the development of their academic potential. School prevention strategies can assist the black family and the community by identifying at-risk youths, monitoring their progress, and intervening with effective programs at critical times during a youth's development. School should use the following:

Conflict Resolution. These techniques teach black males creative problem-solving strategies, ways to voice their opinions, and achievement of mutually acceptable solutions. These conflict resolution programs should be comprehensive and should include moral reasoning, anger control, social skills development, and collaborative problem-solving methods. To practice and understand the techniques, students should engage in role playing, design posters that highlight the skills, and perform appropriate activities.

Conflict resolution concepts should be infused in the curriculum so that teachers can teach these skills in the core curriculum areas.

School-Parent Intervention Team Approach. Parents and schools cooperate to form intervention teams. Teams would consist of administrators, teachers, and parents, organized to plan and implement school policies and programs. They would address a number of risk factors, such as academic failure, lack of commitment to school, and alienation in school.

This approach was originally implemented in two inner-city schools in New Haven, Connecticut, where 99% of students were African Americans and the majority came from single-parent families. Before this strategy was used, poor attendance, low achievement, discipline problems, and high teacher turnover were commonplace. In the year that parent involvement in the schools increased, students improved their grades and academic achievement test scores relative to students in a similar school without the program (Comer, 1988).

Service-Learning Approach. Typically, students combine their academic education with unpaid activities, such as working with the elderly or the homeless. This provides the opportunity for the student to combine practical experience with academic education. It also addresses risk factors, such as alienation and lack of commitment to school, and provides the opportunity to participate in positive activities. It can also increase the bonding with the school and the community.

Field Trips. Students get firsthand experiences of the human and tragic consequences of delinquency. These experiences sensitize youths to the horrors of violence, murder, drug use, and other forms of delinquency. Field trips should include visits to trauma centers, drug rehabilitation centers, morgues, and prisons. These trips should start at a young age before black males engage in delinquency.

The Peer Group

Peers are very influential in the lives of black males, especially as they become adolescents. Peers exert a tremendous amount of influence and control on youths to conform to group values and norms. Peer pressure can have positive or negative impact on young people. Research has shown that delinquency is often committed in small groups, a process called co-offending (Reiss, 1988). This is particularly true of black youth gangs. Because peers are important to black males, peers can be used to promote law-abiding behaviors among them. Schools and the community should provide the following:

Peer Counseling. Peers can assist troubled youths with their problems. Schools should train black students as peer counselors or facilitators to help other black youths cope with social, emotional, and practical problems.

These counselors should have skills in active and empathetic listening and feedback techniques.

Peer Leadership Groups. An effective means of encouraging leaders of delinquency-prone groups to establish friendships with more conventional peers. Crime prevention programs that educate youth on how to prevent juvenile violence and crime and provide opportunities for youth to actually work on solving specific community delinquency problems are another effective way of encouraging peer leadership.

Mentoring. Should be used for black males at risk for delinquency. These programs should involved volunteers, who are supportive and nonjudgmental and can act as role models. The mentoring should address risk factors such as alienation, academic failure, and association with other delinquents, as well as prosocial behavior. College students can be used as mentors. Mentoring should start very early—fifth and sixth grades, for example. Mentors should meet weekly with those they mentor and provide social support, encouragement, and motivation.

The Community

Children do not choose where they live. Children who live in fear of drug dealers, street violence, and gang shootings cannot enjoy childhood. They are dependent on parents, neighbors, and police to provide a safe and secure environment in which to play, go to school, and work. Black communities can benefit from a number of community-level intervention:

Neighborhood Resource Teams. Composed of community police officers, social workers, health care workers, housing experts, and school personnel. Teams can be established to ensure that a wide range of problems are attacked in a timely and coordinated manner. This can also serve as a referral service for black youths.

Workshops. The black community might conduct delinquency prevention festivals, symposiums, or conferences for black males, especially for those at risk. Workshops can use rap music, role playing, and talent competition to emphasize the importance of conformity.

Delinquency Prevention Awareness Week. This occasion can be marked every year by providing a series of activities such as lectures, rap sessions, films, and workshops. This can be extended to an awareness month with demonstrations against gangs, drugs, and crimes.

Information Dissemination. Black community groups should inform neighbors in simple language about the debilitating effects of drugs, gangs, and violence. They should also use the media, radio, television, magazines, and billboards as vehicles for delinquency prevention messages. Black male volunteers can be recruited to get involved with the media projects by making posters, presenting plays, and speaking on the radio and television.

Consciousness-Raising Strategies. Calling attention to the problems of crime and delinquency helps to encourage parents and members of the community to participate in their solution. The African American community should organized anticrime conferences, youth marches, and public meetings in communities to emphasize the black community's responsibility in fighting crime and delinquency. These activities should be held in places that are accessible to all members of the community, such as community centers, street corners, and public parks, rather than in expensive hotels.

Parent Advisory Committees. These can be created to lobby boards of education to include culturally specific delinquency prevention models in school curriculum. These committees should make contact with the superintendent or Parent Teachers Association and school curriculum committees to coordinate efforts of delinquency prevention programs.

Community Action Teams. Representatives from schools, businesses, parents, youth, and religious groups can develop long-term and comprehensive approaches to problems in the community. Such teams can be involved in job creation and training programs, youth recreation, block teams, neighborhood watch, citizen's awareness, and antidrug and antigang activities.

Community Planning Teams. Representatives from the criminal justice system, the juvenile justice system, mental health, child welfare, recreation, housing, religious institutions, parent groups, and education can be encouraged to form a partnership to develop a comprehensive approach to solving the problem of delinquency among black males. These teams can develop plans of action to implement and evaluate risk-reduction strategies for black males.

Joint Ventures With Businesses. Youth benefit from structured opportunities to develop skills and contribute to the community during nonschool hours. This is particularly important for at-risk youth, who have lower levels of personal and social support.

Youth Training and Employment. Such programs are intended to increase a youth's participation in the labor market. These programs should target at-risk African American males and should include job training skills, job readiness skills, life skills, career planning, and employment counseling. These programs should also help the youths to acquire jobs, especially summer jobs.

Afterschool Programs. The goal is to help prevent black males from associating with delinquent peers or gang members. These programs should be structured and operated by black community volunteers who can provide guidance, leadership, and mentoring. Programs include sports, music, crafts, clubs, and summer camps. The programs should maintain a high participation rate by aggressively recruiting black males in schools and gangs.

SUMMARY

Delinquency prevention programs need to start early in life to counteract the onset of delinquency. Programs starting in the elementary years will be most effective. Prevention programs should be designed to intercept or short-circuit youths on the path to delinquency. Tackling the complex problem of delinquency among African American males will not necessarily produce immediate results. Long-term results are usually built on short-term efforts and successes. The best delinquency prevention programs are comprehensive and focused on multiple risk factors. This means that to effectively reduce delinquency, programs must focus on all the institutions that affect a young person's life.

CHAPTER 20

Delivering Comprehensive Services to High-Risk African American Males

MARY NAKASHIAN
PAULA KLEINMAN

There is a crisis in the lives of many African American men. Too many of their lives are marked by unemployment, criminal activity, and substance abuse. On an average day in the United States in 1990, one in every four African American men age 20 to 29 was involved with the criminal justice system, that is, in prison, in jail, or on probation/parole (Mauer, 1990).

Because there is a close association between drug abuse and criminal justice involvement (Elliott, Huizinga, & Ageton, 1985; National Institute of Justice, 1995), it is not surprising to find high rates of drug dependence among the most vulnerable African American men.

During adolescence, the use of addictive substances rises sharply: About 25% of eighth graders say that they have drunk alcohol within the past month, 14% report having used an illicit drug or an inhalant within the past month (Johnston, O'Malley, & Bachman, 1995), and 43% say they have at least one friend with a serious drug problem (National Center on Addiction and Substance Abuse, 1996).

Early use of substances is strongly predictive of later substance abuse (National Center on Addiction and Substance Abuse, 1994; Robins & Przybeck, 1985), underscoring the critical importance of substance abuse prevention for children and adolescents, especially for African American boys. Apart from the positive reasons to pursue prevention, effective prevention strategies, especially for African American men, make sense because of the astronomical social and economic costs of substance abuse and addiction.

What follows are suggestions for developing and operating effective delinquency and drug prevention programs, based on the authors' experience in designing, implementing, and evaluating the national prevention program, Children at Risk (CAR), which was conceived and developed by the National Center on Addiction and Substance Abuse (CASA) at Columbia University,[1] and especially how the program was implemented in one city, Savannah, Georgia. The CAR program in Savannah was based on the Seven Principles of Nguzo Saba and was called *Uhuru,* a Kiswahili word for freedom.

THE CHILDREN AT RISK (CAR) PROGRAM MODEL

The CAR model was based on the integrated theoretical explanation of drug use and delinquency proposed by Elliott et al. (1985). This explanation integrates three theories: strain theory (Cloward & Ohlin, 1960; Merton, 1957), social control theory (Hirschi, 1969), and social learning theory (Akers, Krohn, Lanza-Kaduce, & Radosevich, 1979; Bandura, 1977). The integrated theory assumes that both conventional and deviant behaviors are socially learned and that the learning process is governed by exposure to social learning role models and experiences, and by the anticipated or real rewards and punishments of various behaviors (Elliott et al., 1985).

Through a coordinated and intensive program based on the integrated theory, the CAR model sought to reduce risk factors for delinquency and drug use by improving youths' attachment to prosocial individuals and institutions, reducing their bonds to deviant norms and groups, increasing their opportunities to achieve positive goals, and decreasing their opportunities for exposure to negative experiences.

CAR was a national research and demonstration program of CASA, supported by funds from several national foundations and the U.S. Department of Justice. The demonstration ran from 1992 to 1995, with sites in Austin, Texas; Bridgeport, Connecticut; Memphis, Tennessee; Newark, New Jersey; and Savannah, Georgia. The programs in Austin, Bridgeport, and Savannah continue to operate, using local funds.

SAVANNAH, GEORGIA

The city of Savannah is a study in contrasts. Since 1970, it has spent more than $270 million on capital improvement programs and has authorized millions of dollars in tax-free or low interest loans to large and small business. In recent years, Savannah has turned to its potential as a tourist attraction in order to bolster municipal income and increase its base of service-sector jobs. However, Savannah also has a more disturbing aspect. In 1991, the Savannah Police Department produced a study that linked the location of crimes committed in the city with the occurrence of other social ills. The study found that the 4-square-mile Area C, with 26,975 people or 19% of the city's population, accounted for 32% of its homicides, 41% of its robberies, 43% of its aggravated assaults, and 43% of its drug and sex offenses.

In 1990, there were 1,565 incidents involving juveniles in Savannah. Of all 1991 juvenile filings, 81% of the individuals charged were black males. Moreover, 75% of theft, 84% of stolen property, 78% of battery, and 90% of assault case filings in juvenile court involved perpetrators between age 13 and 16.

When CASA approached officials in Savannah in 1991 about participating in the CAR program, local leaders saw CAR as an opportunity to improve these dire statistics.

A FRAMEWORK FOR SERVING AFRICAN AMERICAN BOYS

Programs serving African American males should operate within a framework that includes four characteristics: They should be targeted, comprehensive, coordinated, and integrated; they should also be locally planned and directed. Each of these characteristics is summarized here. In the next sections, observations are made regarding their application within an African American context.

First, several types of targeting are important. Programs should focus on a particular, well-defined neighborhood. In addition, we found it helpful for programs serving elementary and middle school students in particular to select a target school within the neighborhood. Finally, it is especially important for programs to target which children and families it will serve.

Second, early in planning, community organizations, residents, and public agencies should specify what they mean by comprehensive and list those services that will be available to all participants. CASA decided on the following components: case management, education services, afterschool and summer activities, mentoring, incentives, family services, community policing, and juvenile justice intervention.

Third, it is important that programs be organized in a way that makes sense to children, parents, and service providers. In too many American communities, families are left to negotiate a myriad of services and agencies so that services, although available, operate either in isolation or at cross-purposes to each other.

Fourth, special attention should be paid to assure that the programs support the values and cultural backgrounds of the neighborhoods they serve. For programs to be locally driven, they have to focus on a neighborhood that falls within the natural boundaries of a community.

Programs Should Be Targeted

The Neighborhood

Building on the traditional African value that the community is a family, programs seeking to improve the lives of children and their families should focus on a particular neighborhood. Sometimes, the neighborhood coincides with a school district, a community board, or a police precinct, and sometimes it will need to be created for the purposes of this program. In either case, there should be consensus among neighborhood residents, service-providing agencies, and public officials as to the boundaries for a program. In Savannah, for example, Area C emerged as a priority both for public officials concerned about crime and for social service agencies and residents concerned about poverty, poor health, and crime. In many cities, there are neighborhoods that have a particular identifying characteristic that marks them as a community. Frequently, that characteristic has to do with race or ethnicity, but it is possible for neighborhoods to be known for other characteristics.

The School

For programs serving African American boys, we found it helpful to select a target school within the neighborhood. Particularly with younger children, their schools are located in their community. Children attend school with their siblings and their friends. Children and their parents can walk to school for meetings or activities. Increasingly, schools are a center for services such as health clinics or adult education programs, and they serve as the base for supplemental academic and recreational activities for children.

Schools, along with the lead agency and the police, became the major collaborative partners in operating their CAR programs. One critical role for the school was to identify children as potential participants in the program. Using information supplied by counselors or administrators, case managers employed by the lead agency made home visits to the child and parent for purposes of recruitment. In CAR, this strategy ensured that school staff became involved with the program in a meaningful way from the start. Once children were recruited into the program, school staff and case managers were well-positioned to collaborate on behalf of children. Case managers, responding to concerns expressed by school staff, were able to meet with a family at home on a weekend or during the evening. In this way, school staff came to view the program as helping them with students rather than as one of several "outside" programs sitting in their schools.

If a program serving African American boys focuses its attention on one neighborhood school, it is possible for that school to become a hub of community activity and an extended family to community residents. In Savannah, the Uhuru program provided a comprehensive way for the school to reach its high-risk students. The school made space available for weekly case conferencing meetings among the Uhuru Family Advocates (called case managers or family mentors in other locations), the mental health therapist, the Uhuru police officers, and school staff to discuss service strategies for particular youth and their families.

The Children and Their Families

It is important for programs to decide which children and families it will serve. Frequently, comprehensive community-based interventions operate on the assumption that all residents of the community should have access to the same broad array of services. This approach leads to two kinds of problems: Either the program becomes "watered down" in an attempt to give something to everyone, or the program enrolls everyone until it runs out of room, after which no one else is allowed in. We recommend that organizations and individuals set standards for who their participants should be—should they be the most vulnerable children and families, who need very intensive services, or should they be families who need only a modest amount of support to get back on their feet?

Although these decisions are very difficult and frequently cause tension among direct service staff, they have been extremely helpful in matching resources to needs. By improving the capacity to match programs with people, it is possible to serve both those who need help the most and those who need it to a lesser degree.

There are some techniques we have found helpful in resolving the problem of standards. For example, once a particular youth is recruited into the program, it is important that his or her family be considered as participating as well. This approach builds on the natural relationship of child to family and does not isolate one family member from the others. It also sets the stage for building on family strengths and developing the family's capacity to resolve its problems. However, this strategy has important implications for staffing and management decisions. Staff-to-participant ratios should be built on the assumption that a case involves more than one individual and spans more than one generation. Staff qualifications, supervision, and training should reflect the family-focused nature of the work.

Another way to address the problem of eligibility guidelines is to be sure they are appropriate to program participants. If a program has decided to serve the "most at risk" young African American males, the standards should make sense for that population. Although criteria will vary across programs and communities, we recommend some broad principles for use in identifying participants. First, for young boys in particular, the program should span a narrow age range and school grade level. The CAR program, for example, selected children age 11 to 13 who were in sixth or seventh grade. Children had to meet both age and grade standards. Second, the criteria should draw from studies and research that offer guidance. We drew on a body of research that led us to select three categories of risk indicators: school risk, personal risk, and family risk. Each category included several specific behaviors, and children were eligible if they had exhibited those behaviors.

Programs Should Be Comprehensive

General Considerations

The concept of comprehensive services is overused in rhetoric and under-applied in action. In some ways, defining services fulfills the same function as targeting the program. It forces people to make systematic decisions that have implications for who receives services, who provides services, who influences policy decisions, and who gets resources.

Too often, programs are shaped based on the requirements of funding sources or the expertise of the service provider. Although program elements are frequently dictated by outside sources such as funding streams, a local agency can bring together a range of people to develop shared goals, expectations, and strategies. Even within program limitations, people can be given more control over services offered to their community. This process can also help identify people or agencies who have been omitted and reach out to them early in the process of program design. In Austin, for example, CAR staff from police, school, and social agencies participated in a weekend retreat to discuss their goals and expectations for children and families. During this weekend, they did not talk about the CAR program itself; rather, they used the time to help everyone return home willing to work with each other in a new way.

At the national level, CASA designed the CAR program to include case management, education services, afterschool and summer activities, mentoring, incentives, family services, community policing, and juvenile justice intervention. In each CAR community, local agencies decided how these components would be delivered.

Criminal Justice Participation

The role of criminal and juvenile justice agencies in programs serving African American males is important to note. In our experience, although police involvement has been a striking feature of the strongest CAR programs, we also learned that such involvement is not possible unless the police department is otherwise committed to community-oriented policing. Bringing police into program planning, design, and management provides a forum for them to meet with community residents in a new way. Police can be effective in helping social service programs broaden their potential for success by adding an important community wide dimension. While case managers and service providers work with individual families, police work with residents to identify and resolve larger safety problems in the neighborhood. Thus, the service intervention occurs within the context of a community-wide social service and public safety initiative.

Police involvement in programs serving young African American males is particularly important and delicate. The police have the potential to create a sense of community security, safety, and protection that is important for boys and young men—and essential for communities—to thrive. However, relationships between police and African American boys have traditionally been tense and hostile. Many police officers in urban areas do not live in the community where they work, and they frequently do not represent the racial, religious, or ethnic character of the areas they patrol. Residents of African American communities often feel police view everyone in their neighborhood with suspicion, make little attempt to arrive at a solution other than arrest, and are not effective in solving the problems residents feel are the most pressing.

Innovative Strategies for Improving Criminal Justice/Community Relationships

One of the challenges, and opportunities, in operating a program aimed at African American males is finding ways to change these relationships. There are strategies that seem to have shown some success. First, police can be involved at the early stages of program design. For example, the police often have arrest and crime data that will help residents and social service agencies determine the boundaries of the target neighborhood. They also have important information about the most troublesome criminals in the area as well as the most difficult "sore spots" of the neighborhood.

Second, police can organize their patrol routes and schedules around certain program activities. Third, police can participate in program activities with individual children and families. In Savannah, police served as mentors for some Uhuru children and as role models for all of them. There were two Uhuru officers stationed at the target school. Both were African American, and they drew from their own life experiences in teaching lessons about anger management and self-esteem. Fourth, police can pair with program staff in solving particular family problems. If the program can generate trust between the community-based program staff and the police, they can make joint home visits to families, and working in the home with the family, peacefully resolve a family crisis that would otherwise explode into a criminal justice case.

Police, community residents, and local businesses do agree on specific neighborhood problems. There may be an abandoned building where drug dealing takes place, a street known for dangerous speeding, or a liquor store known as a place where adults hang out, drink, and intimidate residents. As part of a community-based program aimed at preventing substance abuse among children, the residents, businesses, social agencies, and police can work together to identify and prioritize neighborhood problems and plan ways to address them.

As noted earlier, for police involvement to be effective, it is important that the police department be interested in community policing, or problem-oriented policing. If this is the case, it is equally important that the program involve the police in multiple ways and not limit their involvement to settling disputes. For example, police should attend regular case conference meetings (these are meetings of all agencies involved with families in the program, during which each child and family is reviewed and actions determined).

Programs Should Be Coordinated

Programs have to be organized in a way that makes sense to children, parents, and service providers. One way to coordinate diverse program activities is through the use of a theme. In Savannah, the Afrocentric theme was a powerful tool in making the program logical not only to those it served but also to the larger community. The use of a theme, and the word Uhuru itself, provided a coherence across the components of the program, unified diverse staff responsibilities, and framed the program and its services for participants.

Although use of a theme sets the stage for improved program coordination, coordination requires other activities as well. One way to enhance service coordination is to co-locate services. Co-location has been used in the social service field to refer to the delivery of multiple services at one location. Co-location does not automatically lead to sharing, but it can help. A common location can supply a continuity to program activities as well as serving as a social setting. If the program has been carefully targeted, either a neighborhood center or a school will host activities. In particular, if a school is involved with the program, it can provide an excellent setting for activities. For example, the police department in Savannah stationed two Uhuru officers at Hubert Middle School, where they also taught several classes each day. At the school, the officers learned about Uhuru children informally from teachers, social work staff, or case managers. They also had a better understanding of children and families to share with the colleagues responsible for patrolling the neighborhood.

Effective coordination requires that staff serving African American boys coordinate an array of community resources—social agencies, schools, law enforcement, families, businesses, and churches. Bringing these diverse systems together can be trying and frustrating. When developing new programs, it is useful to identify existing coordinating bodies and try to build on them wherever possible. If these bodies have endured for some time, the chances are good that they have developed effective working relationships and resolved the legal and philosophical differences that lead to the downfall of so many collaborative initiatives.

In Savannah, coordination was enhanced by the particular role of the Youth Futures Authority, a public corporation representing many city agencies and endowed with legal authority and certain administrative powers. The authority provided a collaborative structure for CASA and staff in Savannah to use in designing and managing Uhuru. For example, Uhuru staff were experiencing problems securing immunization records for children so that they could attend summer camp. Attempts to solve the problem child by child were time consuming and only minimally successful. When staff raised this concern with the authority, policymakers from the relevant agencies quickly agreed on a procedure that expedited the release of these records so that children could attend camp.

Programs Should Be Locally Planned and Delivered

A Shared Vision

In planning for the Uhuru program, the Youth Futures Authority and an interagency task force developed a vision statement that guided its work: "Our vision is a city in which all neighborhoods are free of drug trafficking, crime, alcohol, and other drug abuse and addiction, and drug- and alcohol-caused health problems." In developing this vision, the leaders in Savannah, drawing on the Nguzo Saba principles of *nia* (purpose), *ujima* (collective work and responsibility), and *kujichagulia* (self-determination), felt strongly that the long-term well-being of the community required a system by which the African American community could both govern its behavior and assess its growth and development. Indeed, they contended that it is the absence of this commonly held value system that contributes to the community chaos, family dysfunction, and underachievement that exists in Area C.

The vision statement offered a framework within which agencies and individuals could consider their roles in Uhuru. A more subtle effect of the vision statement was to serve sometimes as the only issue on which everyone could agree. By providing one area of common understanding, the vision prevented people from concluding that differences among themselves could never be resolved.

Specific Programs and Activities

Once a community has established a vision for its members, programs and activities can be designed that both validate children's African heritage and at the same time offer ways to integrate it with contemporary American urban life. In Savannah, both the Youth Futures Authority executive director and the Uhuru project coordinator emphasized that the values and goals of the Uhuru project coincided with middle-America values. The Afrocentric concepts underlying Uhuru were incorporated into the *kuumba* (creativity) program offered after school and on weekends. The goal of the kuumba program was to provide a special activity in a contemplative and supportive atmosphere where Uhuru participants could release stress and share insights about who they were and what they had accomplished. It is important that these and other program activities use Afrocentric themes to improve academic performance at the same time as they enhance children's social and emotional development.

Because so many African American youth have been labeled "at risk," the Rites of Passage Enrichment (ROPE) program in Savannah was developed as an activity that combined an African-centered curriculum with appropriate youth-oriented development activities. Working in groups with an Uhuru family advocate, each participant was expected to complete oral and written assignments; participate in physical, intellectual, social, and spiritual developmental activities; and take part in a transformation ceremony on completion of the rites program. The program provided youth with a $10 incentive for each week of perfect attendance at afterschool activities.

In Savannah, one Uhuru family advocate was interested in photography. Using the Nguzo Saba principle of *kujichagulia* (self-determination), he engaged several Uhuru youth, mostly young boys, into a group called the Kujichagulia Shutter Bugs. The boys learned the art of photography and used this skill to record their own experiences and the experiences of their friends. The Shutter Bugs started by creating video and photo journals for Youth Futures Authority projects. Then, they received a grant from a community organization to videotape projects of other agencies as well. More recently, they have contracted with civic groups to photograph and videotape other meetings and events. The experience of the Shutter Bugs has taught young African American males an important and valued skill, enabled them to record and memorialize positive events in their community, and provided them with entrepreneurial and business skills.

Drawing from the Nguzo Saba principles of *ujima* (collective work responsibility) and *ujamma* (cooperative economics), and with support from family advocates, several youth started two entrepreneurial businesses to earn money and serve the community. The girls crafted barrettes and hair bows for sale to residents. The boys began a lawn and landscaping business, selling their services to local corporations and city agencies. The lawn and landscaping business was a particular success, providing a needed service to companies in the neighborhood and a source of earned income for the children. Moreover, it served to improve the community environment, as property was well groomed and maintained.

LESSONS AND CHALLENGES

The CAR program stressed involvement by citizens and community connections by service providers. Savannah was able to use the African theme of community responsibility for its citizens, especially its children, as the keystone on which all individual program activities were built. The Savannah program also illustrated the power of a clear, shared vision statement to inform daily operations. Whereas all CAR sites included afterschool programs, recreational activities, and community-oriented policing, the nature of Savannah's programs in each of these areas was unique. All Uhuru partners, from frontline service staff and police officers to agency heads, were able to explain the Uhuru approach, relate it to the vision statement, and translate it into interactions with children. In doing so, these African American adults became role models for the young African American boys in their communities.

The Savannah experience also demonstrated that an Afrocentric approach can work in modern American society. At the beginning of program planning, staff in Savannah had to convince Uhuru's national funders that their approach was consistent with both the CAR model and with important values shared by all Americans. After several meetings, visits, and telephone conversations, that agreement was reached and the program was funded. Once that agreement was reached, the program itself went through start-up and ongoing operations especially smoothly.

Another important lesson from the Savannah approach is that it is possible to define African American communities in terms of their resources, their strengths, and their potential. One common mistake is to assume that poor communities are packages of negatives without internal resources, strengths, or order. Uhuru's vision of larger community connections, community order, and community cohesiveness was a notable element of the program.

Community-based strategies aimed at African American youth are not easy to operate. In particular, approaches that try to integrate the social services and criminal justice systems pose enormous challenges. Program organizers must mobilize their neighborhoods to convince residents that they have some control over their lives, that they can improve their neighborhoods, and that they can keep children away from drugs and crime. They also have to use community vision to leverage financial support and/or in-kind services from local foundations, government agencies, businesses, and service providers.

There are several questions concerning the future of programs like Uhuru. First, Savannah was fortunate to build on a preexisting citywide collaborative agency that had been established to improve outcomes for children. Savannah was further enriched by the presence of a strong, charismatic African American leader who was widely respected among community residents, officials, and researchers. He not only set and communicated the vision for the Uhuru program, he also served as a role model for individual African American boys. Community-based programs always struggle with how to carry on after the departure of a strong and influential leader. Savannah has not yet had to face that challenge.

Second, the Afrocentric approach is powerful because it touches a common tradition among a group of people. If the Uhuru experience is to be applied in neighborhoods that are composed of different ethnic groups, unifying visions and common traditions must be found that reflect the experiences of those groups. Although the concept of shared vision and building on common tradition might be exportable, in many cases the vision itself and the programs that grow out of it will be different from Uhuru.

Third, as with any complex social service intervention, we know that the final results will be mixed. The outcome findings for CAR show reduced drug use among CAR participants 1 year after completion of the program. These findings apply to use of gateway drugs, use of stronger drugs, and drug sales (Harrell, personal communication, June 1997). However, turning the tide for high-risk boys living in troubled families in crime-ridden neighborhoods is an enormous struggle.

Fourth, programs aimed at young African American males cannot be undertaken in isolation. African American communities that are successful in running programs like Uhuru must also tackle broader concerns such as lack of jobs, inadequate transportation, and economic development. Therefore, attention must be paid to the larger environment within which an individual program operates.

Fifth, one of the most challenging elements of community-based strategies aimed at high-risk youth—and one of the most important in a program aimed at African American boys—is how to work effectively with the child's family. Even within a program employing Afrocentric principles that place high value on the importance of family, it is easy to "fall back" into focusing exclusively on the child or children. In many ways, the harder but more fundamental challenge is how to work effectively with parents or other family members to support them in raising young boys to become healthy men.

Although these suggestions will not suffice to transform the many negative circumstances facing young African American males in the United States, they do provide guidance to organizations that seek to assist them.

NOTE

1. The National Center on Addiction and Substance Abuse (CASA) at Columbia University is a think/action tank that brings together all the professional disciplines needed to study and combat all forms of substance abuse as they affect all aspects of society. Among the strategies used by CASA to fulfill its mission are to assess what works in prevention and treatment in clinical settings and in communities and to provide those on the front lines with the tools they need to succeed. CASA's division of Program Demonstration designs, oversees, and evaluates community-based interventions aimed at preventing or reducing substance abuse. CASA's first demonstration program was Children at Risk (CAR).

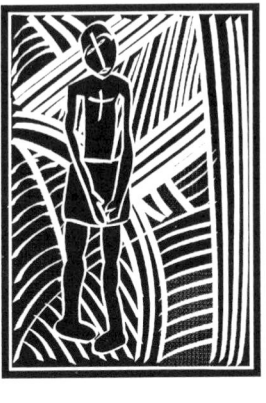

PART VI

Employment and Economic Security

The majority of problems confronting black America can be traced to the economic difficulties of African American males (Bowman, 1993; Sherraden, 1991; Wilson, 1987). As a group, they earn approximately 60% of the income of white males (U.S. Bureau of the Census, 1997), their families possess only one tenth the net worth of white families (U.S. Bureau of the Census, 1995a), and half of all their children are poor as compared to about 16% of white children (U.S. Bureau of the Census, 1991b). Such discrepancies in incomes and assets of whites and blacks should come as no surprise: African American males have experienced a very different employment history than white males. Their long history of slavery, during which they were neither paid nor allowed to create assets, was followed by periods of unemployment and/or underemployment.

But didn't things get better? Although the economic fortunes of African American males did improve in the 1960s and 1970s, they have worsened since the 1980s (Bound & Freeman, 1992; Gittleman & Howell, 1995). For example, in 1970, the unemployment rate for African American males was one and a half times that of whites; by 1990, it was over two times higher (Walker, Spohn, & Delone, 1996). And even such unpleasant statistics as these do not tell us the whole story. First, unemployment figures do not include discouraged workers who have given up and are not looking for work, and second, they fail to include part-time employees who want full-time jobs but cannot find them (Walker et al., 1996). Hence the situation is even worse than most demographics would have us believe, lending credence to the assertion that a greater proportion of African American males may currently lack regular employment than at any time since the Great Depression of the 1930s (Hacker, 1992).

Despite an array of diverse social programs to improve the economic status of black America, unemployment and poverty have doggedly pursued African American males. A plethora of unflattering arguments have been put forth to explain the persistence of their fiscal difficulties: the possession of a problematic culture (Liebow, 1967), inherent low IQs, (Herrnstein & Murray, 1994), and welfare policies that promote immorality and laziness (Murray, 1984). Too many Americans, unfortunately, adhere to such insidious explanations of African American male poverty and unemployment. This reality coupled with the mean-spirited political climate of the 1980s, has resulted in significant numbers of African American men being left out of America's economic picture, and a concomitant growth in those succumbing to economic despair.

More enlightened and less mean-spirited explanations for the financial instability of African American men suggest that two major events have taken place. Both suggest that the problem of African American male unemployment, albeit difficult, is not insurmountable. First, the industrial sector of our economy has experienced substantial losses in the numbers of men it can now support (Wilson, 1987). And second, given the erosion of the industrial sector, many entry-level jobs that were historically available to the semi-skilled and the poor have been eliminated (Gittleman & Howell, 1995; Wilson, 1987). This second observation is perhaps more easily addressed by the readers of this text than is the first. That is, the creation of jobs is sometimes beyond the scope of many of us, whereas preparing African American males for those jobs that do exist is often within our realm of influence.

It is the goal of this section to assist African American males with employment and career opportunities, as well as with creation of assets. Undoubtedly, there is much validity to the argument that micro interventive efforts often fail to deal directly with the large sociopolitical and economic variables that are the root cause to most of the problems experienced by African American males (Wilson, 1990). Still, as was noted in the introduction to this text, "we must do what we can," and there is much that can be done. We must intervene with African American males on all levels to improve their economic realities and those of their families. The three chapters included in this section enhance significantly our understanding of possible steps that might be taken and thereby serve to guide our actions in this most important effort.

CHAPTER 21

Career Counseling With African American Male College Students

FREDERICKA HENDRICKS

R apidly changing demographics and increasing technological advances in society dictate that college graduates be prepared to meet the demands of the 21st-century workplace. Data from the 1990 census indicate that people of color are clustered in occupational industries that are declining, such as manufacturing, production, and agriculture (Okocha, 1994). This is of particular concern because African American males are among the most underemployed and unemployed groups in the nation (Leonard, 1985). In addition, the U.S. Department of Labor (1997) reports that the majority of African American men were employed as correctional officers, security guards, cooks, motor vehicle operators (bus drivers, truck drivers, etc.), janitors, laborers, groundskeepers, and mechanics. Many of these occupations offer low pay, require little training or skills, and offer little chance for advancement (Hargrow & Hendricks, in press). Washington and Newman (1991) found that African American males "sustained greater losses in higher education participation rates than any other racial or gender group" (p. 19). Therefore, it becomes critical that we maximize the potential and assist those African American males who are enrolled in our colleges and universities.

How can we better prepare African American males for economic security and stability in employment? We can begin to counsel them about the world of work early in their college career. In a study of attitudes, skills, and behaviors of black university students, Noldon and Sedlacek (1995) found that black freshmen entering the university reported a need for career guidance and career skills. In a related study, Hargrove and Sedlacek (1995) compared the initial counseling interests of black freshmen in 1984 and 1994. They found that regardless of the year the students entered, students were more interested in seeking counseling for educational/career concerns than emotional/social concerns. There were countless times while working in a university career center that I heard "I wish I had come over here sooner" or "I didn't know you had all this stuff (meaning information) over here." Many students do not take advantage of career services until the end of their college career, when they need help writing a resume or need to research a potential employer. Overlooked and underused, any type of service that has the word *counseling* in it sometimes causes students to stay away.

What is career counseling, and how can it help African American male college students? Career counseling is a service that most colleges and universities provide at no additional or minimal cost to the student. Career counseling is about preparation; it is about self-knowledge and knowledge of the world of work. Jobs that offer economic security are available to those who are prepared. Career counseling can help any student, but it can be especially empowering to African American males because it will provide them with transferable life skills. African American males in particular can be proactive when planning for their occupational futures. Perry and Locke (1985), in their discussion of the career development of black men, stated,

> Both career exploration and career planning by black men occur in the context of a limited opportunity structure. . . . Programs planned to address effectively the career development needs of black males will inevitably be characterized by advocacy, proactive services, and outreach. (pp. 108-109)

It is important to define how I am conceptualizing career development. Career development is a lifelong process, it encompasses much more than an individual's career. Career development is a term that consists of much more than developing skills for an ideal occupation. Career development is proactive, dynamic, contextual, interactive, and lifelong. Once conceptualized in this way, it is easier to discuss how the career counseling process is a part of the college student's development. It also becomes easier to examine strategies and interventions to guide and enhance the student's occupational development. Wolfe and Kolb (1980) have illustratively described career development in the following manner:

Career development involves one's whole life, not just an occupation. As such, it concerns the whole person, needs, and wants, capacities and potentials, excitements and anxieties, insights and blind spots, warts and all. More than that, it concerns him/her in the ever-changing contexts of his/her life. The environmental pressures and constraints, the bonds that tie him/her to significant others, responsibilities to children and aging parents, the total structure of one's circumstances are also factors that must be understood and reckoned with. In these terms, career development and personal development converge. Self and circumstances, evolving, changing, unfolding in mutual interaction—constitute the focus and the drama of career development. (pp. 1-2)

This chapter is designed to provide the reader with ways to effectively counsel African American male college students for life career development and demonstrate how career options and opportunities can be explored. Strategies for enhancing the career development and success of African American males are discussed. A case example is also presented to help the reader conceptualize how various strategies can be used.

CAREER DEVELOPMENT AND THE AFRICAN AMERICAN MALE COLLEGE STUDENT

Traditional models of career development have been strongly influenced by white middle-class American culture. The primary characteristics of this culture emphasize rugged individualism, verbal communication, a linear approach to problem solving, a nondirective approach to counseling, a preoccupation with long-term goals, and an adherence to time schedules (Sue & Sue, 1990). This is reflected in the way many counselors do career counseling. Boykin (1983) outlined distinct cultural characteristics of African Americans, which include (a) a person-to-person focus, (b) preference for oral and auditory modes of communication, (c) interdependence and communalism, (d) a response to whole or gestalts, (e) a flexible time perspective, (f) heightened awareness of nonverbal communication, and (g) a valuing of personal distinctiveness. Many of these African American cultural characteristics are in direct contrast to the characteristics associated with middle-class white America. Therefore, it becomes plausible to maintain that conventional career counseling frameworks that have worked for white college students may not be suited to the experiences of African American college students, males in particular. Researchers (Cheatham, 1990a; Dillard,

1980; Leonard, 1985; Miller, 1974; Warnath, 1975) of vocational theories have found that many of the traditional career theories may be limited in their applicability for the African American male because:

1. Many of these theories rest on the assumption that an occupation provides the individual with an opportunity for self-expression and intrinsic contentment (Warnath, 1975).

2. Career theories and models generalize concepts and constructs based on white male behavior to ethnic and economic subgroups (Miller, 1974).

3. Most theories and models assume that equal opportunities exist for individuals to attain their career goals (Williams, 1972).

The problem with many of the traditional models and theories of career development is that they ignore situational variables that may decrease aspirations or limit an individual's opportunities for career mobility. It is important that counselors and students are aware of the existence of internal corporate structures that may impede career mobility (as evidenced by the infamous Texaco case). Ideally, theoretical models of career development should integrate cultural perspectives into their frameworks. Cheatham (1990a) has proposed a heuristic model of African American students' career development, which accounts for unique cultural characteristics, such as those discussed by Boykin (1983), and acknowledges the impact of white Eurocentric factors on the career development process of African American students. He contends that the "reciprocity between Afrocentric and Eurocentric experiences is a critical determinant in the career development of African American students" (p. 342). The acknowledgment of both Afrocentric and Eurocentric perspectives allows the counselor to view the student contextually and plan interventions that are most appropriate for that individual. Career counselors working with African American male college students may use a combination of traditional interventions, such as the *Self-Directed Search* (Holland, 1970) or the *Strong Interest Inventory* (Strong, Hansen, & Campbell, 1994), and nontraditional interventions, such as an African American career panel. The important factor to consider in counseling African American male students is how race, socioeconomic background, institutional barriers, current environment, and gender have affected their career aspirations and development.

Life-career development (see McDaniels & Gysbers, 1992) is a concept that attempts "to extend career development from the traditional occupational perspective to a life perspective in which occupation (and work) has meaning" (p. 9). McDaniels and Gysbers (1992) define life-career development as "self-development over the life span through the interaction and integration of the roles, settings, and events of a person's life" (p. 10). Specifically, consideration is given to the individual's (a) *life roles* (learner, brother, son, spouse, and so on), (b) *life settings* (school, home, church, community, workplace), and (c) *life events* (graduation, job entry, marriage, retirement). Furthermore, the authors recognize that race, gender, religion, and ethnic orgin have a profound effect on the career development of clients. They encourage counselors not to ignore these variables but to use them in the counseling process to gain a better understanding of the individual.

STRATEGIES FOR CAREER COUNSELING AFRICAN AMERICAN MALE COLLEGE STUDENTS

For effective career counseling to occur, the basic components of career planning must be employed during various phases of the counseling process. The career exploration and planning process has three interconnecting components: self-knowledge, knowledge of the world of work, and knowledge of career skills/actions. This process is depicted in Figure 21.1.

A Career Counseling Framework

During the initial and/or subsequent sessions, the developmental counseling framework posited by McDaniels and Gysbers (1992) is recommended. The counselor can tailor the basic framework to work with the university population. First, the counselor attempts to identify, clarify, and specify client goal(s) or problem(s). During this phase, the counselor describes the counseling process and the responsibilities of the client. Client information is also gathered during this initial phase. Questions that counselors need to ask are these:

1. What is the student's motivation for seeking career help? Did he seek career counseling on his own, or was he referred?

2. Why did he choose to come to college?

3. How does the client view himself, others, and his environment?

Knowledge About the World of Work	Self-Knowledge	Career Skills and Action Steps
Occupational information from others or written resources	Family occupational history and influence	Goal setting
	Interests	Information gathering
	Abilities	Problem solving
Computer-generated information	Skills	Decision making
	Values	Resume writing
	Personal barriers	Interviewing skills
Experiential learning	Situational barriers	Networking
	Decision-making style	
	Personal style	

Figure 21.1. The Career Exploration and Planning Process Components

4. What is his worldview? How does he view his life roles, settings, and events in three time perspectives (past, future, and present)? What words, phrases, or language does he use to represent his views?

5. Are there any identifiable or underlying themes the client uses to dictate or orient his behavior?

6. What is the client's current environment like? What is his current academic status and standing?
   - major
   - year in school
   - grade point average
   - honors courses taken or currently enrolled in
   - living arrangements
   - part-time or full-time status
   - married or single
   - siblings on campus

7. Are there barriers (either personal or situational) currently operating in his life?

8. What decision-making style(s) does the client use?

9. What extracurricular activities does the client engage in?

The counselor may also consider using some assessment/testing for exploration to help conceptualize client behavior and personality style (while always interpreting results with cultural caution). The counselor will then be able to draw conclusions about the situation and move into the next phase of the counseling process, which consists of problem resolution and meeting client goals. To accomplish this, both the client and counselor must be active in the counseling process. McDaniels and Gysbers (1992) also suggest the use of the Life Career Assessment (see Gysbers & Moore, 1987) as a strategy for gathering pertinent client information in a structured, cohesive manner. Once relevant client information has been gathered, the counselor provides relevant occupational or academic information. The client, with the counselor's help, explores his interests, values, and skills. The counselor develops an individualized career plan and constantly evaluates the client's progress. If the problem is solved or the goals of the client have been met, the counseling relationship is ended. If the problem still exists or goals have not been met, the counselor needs to recycle through the phases he or she believes will be most beneficial to the student.

CAREER INTERVENTIONS

As mentioned earlier in the chapter, a combination of traditional interventions and nontraditional interventions, which recognize the uniqueness of the African American client, will be most effective and beneficial. In addition, following Leonard's (1985) suggestions, it is recommended that counselors working with African American males should specifically engage in the following:

1. Guide the young men through stages of systematic career exploration and choice.

One way this step could be accomplished is through a computerized career exploration program, such as the *System of Interactive Guidance and Information.*

2. Expose them early to a variety of careers and heighten their awareness about the world of work.

This can be done in a variety of ways: a career explorations class, an interest inventory, an occupational card sort, exposure to African American males in various professional occupations, or attendance at a career fair on campus, even when they are not actively job hunting.

3. Help them develop vocational sophistication and coping skills.

This can be achieved by discussing foreseeable barriers, the reality of racism in the workplace, and the importance of transferable and leadership skills in the workplace. Another concrete way vocational sophistication can be heightened is by preparing students for an interview by conducting a videotaped mock interview.

4. Foster the growth of a positive self-concept.

This can be accomplished by creating a nonthreatening, open environment in which the student is able to realistically evaluate his interests, abilities, and goals.

5. Clarify work-related goals, values, and options.

It is important that a student has a sense of what he wants from a career. Therefore, work-related values need to be explored. For example, does he want autonomy or interdependence? Prestige or power? Flexible work hours or set times? Does he want a career that is socially conscious or morally fulfilling?

6. Teach decision-making and problem-solving skills.

The process of clarifying (No. 5) his values and goals will help him with his decision-making and problem-solving skills.

7. Encourage and support positive attitudes about work and career opportunities.

This may require that the student engage in paid or volunteer work experiences during the school term or internships during the summer months.

Because my definition of career development requires proactivity, interventions that empower and reach students before there is a crisis or problem are important. For instance, an example of a proactive intervention is the following: A student enrolled in a career explorations class or working individually with a counselor is required to develop his resume even though he has no use for it at the present time. The act of having him write out and prepare his resume before he needs it is a proactive intervention. Thus, when the time arises for a job or summer internship interview, the student will have already developed his resume, and it will need only minor modifications.

Outreach services are wonderful ways to expose students to the ideas of career development and planning. Some outreach activities require counselors to leave their offices and become visible on campus. The office responsible for career services on campus can sponsor special programs tailored for African American males. Below are example programs that can be implemented.

■ *African American Male Career Forum*

African American males from the campus and neighboring community are invited to speak on a variety of careers. This forum can also be occupation specific: for example, the speakers are all lawyers, but each represents a different field (i.e., corporate, entertainment, tax, real estate, district attorney, criminal defense).

■ *Brother-to-Brother*

Mentoring programs in which incoming African American male freshmen are paired with African American male juniors/seniors. The mentor would be a member of the freshman's prospective academic department.

■ *Fraternity Night*

Invite members of black fraternities to come over and explore the career center. Have counselors or paraprofessionals available to look at resumes, give practice interviews, or answer general questions. Relatedly, ask to come to one of their meetings to discuss the career services and opportunities available to them.

■ *Black History Career Month*

During February, highlight African Americans, and in particular males, in nontraditional or unusual career fields. Use the rich history of the African American community as examples—Eldrick "Tiger" Woods, professional golf player; Thurgood Marshall, Supreme Court justice; Langston Hughes, poet; George Washington Carver, inventor.

In addition to the aforementioned special programs, regular avenues should not be overlooked.

■ *Joint Programming/Planning*

Cosponsor programs with other offices, departments, or groups on campus (i.e., Office of Multicultural Affairs, Black Studies Department, Society of Black Engineers, etc.).

■ *Residence Life*

Contact African American residential life assistants and let them know you (or someone on your staff) are available to discuss career planning/skills with their residents.

■ *Advertise*

Career services should be advertised in places that members of the African American campus community frequent, such as the multicultural center or the African American campus newspaper or newsletter.

■ *Internet*

Help students explore job opportunities using the computer. There are also special-interest websites geared toward African Americans.

■ *On-Campus Recruitment Days*

Ensure that African American males go to interviews with companies that recruit on campus.

■ *Resources*

Career information should come from both people and written sources. Counselors should have names of African Americans (alumni, community members, on-campus contacts) who are willing to help students explore career options. Written resources should include positive pictures of and data about people of color.

■ *Career Workshops*

The offering of periodic career workshops allows students to choose a convenient time to learn about career planning. It may also appear less threatening than coming in for career counseling.

■ *Summer Orientation/Parent's Day*

Make sure that career information is available during these times. Allow students and their families to visit and take a tour of the career center.

■ *Career Exploration Course*

A career course early in the student's college career can help the individual maximize his career potential. Counselors can work with advisers to ensure that African American males register for the course.

Interventions that incorporate these strategies and integrate the concepts of life-career development, the counseling process framework, and characteristics often emphasized in African American culture will help foster successful career planning and exploration for the African American male college student.

CAREER COUNSELING CASE VIGNETTE

The Case of Frederick

Frederick is a 19-year-old African American freshman who has come to the university career center because he is unsure about a major. He has talked to his adviser, who referred him to the center to talk to a career counselor. Currently, he is in the Computer Science department. At the end of next semester Frederick will need to declare his major.

Frederick has always liked computers since receiving his first one in 5th grade. Since that time, he has owned four different systems, each more powerful and better than the last. He is the oldest of three children and the only male child. He grew up in a suburb of Washington, D.C. He attended a private, college prep school in Washington, known for its rigorous academics, and graduated cum laude. He chose this university because it had a large Computer Science department, and many of his high school friends were also attending. Frederick's parents were divorced when he was 4 years old, and his father is not directly involved in Frederick's life but is financing part of Frederick's college tuition. His mother has her master's degree in business administration and holds a high-profile government position.

Frederick is a gregarious, talkative young man. He has an exhilarating air of self-confidence that makes him appear more mature than his chronological age. He is well groomed and stylish in his appearance. Frederick thinks he wants to be a computer programmer and work for a company like Microsoft. His grade point average is 3.72. He works for Outreach, the black campus newspaper, plays intramural basketball, and sings bass in the gospel choir on campus.

He says to the counselor, "I'm not really sure that I want to be a computer science major. I really love doing computer stuff, but I'm not sure I can do it for 4 years. I like math, but what kind of job can you get as a math major? I don't want to end up as a high school algebra teacher." He is feeling some pressure from his mom to stay with his current major because she believes the computer science field will offer her son more opportunities. She also believes that he needs to set an example for his younger siblings.

A typical day for Frederick involves waking up late and then subsequently being late for class. He lives at home and commutes to school. His class *schedule is full, and he usually does not get home before 8 p.m. three nights during the week. In addition, he is a Kappa pledge, and pledge responsibilities keep him quite involved.*

Counselor Response to Frederick

Frederick is like many other freshmen in his uncertainty. The first approach the counselor employed was to normalize his feelings and to reassure him it was acceptable to be undecided about his major. The counselor and Frederick then began to devise a career plan. Establishing a career plan and time line allowed the counselor to foster the idea that effective planning takes time and reduce some of the anxiety Frederick was feeling about trying to decide his major. The outline below shows the process the counselor used to help Frederick:

1. Problem identification: Unsure of major

2. Short-term goal: Explore other possible majors/areas of career interest

3. Long-term goal: Decide on a major in a timely fashion

4. Discuss the career exploration and planning process.

5. Gather pertinent background information not discussed previously. To accomplish Step 5, the counselor used the following creative interventions:

The Counselor Asked Frederick to Complete a Career Genogram. Genograms have been traditionally used in family counseling to aid the counselor in conceptualizing how clients function within their family system (Bowen, 1978). By modifying this intervention slightly, the genogram can serve several functions in the career domain. First, it allows for the representation of occupations at generational levels. Levels of education can also be assessed across generational lines. Second, patterns or themes of career choice can be identified within the family. Third, the counselor can look for evidence of family values related to certain types of occupations and work ethic. Usually, in African American culture, familial influences on career choice can be quite powerful.

Completing the career genogram enabled both the counselor and Frederick to view his family's work and educational history. The counselor learned that Frederick's father was a chemical engineer for DuPont. It also became apparent that Frederick's family had a rich educational history, in that his maternal great-grandfather was a dentist in Harlem. On both sides of his family, his aunts and uncles were high-achieving and college educated. Part of being successful in Frederick's family meant obtaining a college degree.

The Counselor Inquired About the Classes Frederick Liked Best in High School and the Subjects He Had Done Well In. As the counselor had hypothesized, Frederick reported liking and doing well in his math and computer classes (receiving As in all).

The Counselor Conducted a Hero Analysis (Heppner, O'Brien, Hinkelman, & Humphrey, 1994). The counselor asked Frederick to talk about the people in his life he admired. He was encouraged to tell what particular attributes or characteristics made this person one of his heros (or heroines). This allowed the counselor to examine important individuals in Frederick's life and to identify how they had an impact on his career choice. Frederick cited Ron Brown, because of his political acumen and savvy; Dr. Deirdre Holloway, his ophthalmologist, for her successful combination of career and family; his mom, for her strength of character and independence; Tiger Woods and Thurgood Marshall, for breaking down the barriers of racism in their fields. The counselor noted that Frederick's heros and heroines were all successful African Americans. This led her to hypothesize that Frederick had a strong racial identity.

The Counselor Wanted to Assess Frederick's Personal Work Experience and Inquired If He Held Any Job on or off Campus in Addition to the Newspaper. The counselor also asked about the nature of his work at the newspaper (i.e., was he a feature writer, opinion writer, sports writer) and if his position was paid or volunteer.

As the counselor was gathering information, close attention was paid to the way Frederick viewed his role as son, brother, and student and the language he used to represent his views.

6. Begin the exploration process.

During this process various interventions were employed to get Frederick to think about his interests, his skills, and the world of work.

▨ The counselor asked Frederick to imagine his ideal job and work setting. What would it look like? Where would it be (inside/outside, east coast/west coast)? What would he be doing? How many people would work with him? What are the values associated with this job?

- The counselor recognized the importance of computers in Frederick's life; therefore, he completed a computerized interest inventory.

- The counselor also had Frederick do an occupational card sort.

- Using the top five occupations Frederick said he liked in the occupational card sort, the counselor had him research the jobs using the *Occupational Outlook Handbook* and the *Guide for Occupational Exploration.* The counselor explained to Frederick that he could use these reference books on his own to find occupational information.

- They also explored Frederick's decision-making style by having him take a decision-making assessment and discussing the ways in which he had made decisions in the past.

Once Frederick had investigated several occupations, he was ready to go further with the process.

7. Action steps

- The career counselor invited Frederick to a career panel designed specifically for computer science majors. She also gave Frederick the name and phone number of an African American graduate student who was working as a programmer in the area. She told Frederick to be sure to ask the student about his perception of the corporate culture for African Americans.

- Because time management appeared to somewhat of a problem, the counselor instructed Frederick to attend a two-part time-management workshop that she was giving for the black fraternities and sororities on campus.

- The counselor also wanted to capitalize on Frederick's strengths, so she had him research companies on the Internet and join a listserv group for black computer science majors. This particular listserv emphasized group unity and collective knowledge.

8. Next Steps

- The process that Frederick was engaged in required many follow-up sessions. During these follow-up sessions, Frederick and his counselor were able to discuss the various interventions. She was able to monitor his progress and evaluate their effectiveness.

- Recognizing the influence of Frederick's mother, the counselor invited her (with Frederick's permission) to join a session with Frederick, to receive an update on his progress.

- The counselor also told Frederick that he might benefit from enrolling in the one-credit career course offered during the summer and fall, which was taught by an African American professor in psychology.

- The counselor encouraged Frederick to consider living on campus next year to minimize the risk of being late to class.

- They explored the possibility of Frederick obtaining a paid internship with a computer company during the summer.

- Finally, the counselor asked Frederick to promise to stop by every year to inform her of how he was doing.

Frederick was a bright and capable student, as evident by his grade point average and personal demeanor; therefore, he was able to benefit from the career counseling process. The counselor was able to make recommendations and suggestions that gave Frederick just enough responsibility without being overwhelming. She recognized the strong influence of the African American culture and community in Frederick's life and attempted to incorporate these influences into the career planning process. She used his interest in computers to motivate him to explore occupational information via the Internet. From a culturally relevant standpoint, she was able to identify potential African American role models and mentors for Frederick, both on and off campus. Most important, the counselor attempted to impress on Frederick that career planning was not limited to his sessions with her but was something he could do on his own by using the resources (both people and written material) around him.

CONCLUSION

In a related article on career counseling, I challenged counselors and career development professionals to use alternative interventions and counseling strategies with African American college students (see Hendricks, 1994). In this chapter, I re-emphasize similar strategies. I also attempted to clearly delineate the steps in the career counseling process. The beauty of the career counseling process is its fluidity and cumulative effects. It is a process whereby one can learn lifelong, transferrable skills such as decision making . and problem solving. Moreover, it is a process that, if done effectively, will encourage positive self-reliance and occupational productivity. A man successfully completing the career exploration and planning process will be able to articulate these three things:

1. This is who I am, these are my interests, values, and goals.

2. These are things I want in a career.

3. This is the way in which I intend to meet my educational and career goals.

I end this chapter with a challenge for practitioners, educators, counselors, and family members to foster the career development of African American men. I challenge you to encourage education, whether it be completing high school, community college, the university, or graduate school. Education and training will be critical in the next century, and I want to see our men prepared to meet its demands in the workplace.

CHAPTER 22

Employment for Young African American Males: Where the Jobs Are and What Employers Want

HARRY J. HOLZER

The problems experienced by young African American males in the labor market are quite well known. Their unemployment rate is disturbingly high, and their attachment to the labor force is often quite weak (Freeman & Holzer, 1986). Their wages lag behind those of their white counterparts, even when they have comparable amounts of education and work experience. If anything, these developments have grown worse over the past decade or two, as some of the progress made toward earnings equalization between whites and blacks during the civil rights movement has been eroded (Bound & Freeman, 1992). Indeed, many social scientists attribute a wide variety of troubling developments in the African American community, such as declining rates of marriage and growing participation in crime, to the growing difficulties young black men have in finding work at rates of pay they consider acceptable (Wilson, 1987).

These difficulties suggest some type of mismatch between the characteristics of young black males and those sought by employers. Perhaps they do not have the skills or credentials that employers seek (in reality or in the employers' perceptions); perhaps they are looking for work in the wrong sectors of the economy or the wrong geographic locations; or perhaps employers simply don't want to hire young black men. But before we can develop the remedies that practitioners can apply to each of these potential problems, we have to determine the extent to which each is true.

In this chapter, I will provide a summary of the characteristics, requirements, and hiring behavior of employers in jobs that they are currently trying to fill. I will focus primarily on jobs for less educated workers, that is, those that do not require workers to have college diplomas. The findings reported here are based on a survey that I recently administered to 800 employers in each of four large metropolitan areas: Atlanta, Boston, Detroit, and Los Angeles; the results appear in much greater detail in Holzer (1996).

After providing the summary, I will discuss below some implications of the findings for practitioners who are seeking to help young black males obtain employment. In particular, I will offer some general suggestions on how to overcome the barriers that these young males currently face in locating the employers and applying for the jobs whose characteristics I summarize below.

WHERE THE JOBS ARE AND WHAT EMPLOYERS WANT

In recent years, some enormous changes have occurred on the demand side of the labor market, that is, in the characteristics of employers and the jobs they seek to fill. Many of these changes have been particularly harmful for young males without college education, who have experienced declines in their earnings of more than 20% (after adjusting for inflation) during the past two decades (Danziger & Gottschalk, 1995). Young *black* males have experienced even greater difficulties, as they have been particularly hard hit by many of the changes that have taken place.

What are these changes and why have they occurred? The most important can be summarized as follows:

The Loss of Industrial and/or Unionized Jobs. The fraction of overall employment in the United States accounted for by manufacturing has declined quite dramatically over the past few decades (from roughly 30% of all nonfarm jobs in 1960 to about 16% today), and the representation of blacks in these jobs has declined even more dramatically (Bound & Holzer, 1993). The fraction of jobs covered by collective bargaining has also declined quite severely (from roughly 35% of private sector jobs in the mid-1950s to about 10% today (Freeman, 1996). These jobs traditionally employed substantial numbers of less educated workers and enabled them to earn wages well above what they could earn in other sectors of the economy. Black males were especially heavily represented in these jobs and earned relatively large premiums for working there; thus, they were more severely hurt when these jobs disappeared.

Rising Skill Demands Among Employers. In all sectors of the economy, we have experienced a declining need among employers for the type of blue-collar work that has traditionally provided jobs for the majority of non-college-educated men, and even within given job classifications, the need for certain types of skills has apparently grown. The reasons for these trends appear to include major technological changes in the workplace, stemming from the development of personal computers, as well as a variety of workplace reorganizations. Growing international trade, with domestically produced goods being replaced by imported ones (or those outsourced to foreign subsidiaries of U.S. companies), appears to play some role in this process, as well, although not a primary one (Danziger & Gottschalk, 1995).

Employer Relocations Away From the Central Cities. Many central city employers, especially those in manufacturing, have chosen to relocate to distant parts of suburban areas. As housing discrimination and residential segregation often limit the extent to which African Americans can move to these areas, their access to relocating jobs becomes more limited. This might be due to difficulties they experience with transportation (especially for those without their own automobiles), limited information about these areas, a lack of social contacts there, and so on (Holzer, 1991; Kain, 1992).

Employer Discrimination. We have growing evidence of employer discrimination against minorities in hiring from a variety of audit studies, in which matched pairs of white and minority applicants with identical credentials apply for the same jobs (Fix & Struyk, 1994). It is at least possible that such discrimination has grown more severe in recent years, as enforcement of federal affirmative action provisions has diminished (Leonard, 1990) and as the fear of crime among whites (which they often associate with young black men) has grown (Freeman, 1992).

Other developments in the American economy have no doubt reinforced the effects of these demand-side changes on the employment and earnings of less educated males. For instance, the declining real value of the minimum wage (i.e., after adjusting for inflation over time) also appears to have lowered the wages of the least skilled. Also, there have been changes on the supply side of the labor market, such as lagging rates of college enrollment in the 1970s and early 1980s, especially among young blacks (Kane, 1994), and an unwillingness of young men to accept jobs with declining wages (Juhn, 1992); these changes reinforce the demand-side developments that have occurred.

But how have the demand-side changes noted above affected the nature and characteristics of jobs currently available to less educated workers, especially young African American males? Below, I list some of my survey findings regarding the characteristics of employers and the jobs they are currently filling in large metropolitan areas of the United States.

1. *Most jobs for less educated workers, including males, are currently in white-collar occupations and in the retail trade and service sectors of the economy.* The traditional blue-collar job in a factory setting, such as working as a skilled craftsmen or assembly line operator, is becoming a rarity. Overall, manufacturing accounts for roughly 20% of new hires in these areas and only about 10% in most central cities. Blue-collar jobs more generally (defined as positions for skilled craftsmen, semiskilled operators of equipment, or unskilled laborers) account for about 30% of all new hires in non-college jobs and about 20% in the central cities. In contrast, jobs in the retail trade and service sectors (which include schools, hospitals, banks, legal or business services, restaurants, and other retail trade establishments) account for almost two thirds of new employment for the less educated, and the occupations that are most frequently filled are clerical, sales, and service positions.

2. *More jobs are available to less educated workers in suburban areas than in the central cities.* About 75% of all the new jobs in these metropolitan areas are located outside the primary central city neighborhoods. An even larger fraction of the relevant population lives outside the central cities, but there is net commuting by suburban residents into the central city areas for employment. After accounting for these commuting patterns, we find fewer jobs available per unemployed worker in the central cities than in the suburbs. As noted above, manufacturing and/or blue-collar jobs in the central cities are particularly scarce.

3. *A large fraction of jobs are filled by informal recruitment among employers, who seek referrals from their current employees and other acquaintances.* Employers generally believe that they can get fairly accurate information about individual applicants from such referrals, especially from the current employees whom they trust and value (Rees, 1966). Therefore, almost 40% of non-college jobs are filled through such recruitment methods, and almost 20% are filled through other informal practices (such as posting help-wanted signs or accepting direct applications from walk-ins without referrals).

Of the roughly 40% of these jobs filled through more formal means, newspaper ads account for about two thirds. The latter are more frequently used for white-collar and skilled blue-collar positions, whereas informal methods are used more frequently in filling less-skilled positions.

4. *Employer skill needs and credentials requirements are quite extensive, even in jobs that do not require college.* For instance, the vast majority of jobs now involve the use of basic cognitive skills (such as reading or writing of paragraph-length material or arithmetic calculations) on a daily basis. Over half of non-college jobs now involve the use of computers. Roughly 70% also involve daily interaction with customers. Indeed, only about 5% to 10% of newly filled non-college jobs do not involve *any* of these tasks on a daily basis. Furthermore, these requirements are quite extensive, even among blue-collar jobs in industrial settings.

The level of cognitive skill implied in these jobs is not necessarily high because many uses of computers (such as running products over a super-market scanner) are very simple and because arithmetic calculations are often limited to fairly basic efforts (such as making change). But they may be sufficiently high that at least some job seekers will not be able to perform these functions well, at least in the eyes of the employer.

Many employers, especially in filling professional or managerial occupations, seek employees who show some evidence of ability to learn and who are capable of performing higher-level cognitive tasks, such as various kinds of problem solving. Others seek skills that are specific to the job for which they are hiring (National Center on the Educational Quality of the Workforce, 1995).

To find employees with the relevant skills, employers seek a set of credentials that signal to them an employee's ability in a variety of areas. The most basic credential, of course, is the high school diploma. Although roughly 80% of new jobs require (or strongly prefer) that applicants have high school diplomas, it is also clear that this is a necessary but not sufficient condition for gaining employment. Thus, employers frequently lament that the diploma indicates little about an applicant's ability to read, write, or learn (National Center on the Educational Quality of the Workforce, 1995), but *not* having one certainly signals an inability to perform these functions.

What other signals of ability do employers then seek among non-college applicants? Roughly two thirds require or strongly prefer that applicants have experience in the particular line of work. About 40% require some type of previous vocational training or skill certification. About three fourths also expect to see some type of reference. Once again, only about 5% of non-college jobs do not require or strongly prefer that applicants have any of the above credentials.

Many of the skills that employers weight fairly heavily in evaluating applicants are frequently referred to as "soft skills," such as verbal/communication abilities and personal attitudes toward work and responsibility. Of course, these are harder for an employer to gauge with any degree of objectivity. Employers rely heavily on personal impressions made in interviews, which are likely to be highly subjective (Moss & Tilly, 1995).

5. *Employers seem quite reluctant to hire applicants with spotty or unstable work histories, especially those whom they suspect of having criminal records.* More than half of employers claim they would definitely not or probably not hire someone into a non-college job with only short-term or part-time work experience in the recent past (as in Ballen & Freeman, 1986). Furthermore, about two thirds claim they would not hire someone with a criminal record.

Of the latter, many employers do not actually check the criminal records of their applicants (which, at least in many states, can be a difficult and time-consuming process). Although some written applications ask about previous arrest records, there is little reason for employers to believe that these responses are always honest. Consequently, they are not likely to hire those whom they suspect of such histories, such as young black males with major gaps in their educational or employment histories.

6. *Blacks and Hispanics are clearly less likely to be hired into jobs that involve daily use of certain cognitive or social skills, as well as those that require credentials such as education, experience, and training.* For instance, blacks and Hispanics represent about 45% of workers hired into non-college jobs that do not require daily use of arithmetic and about 30% of those that do require its daily use; numbers for computer use are comparable. The hiring of blacks is particularly reduced by requirements of specific previous experience or training.

Of course, the extent to which blacks are truly less able to perform the work on jobs with these requirements may be open to question, but, in this case, it is the employers' perception of their ability, rather than their ability in reality, that ultimately matters here. For instance, employers might assume that blacks perform certain cognitive functions less well, based on patterns of speech or residential location; these assumptions may or may not be accurate for particular individuals. This implies a problem of *statistical discrimination,* in which individuals are judged on the basis of average characteristics of people in their groups.

7. *Employers in the central cities obtain about twice as many black applicants as do those in the suburbs. Employers located closer to black residential areas and public transit stops get especially high numbers of black applicants and employees.* These results indicate that geographical locations of employers do matter, and that some are more accessible to central city minorities than others (Holzer & Ihlanfeldt, 1996).

8. *Employers generally seem to prefer Hispanic applicants to blacks and black females to black males. Employers in small establishments and in the suburbs, especially those serving predominantly white customers, seem the most reluctant to hire blacks.* Those blacks who apply for jobs in the suburbs generally have higher skills (such as educational attainment), relative to white males, than those applying in the central cities. Educational attainment among blacks is generally higher than among Hispanics.

Therefore, it seems quite likely that blacks in general, and black males in particular, face more employer discrimination, especially in suburban areas. This is not surprising in some ways, given that employers who choose to locate in parts of the suburbs least accessible to the central city sometimes do so deliberately to get away from the local black population (Kasarda, 1995; Mieszkowski & Mills, 1993). Smaller suburban employers also are less vulnerable to legal action for discrimination because their hiring behavior is monitored less closely than that of larger firms; they face fewer blacks in the relevant "local labor force" on which claims of discrimination are statistically analyzed (Bloch, 1994).

The preference of employers for Hispanics over blacks in jobs that do not require much cognitive or interactive skill, for example, in manufacturing, may reflect the greater presence of immigrants among the former. Immigrants are widely perceived to have stronger work ethics than native-born minorities. Employers also tend to hold more negative views of black males than black females, perhaps because of greater fears about crime or violence (Kirschenman, 1991).

Overall, black males clearly face problems in terms of their skills and credentials, their geographical locations, and stereotypical employer attitudes when they seek employment.

HOW TO HELP BLACK MALES OVERCOME THESE BARRIERS

Given the multiple difficulties that black males face in obtaining jobs, how can practitioners help them to overcome these problems and obtain employment at more acceptable wages? The following suggestions provide some general guidelines, based on the above findings (and more evidence from the literature on employment and training programs).

1. *Young black males need to attain stronger educational and training credentials and send stronger signals of their abilities to perform basic cognitive and social tasks.* As noted earlier, high school dropout rates for

young blacks have declined substantially in the past few decades. Unfortunately, employers no longer interpret the attainment of a high school diploma (especially from high schools in lower-income, inner-city areas) as great evidence of individuals' cognitive abilities.

Of course, it is critically important that young blacks attain these diplomas because failure to do so today sends a very strong negative signal to employers. Indeed, the extremely high rates of criminal activity among young black male high school dropouts (Freeman, 1992) suggests that their labor force opportunities and attachments are both extremely limited. But wherever possible, it is important that young blacks attain additional educational credentials beyond the high school diploma.

The widening gaps in earnings and employment between those with and without college diplomas in our economy overall suggests the benefits that accrue to those who can obtain this degree. Wherever possible, practitioners should help young black males overcome personal financial constraints by making them aware of financial aid options (such as Pell grants) that might enable them to attend these institutions. As early as possible, those who have contact with high school students (whether they be teachers, counselors, or other members of the local community) must also stress the links between academic performance in high school and ability to attend college for those who may not themselves accurately perceive the incentives.

Those who will not obtain a bachelor's degree need to be aware of and pursue opportunities to obtain credentials from other educational or training institutions, such as community colleges or other vocational programs. Any other certification that clearly signals an ability to read/write, perform arithmetic, use computers, and so on could be useful. Counselors might need to make individuals more aware of all local options in this regard.

2. *It is also important for young males to send positive signals of other employment-related characteristics, such as stable early work experience and avoidance of criminal activity.* The school-to-work transition seems particularly problematic for young blacks, and early gaps between themselves and others in employment rates quickly widen over time (Hotz & Tienda, 1995). Thus, helping young black males attain some stable, early private-sector employment experience may enable them to send important signals to their later employers regarding their work attitudes, reliability, and the like.

Recent evidence suggests that modest amounts of work during high school (i.e., 10 to 15 hours per week) have positive effects on postschool employment rates for young people without adversely affecting their academic performance (e.g., Ruhm, 1995). Where such employment has not been quickly or easily attained during or after high school, young black males may need to convince employers that they have spent their time productively and have avoided participation in illegal activities.

3. *Providing job placements, transportation assistance, and job search assistance might enable young black males to more easily obtain such early employment experience, especially in suburban areas where unskilled employment is more readily available.* Young blacks who reside in central-city areas may lack access to employers in the distant suburbs because they lack transportation, but other possibilities include a lack of information about job openings in outlying areas, a lack of orientation to the local geography, a lack of informal contacts in these areas, and a perception of hostility among local whites (which may or may not be accurate).

Practitioners can help young black males become more oriented to the outlying parts of metropolitan areas, to local transportation systems, and to where major centers of employment are located. Local programs that combine transportation assistance (such as van pooling) with job placement activity and counseling (regarding employer expectations of work performance, etc.) are relatively low-cost interventions that might be quite effective for individuals who are relatively employable in terms of basic skills (Hughes & Sternberg, 1992). This is especially true for those placement agencies that develop good personal ties to employers, with a reputation for providing employable applicants who are well matched to the requirements of their jobs.

Assisting individuals with their job search similarly appears to be a low-cost intervention that is modestly effective with certain populations (e.g., Leigh, 1990). As noted above, young black males appear to face major disadvantages in terms of their access to informal referral networks and in more subjective screening formats (such as interviews with employers); thus, any assistance they can obtain on how to obtain such referrals (from acquaintances, teachers, community members, etc.) and how to conduct themselves in these contexts could be quite valuable to them.

4. *Follow-up efforts must also be available to deal with problems young black males will likely encounter after they have been placed in these jobs.* Many employers, both black and white, complain about poor work attitudes and performance among young black males (e.g., Kirschenman & Neckerman, 1991; Moss & Tilly, 1995). Young blacks also are much more likely to be discharged from employment due to absenteeism or other problems in the workplace (Ferguson & Filer, 1986).

Thus, practitioners must be available to counsel young black males about difficult and unexpected situations that will inevitably arise in the workplaces in which they have been placed. Some turnover out of these jobs must certainly be anticipated and dealt with as it occurs.

5. *Job placement practitioners should take note of employers who repeated fail to hire apparently qualified black male job applicants and should consider a variety of options when such employers are identified.* This, of course, is a problematic strategy in many ways. For one thing, it is generally the smallest employers in areas most removed from central cities who are most likely to engage in such behavior; monitoring their behaviors in this regard is quite costly. Furthermore, any placement agency that develops a local reputation for pressuring employers may immediately lose the goodwill among employers that is necessary for successful placements over time.

Nevertheless, the research evidence strongly suggests that young black males will face more discriminatory employer behavior in the suburban areas where more jobs for less skilled workers are available. Given this dilemma, practitioners who try to improve the access of inner-city black males to these suburban labor markets must expect that they will encounter some resistance when they apply for work there, and they should be ready to consider a variety of options (ranging from informal private or public pressure to legal remedies) when this occurs repeatedly.

CONCLUSION

The demand side of the labor market that young African American males currently face has changed dramatically in recent years. The traditional blue-collar industrial jobs that were once plentiful in major central-city areas exist in much smaller numbers today. They have been replaced by largely white-collar and service occupations in the retail trade and service sectors, jobs that are relatively more available in suburban areas. Even jobs that do not require college degrees often involve daily use of a variety of social and cognitive skills, and they usually have major requirements in terms of experience or training credentials. Employers frequently recruit informally for these jobs, use screens that leave much room for subjective judgment, and strongly distrust job candidates with unstable work histories and suspected involvement in criminal activities.

Black males are clearly disadvantaged by many of these developments in the labor market; they face major barriers in terms of their own skill attainment and credentials (relative to those that employers seek) as well as the location and behavior of employers. Practitioners must be aware of, and must address, a wide range of potential labor market difficulties these young males will develop or face at quite early ages. An awareness of the characteristics and behaviors of employers and jobs in major metropolitan areas will help them develop effective strategies for addressing these very important problems.

CHAPTER 23

Building Assets Among African American Males

MICHAEL SHERRADEN

Recently, I had the honor of speaking at a conference on rural development at Tuskegee University, and the focus of my remarks was on African American land ownership. As the reader probably knows, the number of black farmers has declined sharply in the United States, falling by more than 95% since 1954, so that today, fewer than 19,000 black farmers remain. This is a deep tragedy because freed slaves had to struggle very hard, against all odds, for the agricultural land that they eventually owned. It would be an understatement to say that whites never made it easy. As the 20th century draws to a close, the legacy of land owning among rural blacks is all but disappearing. In opening my talk at Tuskegee, I told the audience of

AUTHOR'S NOTE: Portions of the introduction and discussion of race and wealth borrow from my review of Oliver and Shapiro's (1995) *Black Wealth/White Wealth,* which appeared in *Social Service Review.* Some of the historical text on assets and African Americans borrows from my *Assets and the Poor* (Sherraden, 1991). I am indebted to Jami Curley for tabulating data on 1996 federal social expenditures. The section on discrimination in home mortgage relies on Scanlon and Emerson (1997), *Home Mortgage Lending in St. Louis.* Much of the discussion on IDAs in welfare reform and state policy borrows from Grossman and Friedman (1997), *Building Ecoomic Independence Through Individual Development Accounts.* Karen Edwards assisted with IDA design features. For information on youth entrepreneurship programs, I am indebted to Cicero Wilson of the Corporation for Enterprise Development. My colleagues at Washington University, Letha Chadiha and Robert Pierce, provided information on African American family associations and reunions, and Garrett Duncan gave me helpful comments.

agricultural professionals that, in a perverse way, young African Americans males were in fact returning to rural areas, and in record numbers. They could be seen in Alabama, as I saw them, tending seedlings along the highways. But today they are dressed in starchy white uniforms and chained together. Instead of working as independent farmers, they toil as prisoners in chain gangs. Looking at this in a slightly different way, young African American males have themselves become a kind of cash crop for rural communities in almost every state, where new prisons are avidly sought as an economic development strategy. An ever growing number of rural whites earn their livelihoods as prison guards. For African American males, the historical reverberations of these developments—130 years after the end of slavery— are inescapable.

As I walked on the campus of Tuskegee, founded by Booker T. Washington, I recalled his famous "caste down your buckets where you are" speech of 1895, a speech urging blacks to make the most of what they had. Washington was willing to endure the discrimination of whites and focus instead on economic development. This was undoubtedly a prudent strategy at the time, but as rival black leader W.E.B. Du Bois proclaimed, it was not enough. A century later, we can in some measure assess the outcome of this debate, and property ownership is a useful standard by which to gauge the progress of blacks in the United States. As shown in this chapter, progress has been quite limited. When African Americans follow Booker T. Washington's advice to "caste down your bucket where you are," they usually do not come up with very much.

The point of these observations is to emphasize the tenuous hold on property—any kind of property—that blacks have in America, and the deep historical roots of this situation. With few exceptions, not even successful blacks have accumulated much wealth, and poor blacks have almost none at all. In this chapter, we look at the issue of asset (wealth) inequality, consider the effects on African American males, and make suggestions for advocacy, public policy, community development, and individual strategies that focus on asset accumulation. First, let us turn to several key points of American history, property ownership, public policy, and black males.

SLAVERY, RECONSTRUCTION, AND PROPERTY

Perhaps more than any other single idea, America is about the freedom to own property. Thomas Jefferson celebrated small land holding as the foundation not only of a growing economy but also of active citizenship and a strong democracy. Unfortunately, Jefferson exemplified the bigoted foundations of America; he was not troubled by the fact that the land he spoke so passionately about had been stolen from native peoples and worked for hundreds of years by African slaves. Jefferson's vision of who should own property was flawed, but his thinking about the meaning of ownership was brilliant. Today, we know that property ownership leads to many positive outcomes for families and communities.

For most people of African descent on American shores prior to the Civil War, slavery precluded the practice or culture of property ownership. Nonetheless, slaves knew very well the importance of owning land. During the Civil War, there were numerous accounts of slaves marking off plots on the plantations, thinking that the land would be theirs if the South lost the war. So urgent was their desire to become independent farmers, that former slaves sometimes raised crops on contested ground during the war:

> In many instances they took possession of land dangerously near the field of battle, risking their liberty and even their lives. Along the North Carolina coast, when the Union Army had not captured enough ground to "rest their tents upon," freedmen squatted on lands in "No Man's Land," and there grew cotton and corn or made turpentine. (Allen, 1937, p. 44)

But to no avail. When the war was over, with few exceptions, freed slaves were forced into wage labor or share-tenancy agriculture, which was little better than the conditions of slavery. Regrettably, the federal government in Washington and northern troops took the lead in forcing freed slaves out of their claim of ownership and into peonage labor.

Also, there were promises made during the Civil War, believed by many blacks, of "forty acres and a mule" going to freed slaves, but the land was never delivered. It is important to note that 40 acres was only one fourth of the 160 acres that was actually distributed to newly arrived European Americans under the Homestead Act. This is of more than historical interest. My great-grandfather was a homesteader in Kansas; he received 160 acres from the U.S. government; this is how my family got a foothold in the American economy and became part of a community. Millions of white Americans living today have similar backgrounds. One cannot help but wonder how different America would be at the end of the 20th century if land had also been distributed to freed blacks after the Civil War. As Du Bois (1935/1968) later suggested, it "would have made a basis of real democracy in the United States" (p. 602).

During the Reconstruction period, one major institution, the Freedmen's Bank, did seek to encourage savings among freed slaves for land and homes (regular banks were not open to blacks). Frederick Douglass, who accepted a leadership role with the Freedmen's Bank, commented,

> The history of civilization shows that no people can well rise to a high degree of mental or even moral excellence without wealth. A people uniformly poor and compelled to struggle for barely a physical existence will be dependent and despised by their neighbors, and will finally despise themselves. . . . The mission of the Freedmen's Bank is to show our people the road to a share of the wealth and well-being of the world. (Douglass, 1874)

The Freedmen's Bank was successful in increasing black savings and ownership, but it was undermined by the corrupt practices of a white board of directors, and it failed in the depression of 1873-1874. Thousands of blacks lost their life savings and were never repaid. This loss had a devastating effect on the relationship of blacks to financial institutions and the accumulation of wealth. Decades later, Du Bois said that the crash of the Freedmen's Bank cost blacks their trust in saving: "Not even ten additional years of slavery could have done so much to throttle the thrift of the freedmen as the mismanagement and bankruptcy of the series of savings banks chartered by the Nation for their especial aid" (Du Bois, 1903/1970, p. 39). Even Booker T. Washington (1909) could not help but comment, "When they found that they had lost, or been swindled out of all their little savings, they lost faith in savings banks" (Vol. 2, p. 214).

Thus, Reconstruction ended without land acquisition for the vast majority of freed slaves. Looking back, "the tragedy of Reconstruction [was] the failure of the black masses to acquire land, since without the economic security provided by land ownership the freedmen were soon deprived of the political and civil rights which they had won" (Oubre, 1978, p. 197). The remainder of the 19th century was no better. "Black Code" regulations restricted black enterprise (Marable, 1983, pp. 142-143), and intimidation and lynchings were used to shut down black enterprises that might compete with businesses owned by whites (Wells-Barnett, 1892, 1894, 1900/1969).

THE 20TH CENTURY

The 20th century has brought some improvement in the most blatant forms of property discrimination, but as Oliver and Shapiro (1995) document, discrimination in access to home ownership and home insurance has continued, often with the explicit or implicit approval of the federal government. Scanlon and Emerson (1997) comment on these practices:

> For at least the first 60 years of this century, intentional racial discrimination was an explicit requirement of housing and housing finance practices, with the full support of federal law. . . . The existence, and enforcement by federal courts, of racially restrictive covenants and exclusionary zoning laws coupled with discriminatory practices by property insurers, home builders, as well as appraisers and lenders all served to create and reinforce dual housing markets in cities throughout the United States. (pp. 2-3)

During the 1960s, federal law changed dramatically, with the Civil Rights Act of 1964 and the Federal Housing Act of 1968. Nonetheless, studies in the 1970s by the Comptroller of the Currency and the Federal Home Loan Bank Board indicated a strong probability of race discrimination in mortgage credit. Congress responded with the Equal Credit Opportunity Act of 1974, the Home Mortgage Disclosure Act of 1975, and the Community Reinvestment Act of 1977. Despite these very influential laws, there are substantial indications that racial discrimination in mortgage lending continues (Scanlon & Emerson, 1997). Because home owning is typically a first step on a ladder of asset building that proceeds across generations, property discrimination has severely limited wealth accumulation in African American households.

THE WELFARE STATE AND BLACK MALES

A few years ago at a planning meeting held at the United Way of Greater St. Louis, following hours of hopeful discussion about new programs for women and children, a woman from one of the neighborhoods stood and asked, "What about the men-ses? What are you gonna do about the men-ses?" Her very direct inquiry got everyone's attention—the room fell silent—but her question was never answered. This question, in its largest sense, remains unanswered. In America, we have never known what to do about—and we have done almost nothing for—African American males. Young black males are more apt to be seen as "social dynamite" than as potential contributors to society (Sherraden & Adamek, 1984).

The welfare state, that is, all of the policies and programs funded by the federal government, today makes up a huge part—over 60%—of what the federal government spends each year, but very little of this spending reaches impoverished black males. Most of the money, 78.0% in 1996, is not targeted to poor people. Of the remaining 22.0%, almost all of the money is distributed as income transfers or in-kind services. The primary recipients for this "poor people's money" are the elderly, the disabled, and single mothers with children. But young black males, unless they are under 18 and in a welfare household, get little or none of it. Indeed, the categories of federal expenditures that would be the most help to young black males— education and employment—together represent only 2.7% of welfare state expenditures, and only about half of this spending is targeted to the poor. As I have said elsewhere, the welfare state is not about development, it is about maintenance—and the people who are being maintained are not young black males. The vast expenditures and programming of the welfare state have largely bypassed impoverished black males (Mincy, 1994b).

NOT INCOME ALONE BUT ASSETS AS WELL

In discussions of race and poverty, it is common to turn to employment as the fundamental issue (in this volume, see the excellent chapter on employment by Holzer). The goal of employment is to earn a living and therefore be able to support a household. In other words, the primary meaning of employment is the income that it provides. In addition to income, Wilson (1996) writes persuasively about the role of employment in regularizing life, creating a daily pattern of activity and responsibility in families and communities. For Wilson and many other analysts, the absence of employment is the key issue for blacks, and policy responses often emphasize employment. For example, the emphasis in welfare reform (U.S. Congress, 1996) is decidedly on employment (although like most other U.S. social policy, welfare reform will do little to help black males). The central role of employment is undeniable, and all efforts to increase employment should be supported. But at the same time, too narrow a focus on employment and the income it generates can overlook the equally important issue of what people have, their stake in America, their assets.

In the academic world, we have for the most part fallen into this pattern of overlooking assets and assuming that income is all that matters. Poverty and inequality are typically defined and measured in terms of income, and most poverty and inequality research is about income. For many decades, a small industry of poverty researchers has studied income almost exclusively. The central theme of these thousands of studies has been who gets what and how public policy might change that. As the century draws to a close, this largely atheoretical body of research is generating little new understanding and insight. As one alternative, American social scientists are beginning to pay more attention to wealth accumulation as an inequality issue, and proposals for asset building in domestic policy have emerged in recent years (Oliver & Shapiro, 1995; Sherraden, 1991; Wolff, 1995).

RACIAL INEQUALITY IN WEALTH

Property ownership was not a strong theme in discussions of race in America until *Black Wealth/White Wealth* was written by Melvin Oliver and Thomas Shapiro in 1995. Prior to this book, inequality scholars had assumed that the implications of asset accumulation were not different from the implications of income flows, and in the case of poor households, researchers had assumed that asset accumulation was inconsequential and not worth studying. Oliver and Shapiro demonstrate convincingly that these assumptions are wrong and should be discarded. Wealth is a major inequality issue across the entire socioeconomic spectrum, and it has particular bearing on understanding race relations. A fundamental point of *Black Wealth/White Wealth* is that "substituting what is known about income inequality for what is not known about wealth inequality limits, and even biases, our understanding of inequality" (p. 89). For example, looking at wealth discrepancies by race, using the 1987 panel data from the Survey of Income and Program Participation, the median income of whites is $25,384 and of blacks is $15,630 (a ratio of less than 2:1), but turning to wealth, the median net worth of whites is $43,800 and of blacks is a disturbingly low $3,700 (a ratio of more than 11:1). At poverty-level incomes, the median net worth of whites is $2,173, but for blacks, it is zero. Among single-parent families with children, whites have a median net worth of $4,010; for blacks, it is zero. Perhaps more worrisome, the median net financial assets (cash, checking, savings, stocks and bonds, less credit card and other cash debts) of whites is $6,999 and of blacks is zero or negative. In fact, 60.9% of all black households have zero or negative net financial assets, and nearly three quarters of all black children grow up in households with no net financial assets.

Why have blacks been less able than whites to accumulate assets? The most obvious answer is that blacks have always earned less than whites, and these earnings shortfalls have resulted in less savings, less investment, and less asset accumulation. With the passage of generations, the differential in wealth by race becomes large. But as indicated above, it is also true that social and economic institutions have systematically blocked asset accumulation among African Americans, from slavery to the present (Sherraden, 1991, pp. 131-139). Oliver and Shapiro (1995) offer three explanations. The first they call the racialization of state policy. Under this heading, they discuss institutional and policy factors that affect home equity accumulation, such as racial patterns in residential location, discrimination in mortgage loan approvals, loan interest rate differentials, and inequalities in city services (not mentioned are home insurance costs, which also differ significantly by race). The extent of this discrimination, which goes on day by day, year after year, is literally astounding, and these factors combine to limit equity accumulation for black homeowners severely. The second explanation is the economic detour, an analysis of why blacks have not built enterprises to the same extent as other racial and ethnic groups in America. Self-employment for African Americans, say Oliver and Shapiro, is fundamentally different because the market for black businesses has been largely restricted to black customers. The third explanation is the sedimentation of racial inequality, which refers to the additive effects of asset inequality, generation after generation. This historical transmission of wealth inequality places most blacks in a precarious life position, where limited inheritance often undermines achievement. Looking at the three themes together, and borrowing again from Booker T. Washington's language, we could summarize by saying that African Americans will not achieve economic and social equality until they are able to caste down their buckets in the same waters as everyone else. As Ida B. Wells recognized following Reconstruction, racial discrimination is not merely a social matter but a strategy used by whites to limit asset accumulation among blacks. In a word, racial discrimination is fundamentally about property.

WHY DO ASSETS MATTER?

Mainstream economic thinking views assets as a storehouse for future consumption, but nothing more. Elsewhere, I have suggested that this thinking is inadequate. I have hypothesized that assets give people a stake in the future, a reason to dream and to invest time, effort, and resources in creating a future for themselves and their children. Assets also connect people both economically and socially to others in the community (Sherraden, 1991). In sum, "when people control key assets, they have a sense of ownership, power, and hope for the future that profoundly affects the way they conduct their lives" (Oliver, 1997, p. 8).

We are becoming aware that the presence of assets, perhaps especially in poor households, is likely to have a wide range of positive outcomes. A review of 25 studies that speak to social and economic effects of asset holding finds generally positive impacts (Page-Adams & Sherraden, 1996). If additional research confirms these results, assets would appear to be on the short list for promising strategies in domestic policy.

ASSET BUILDING FOR ALL AMERICANS, INCLUDING AFRICAN AMERICAN MALES

I am suggesting a simple but often overlooked idea: that African American males must accumulate wealth if they are to take control of their lives, have resources to solve problems, develop to their fullest potential, support families, and contribute to the community. In the late 20th century, this message has been offered occasionally by black separatists and community economic development specialists, but they have been in a minority among the black leadership. A majority of black leaders have been more attuned to civil and political rights and the income supports of the welfare state. How can asset building among African American males be promoted? There are many possible answers to this question; some are discussed below.

Public Education and Advocacy. Given the grave injustices of property and race in America, I believe that public education and advocacy regarding asset inequality are necessary. As a fundamental strategy, it is essential to put property at the center of understanding in discussions of the history of blacks in America. For the most part, this has not occurred in the past, perhaps because we have been too preoccupied with income, as if this were all that mattered. The key property issues for blacks are the economic cost of slavery itself, the loss of funds in the failure of the Freedmen's Bank, and continuing barriers to business and residential property ownership. These are huge economic issues. They should be spelled out and repeated again and again until they can no longer be ignored. Indeed, one suspects that the American people have been able to ignore them for so long only because they are too big, and the implications too sweeping, to contemplate.

What should be the primary goals in advocacy? Proposals for reparations for slavery and compensation for the funds lost by the Freedmen's Bank are in my view well justified, and they should be pursued vigorously. However, it is unlikely that the American people are going to vote anytime soon for a massive redistribution of assets to blacks. Reparations and compensation should nonetheless be pursued for two main reasons: as a mechanism to educate the public about this overlooked dimension of African American history and to set out a radical political position. One day, it may be achieved, but even if it is not, it will lay the groundwork for other asset-building proposals that may be more politically acceptable.

At this point, creativity is required. Although the American people, acting through the U.S. government, will be reluctant to offer mass compensation to blacks, they may be more open to strategies that are targeted to specific purposes and build assets over time. For example, consider the possibility of educational savings accounts started at birth for all black children, with some degree of public funding—or perhaps more politically acceptable, educational savings accounts for all children in America, but with very progressive funding for accounts of the poor. Consider the possibility of a program of economic education and entrepreneurial training in predominantly black schools, with real funds used for investment decisions, and businesses started in the schools and then transplanted to the community. Consider special savings accounts for all children in foster care so they would have a realistic opportunity for a successful transition to adulthood. Consider the possibility of subsidized savings and investment clubs in prisons so that prisoners would have a better understanding of mainstream and legitimate economic matters, as well as some assets, when they are released. More creative still, consider the possibility of stock ownership by prisoners in the private companies that today run many of the prisons; this would be a bold extension of employee stock ownership plans, and the effect on prisoner behavior would likely be quite positive. There are hundreds of other possibilities. The point is to bring asset accumulation into the daily patterns of as many African Americans as possible. Continual advocacy must be combined with asset-building proposals that are goal oriented and can attract a broad range of political support.

In sum, both radical advocacy and creative asset-building strategies are necessary. Regardless of one's political orientation, there is plenty of work to do. The key point is to introduce asset building into a broad range of discussions and settings where it does not today appear.

Public Policy and Individual Development Accounts. In the limited space of this chapter, I focus primarily on one asset-building policy mechanism–individual development accounts, or IDAs (Sherraden, 1988, 1989, 1990). An IDA is like an individual retirement account (IRA) except that it can begin as early as birth; it can be targeted to a specific population; savings can come from any source (i.e., not limited to earned income); savings should be matched progressively (i.e., higher matches to those with less income and wealth); the matching partners can be public, nonprofit, or private; and the purpose of the account can include education, home ownership, and business capitalization. An IDA is a desirable policy mechanism because it is simple and easily understood; it is popular with a broad range of the American people; and it is flexible and adaptable to a broad range of purposes and circumstances.

Federal IDA Policy. Among the early supporters of asset building were Jack Kemp, when he was Secretary of Housing and Urban Development, and then-Rep. Mike Espy, D-MS, who strongly advocated for IDAs within the Congressional Black Caucus and in the House of Representatives. IDAs were proposed by President Clinton as early as 1992 and were included in his 1994 welfare reform proposal. In the Congress, legislation for IDAs has been introduced since 1991 and was sponsored by Senators Coats, R-IN, and Moseley-Braun, D-IL, in the *Assets for Independence Act* in the 104th Congress (U.S. Senate, 1995), calling for a $100 million demonstration of IDAs over 4 years. IDAs and other asset-building proposals have broad bipartisan support and the co-sponsorship of black legislators of every political orientation, ranging from Maxine Waters, D-CA, to J. C. Watt, R-OK. All of these federal asset-building initiatives should be supported by every organization working with young black males.

IDAs in Welfare Reform. In the past, welfare recipients have not been able to accumulate more than a small amount of savings or they would lose eligibility. This counterproductive policy is being changed. IDA provisions are included in the Personal Responsibility and Work Opportunity Act (U.S. Congress, 1996); states can specify that they have an IDA program in their Temporary Assistance to Needy Families (TANF) state plans. The legislation specifies that only earned income (and matching funds) can be saved in IDAs; it designates not-for-profit community-based organizations as custodians of IDA accounts; and it permits IDAs to be used for education, home ownership, and small business capitalization. At this writing, 24 states have indicated in their TANF plans that they will allow IDAs to be created for families receiving assistance. IDAs in welfare reform present an unusual opportunity to work with children and adolescents. IDA programs can reach out to youth participants to open college savings accounts and start businesses. States can disregard the savings, assets, and income of children when determining the eligibility of their parents to receive government assistance.

States do not have to dedicate TANF dollars to IDAs to have a positive impact. The legal structure of an IDA can be used to catalyze involvement of nongovernmental sources of funding, such as employers, foundations, financial institutions, and religious institutions. For example, the National Congress of Black Churches is interested in IDA development, as are a number of United Ways around the country.

Another option for states is to require employers to contribute to the IDAs of welfare recipients whom they hire as employees and for whom they are receiving a wage subsidy. The full employment plans of Massachusetts, Mississippi, and Oregon have this provision. In these states, employers have already hired many welfare recipients and are putting aside up to one dollar per hour in wages into an IDA for training and skill development of the workers.

State IDA Policy. Welfare recipients generally make up only about 23% of the poor, and states should not limit IDAs to the welfare population. Black males who are poor could also benefit from IDAs. State policy should be patterned on the proposed federal IDA legislation to take advantage of this potential opportunity for funding. Sliding-scale matches, usually for households with income up to 200% of poverty, ensure that participants with different income levels can accumulate assets to meet life goals. States can consider a range of options for matching IDAs and encouraging the private sector to contribute to IDAs.

State Tax Incentives to Account Holders. These can include deductibility of savings in IDAs and exemption of earnings in the accounts. For low-income account holders, refundable tax credits, perhaps on a sliding scale, would be desirable. Iowa has pioneered this model, although with very small incentives. To be successful, tax credits should be at least 50% for the very poorest IDA participants. Experience in Iowa also suggests that states should provide some program operating expenses to community organizations who run IDA programs.

State Tax Incentives to Individual and Corporate Contributors to IDAs. States such as Colorado, Missouri, Pennsylvania, and Virginia have proposed this model. States that already have a Neighborhood Assistance Tax Credit Program (NAP), which provides a tax credit to contributors to community development organizations, can merely adapt this model for IDA funding. In Missouri, for example, pending legislation calls for $4 million in tax credits to IDA contributors. The tax credit would be 50%, and contributors would also be eligible for a federal income tax deduction because the money would be contributed to a nonprofit organization, thus making their total tax benefit

70% or more of contributed funds. This is extraordinary leverage for private donations, and the success of NAP in Missouri and other states suggests that this mechanism can generate private financial participation.

Community Development Funds, Low Income Housing and Home Ownership Funds, Scholarship Funds, Job Training Funds, and Microloan Funds for IDA Matches. Numerous existing funding streams to the states are candidates for IDA matching funds because IDAs are an effective mechanism for achieving goals in home ownership, education, job training, and microenterprise development.

States that adopt IDAs should include requirements and funding for monitoring and evaluation so that successes can be readily transferred from one state to another. If the IDA model is community based, then states should also provide at least modest support to community development organizations that create and administer IDA programs. One model, as in the Missouri tax credit legislation, is to allow up to 20% of all funding to be used for administration, with the remaining 80% or more available for IDA matching funds (State of Missouri, 1997). At this writing, over 30 states have enacted IDA programs in different forms (sometimes with variations on the name: Individual Asset Accounts, Individual Education Accounts, Family Development Accounts). Most of these are currently in the planning stages or are just getting under way. Because state IDA programs are typically community based, all organizations that work with young black males—schools, churches, sports associations, child welfare agencies, youth clubs, and juvenile justice agencies—should consider adding IDAs to their programming.

Asset Building in Community Development. Asset building is an emerging theme in community development (Sherraden & Ninacs, 1998). Community innovations in home ownership, micro enterprise, and savings clubs have expanded rapidly in recent years. Signaling this change in direction, the Ford Foundation has recently consolidated four antipoverty programs into a large new division under the heading of Asset Building and Community Development. The new program "is particularly interested in building assets— whether they are educational, financial, or control over natural resources— that can be passed from generation to generation" (Oliver, 1997, p. 8). Other foundations are beginning to follow this lead, so that resources for asset building in community development are likely to increase. IDAs are part of this trend. Design principles for IDAs should include the following. The purpose for establishing an IDA program should reflect the needs and life goals of the participants. The IDA program should be kept as simple as possible. The program should allow for adequate accumulation of savings to achieve a meaningful financial goal within 2 to 3 years. An economic literacy curriculum should accompany the IDA program. IDAs should be housed in a local financial institution that is committed to working with program staff and participants. Accounts should be interest bearing and free of any bank charges for the participant. More information on IDA design in community projects can be found in Grossman, Sahay, and Friedman (1996). Edwards (1997) describes several community IDA projects in detail and gives contact information. The web pages of the Corporation for Enterprise Development in Washington and the Center for Social Development at Washington University in St. Louis provide additional IDA information and resources.

Working With Individuals and Groups. Most of the chapters in this book focus on working with individuals or small groups, whereas the current chapter is mostly about advocacy, public policy, and community development. This does not mean that asset building is a "big idea" that is not directly relevant to working with individuals and small groups. Far from it. As examples, several different approaches to addressing asset inequality and wealth building are discussed briefly below.

Economic Education. One of the first things that should be done in working with young African American males and other low-wealth groups is to educate them in economic fundamentals. This should begin with personal economic concepts and strategies, covering the basics of income, budgeting, consumption, credit, saving, and investments. This knowledge is seldom covered in schools and is not present in most impoverished households. There are many innovative ways to engage young people in such economic literacy training. "Hands-on" projects are generally more effective than classroom study. A wide range of curriculum materials have been prepared by financial institutions, state governments, nonprofit organizations, and school systems.

Young black males should also have an appreciation of the history of race and assets and ongoing causes and consequences of asset inequality. Reading Oliver and Shapiro (1995) would be a good start. Let young black males learn from Ida B. Wells how a young couple, her close friends, were persecuted and the man eventually killed by whites simply because he owned a business. Let them learn from Charles Oubre about the inside dealings by whites and the loss of savings by blacks in the failure of the Freedmen's Bank. Let them learn from studies by the U.S. Federal Reserve about discrimination in home mortgage lending. If the texts are too complicated for young or poorly educated readers, then summaries, stories, tables, videos, overheads, and so forth can be obtained or created especially to get the materials across.

Community, Family, and Self-Assessment. In making the history and sociology of asset ownership directly relevant to young African American males, it will be useful for them to undertake assessments of asset ownership for their community, their family, and themselves. Depending on the educational level of the young men, different types of information and assessment tools can be developed for this purpose. The important messages in these exercises are that blacks, on average, have less than one tenth the net worth of whites and that this has direct relevance in their own lives, day in and day out.

Savings Groups and Investment Clubs. Modeled on grassroots experiences in impoverished nations, savings groups have been introduced into the United States (Keeley & Weiss, 1993). To date, most of these groups have been organized with welfare mothers and other low-wealth women. Savings clubs should also be initiated with other segments of the population, including young black males. A similar and much more common phenomenon is investment clubs. These number in the thousands, and they have their own associations that suggest guidelines and provide materials. Investment clubs serve both male and female membership, but they are concentrated among middle-class white households. This model, and the resources that have been developed for it, should be adapted to all low-wealth groups, including young African American males. Savings and investment clubs can be set up by any type of informal group or through formal organizations such as schools, youth organizations, sports teams, churches, social service agencies, and financial institutions.

Youth Entrepreneurship. African Americans have been systematically blocked from business ownership in the United States, and a culture of entrepreneurship has been slow to develop. Oliver and Shapiro (1995) warn that business ownership has been an economic detour for many African Americans because whites tend not to shop at black businesses. Nonetheless, business ownership will be essential if blacks are to accumulate their share of America's wealth. Black businesses tend to employ blacks, and although it is not the conventional wisdom, a strong emphasis on entrepreneurship could have a significantly positive impact on employment opportunities for young black males.

Youth entrepreneurship programs provide business and financial training to young people from the preteen years to adulthood. The programs are aimed at enabling participants to start and operate a business of their own. They operate in a wide variety of sites, including public schools, community centers, churches, community colleges, and universities. The oldest program,

Junior Achievement, was founded in 1919, and today, there are at least 15 national programs, 15 regional programs, and a large number of local programs. Junior Achievement alone enrolled 1.8 million young people in 1994. Although good evaluations have not been carried out, anecdotal reporting indicates that youth entrepreneurship programs generate not only an opportunity to earn money but also excitement, pride, and improved educational attainment. Program staff report that youths of all backgrounds can be taught the skills and attitudes required for business success.

More entrepreneurship programs for young black males are beginning to emerge. Expanding from its traditional white and middle-class base, Junior Achievement has taken steps to bring business savvy into the lives of urban minorities. Some corporations have instituted special business training programs in high schools. One of the most effective is the Financial Training Institute, spearheaded by Shearson/American Express, that serves mostly urban minority high school students, working in cooperation with local banks. In some cases, banks open branch offices in the schools as training centers. This program has the backing of the Office of the Comptroller of the Currency (OCC) and is expanding to more cities. In St. Louis, the OCC has approached the Center for Social Development at Washington University about the possibility of including IDAs with the Financial Training Institute.

Overall, there is evidence that youth entrepreneurship programs create opportunities for youths, open doors, successfully compete with street gangs, and improve educational motivation and performance. The program design is popular with business people and politicians, and it is an excellent focal point for mentors and volunteers.

Family Associations and Reunions. A vital institution for many African Americans is the family association and/or reunion, wherein extended family members renew kinship ties and maintain a network of support. The primary emphasis is usually social, but in some family association and reunion groups, economic aid, most often a fund for college education, is part of the support that is available. Family associations and reunions lend themselves to becoming centers of wealth building through periodic deposits, investments, and gradual accumulation. One mechanism would be the IDA (perhaps called the Family Development Account or some other name). The family can set up IDAs and begin deposits into accounts of all its children beginning at birth. Family fund-raisers can be used to strengthen family ties and generate deposits into IDAs for the next generation. The potential of family reunions as a vehicle for asset building is awaiting creative solutions that fit the circumstances and goals of each family group. The Family

Reunion Institute at Temple University holds a periodic conference on African American family reunions, and one of the usual sessions is on family economics, resources, and investments.

CONCLUSION

In closing, permit me to say a personal word on how I think about my work on asset building. As a personal compass, I have an image that guides me. The image is from 1870: An African American male, freed from slavery by the Civil War, is plowing a field under a blue sky. The 40-acre farm is his; he owns it outright. Across the field is a cabin where his wife is feeding chickens, watering seedlings of fruit trees, mending a gate, and tending her newborn child. They have a place to raise their family. They have a stake in the American economy, which they and their ancestors did so much to develop. They have neighbors on every side who also own their land; they are part of a community. This image fundamentally changes America; it assumes that freed slaves were given 40 acres and a mule after the Civil War, got a foothold in the American economy, and gradually recovered from the devastation of slavery. This could have happened, but it did not.

So I have another image; this one looks forward rather than backward. By the year 2020, I picture every child in America, including every black child, with an IDA for education. Every adult who wishes to own a home has a realistic opportunity to do so. The home ownership rate in the United States is 80% (up from 66% today), and there is no difference in home ownership by race. Discrimination in mortgage lending and property insurance has disappeared. Businesses both large and small are owned by men and women of every color. Stocks and bonds are owned by all Americans. This image also fundamentally changes America; it assumes that we begin today to undertake asset building for all young Americans, regardless of color.

References

Abrahamse, A. F., Morson, P., A., & Waite, L. J. (1988). *Beyond stereotypes: Who becomes a single teenage mother?* Santa Monica, CA: RAND.

Achatz, M., & MacAllum, C. A. (1994). *Young unwed fathers: Report from the field.* Philadelphia: Public/Private Ventures.

Ackerman, M. D., Montague, D. K., & Morganstern, S. (1994, March 15). Impotence: Help for erectile dysfunction. *Patient Care*, pp. 22-26.

Acosta, F. X., Yamamota, J., & Evans, L. A. (1982). *Effective psychotherapy for low-income and minority patients.* New York: Plenum.

Adalist Estrin, A. (1994). Family support and criminal justice. In S. L. Kagan & B. Weissbourd (Eds.), *Putting families first: America's family support movement and the challenge of change.* San Francisco: Jossey-Bass.

Adalist Estrin, A. (1995). Strengthening inmate-family relationships: Programs that work. *Corrections Today, 57*(7), 116-119.

Adams-Tucker, C., & Adams, P. (1984). Treatment of sexually abused children. In I. R. Stuart & J. G. Greer (Eds.), *Victims of sexual aggression: Treatment of children, women, and men* (pp. 57-74). New York: Van Nostrand Reinhold.

Adebimpe, V. R. (1981a). Hallucinations and delusions in black psychiatric patients. *Journal of the National Medical Association, 73,* 517-520.

Adebimpe, V. R. (1981b). Overview: White norms and psychiatric diagnosis of black patients. *American Journal of Psychiatry, 138,* 279-285.

Akbar, N. (1981). Mental disorder among African-Americans. *Black Books Bulletin, 7*(2), 18-25.

Akbar, N. (1991a). Mental disorders among African Americans. In R. L. Jones (Ed.), *Black psychology* (3rd ed., pp. 339-352). Berkeley, CA: Cobb & Harris.

Akbar, N. (1991b). *Visions for black men.* Nashville, TN: Winston-Derek.

Akers, R. L., Krohn, M. D., Lanza-Kaduce, L., & Radosevich, M. (1979). Social learning and deviant behavior: A specific test of a general theory. *American Sociological Review, 44,* 635-655.

Albrecht, S. (1992, June). Criminal aliens: What every officer should know. *Law and Order,* pp. 79-81.

Alexander, R., & Curtis, C. M. (1995). A critical review of strategies to reduce school violence. *Social Work in Education, 17,* 73-82.

Allen, J. S. (1937). *Reconstruction: The battle for democracy, 1865-1876.* New York: International Publishers.

Allen, W. R., Epps, E., & Haniff, N. Z. (1991). *College in black and white: African American students in predominantly white and in historically black public universities.* Albany: State University of New York Press.

Allen-Meares, P., & Burman, S. (1995). The endangerment of African-American men: An appeal for social work action. *Social Work, 40,* 268-274.

Allen-Meares, P., Washington, R., & Welsh, B. (1996). *Social work services in schools* (2nd ed.). Needham Heights, MA: Allyn & Bacon.

American Cancer Society. (1994). *Cancer facts and figures for minority Americans.* New York: Author.

American Cancer Society. (1997). *Cancer statistics 1997.* New York: Author.

American Psychiatric Association. (1987). *Diagnostic and statistical manual of mental disorders* (3rd ed., rev.). Washington, DC: Author.

American Psychiatric Association. (1994). *Diagnostic and statistical manual of mental disorders* (4th ed.). Washington, DC: Author.

Anderson, E. (1993). *Drugs and the inner-city family.* Washington, DC: Urban Institute.

Anderson, R. (1994). *Atlas of the American economy: An illustrated guide to industries and trends.* Washington, DC: Congressional Quarterly Press.

Anderson, R. M., Herman, W. H., Davis, J. M., et al. (1991). Barriers to improving diabetes care for blacks. *Diabetes Care, 14,* 605-609.

Angel, I. L., & Hogan, D. P. (1991). The demography of minority aging populations. In L. K. Harootyan (Ed.), *Minority elderly: Longevity, economics, and health. Building a policy base* (pp. 1-13). Washington, DC: Gerontological Society of America.

Asante, M. K. (1980). *Afrocentricity: The theory of social change.* Buffalo, NY: Amulefi.

Asante, M. K. (1987). *The Afrocentric idea.* Philadelphia: Temple University Press.

Ascher, C. (1992). Programs for African American males . . . and females. *Phi Delta Kappan, 73,* 777-782.

Ash, P., Kellermann, A., Fuqua-Whitley, D., & Johnson, A. (1996). Gun acquisition and use by juvenile offenders. *Journal of the American Medical Association, 275,* 1754-1758.

Astor, R., Behre, W., Fravil, K., & Wallace, J. (1997). Perceptions of school violence as a problem and reports of violent events: A national survey of school social workers. *Social Work, 42,* 55-68.

Astor, R., Behre, W., Wallace, J., & Fravil, K. (1998). School social workers and school violence: Personal safety, violence programs, and training. *Social Work, 43,* 223-232.

Astor, R., Meyer, H., & Behre, W. (in press). Unowned space and time in high schools: Mapping violence with students and teachers. *American Educational Research Journal.*

Astor, R. A. (1998). School violence: A blueprint for elementary school interventions. In E. M. Freeman, C. G. Franklin, R. Fong, G. Shaffer, & E. M. Timberlake (Eds.), *Multisystemic skills and interventions in school social work practice* (pp. 281-295). Washington, DC: NASW Press.

Atkinson, D. R., Morten, G., & Sue, D. W. (1993). *Counseling American minorities: A cross-cultural perspective.* Madison, WI: Brown and Benchmark.

Azibo, D. A. (1989). African-centered theses on mental health and a nosology of black/African personality disorder. *Journal of Black Psychology, 15*(2), 173-214.

Baker, F. M. (1982). The black elderly: Biopsychosocial perspective within an age cohort and adult development context. *Journal of Geriatric Psychiatry, 15*(2), 227-239.

Baker, F. M. (1985). Group psychotherapy with patients over 50: An adult development approach. *Journal of Geriatric Psychiatry, 17*(1), 79-101.

Baker, F. M. (1987). The Afro-American life cycle: Success, failure, and mental health. *Journal of the National Medical Association, 79*(6), 625-633.

Baker, F. M. (1994a). Psychiatric treatment of older African Americans. *Hospital and Community Psychiatry, 45*(1), 32-37.

Baker, F. M. (1994b). Suicide among ethnic minority elderly. *Journal of Geriatric Psychiatry, 27*(2), 241-264.

Baker, F. M. (1995). Misdiagnosis among older psychiatric patients. *Journal of the National Medical Association, 87*(12), 872-876.

Baker, F. M., Lavizzo-Mourey, R., & Jones, B. E. (1993). Acute care of the African American elder. *Journal of Geriatric Psychiatry and Neurology, 6*(2), 66-71.

Baker, F. M., Robinson, B. H., & Stewart, B. (1993). Use of the Mini-Mental State Examination in African American elders. *Clinical Gerontologist, 14*(1), 15-29.

Baker, F. M., Vellie, S. A., Friedman, J., & Wiley, C. (1995). Screening tests for depression in black and white patients. *American Journal of Geriatric Psychiatry, 3*(1), 45-51.

Ball, A. (1995). Text design patterns in the writing of urban African American students: Teaching to the cultural strengths of students in multicultural settings. *Urban Education, 30*(3), 253-289.

Ballen, J., & Freeman, R. (1986). Transitions between employment and nonemployment. In R. Freeman & H. Holzer (Eds.), *The black youth employment crisis.* Chicago: University of Chicago Press.

Ball-Rokeach, S. (1973). Values and violence: A test of the subculture of violence thesis. *American Sociological Review, 38,* 736-749.

Baly, I. (1989). Career and vocational development of Black youth. In R. L. Jones (Ed.), *Black adolescents* (pp. 249-265). Berkeley, CA: Cobb & Henry.

Bandura, A. (1977). Self-efficacy: Toward a unifying theory of behavioral change. *Psychological Review, 84,* 191-215.

Baquet, C. R. (1988). Cancer prevention and control in the black population: Epidemiology and aging considerations. In J. S. Jackson (Ed.), *The Black American elderly: Research and physical and psychosocial health* (pp. 50-68). New York: Springer.

Barber, J., & Munn, A. (1993, March). *Male involvement.* Symposium conducted at the Annual Conference of the Indiana Council on Adolescent Pregnancy, Indianapolis, IN.

Barth, R. P., Claycomb, M., & Loomis, A. (1988). Services to adolescent fathers. *Health and Social Work, 13,* 277-287.

Bartollas, C., & Miller, S. (1994) *Juvenile delinquency in America.* Englewood Cliffs, NJ: Regents/Prentice Hall.

Battle, S. F. (1988/1989, Summer/Winter). African-American male responsibility in teenage pregnancy: The role of education. *Urban League Review,* pp. 71-81.

Baugh, J. (1983). *Black street speech: Its history, structure, and survival.* Austin: University of Texas Press.

Beam, J. (1986). Brother to brother: Words from the heart. In J. Beam (Ed.), *In the life: A black gay anthology* (pp. 230-242). Boston: Alyson.

Belcastro, P. A. (1985). Sexual behavior differences between black and white students. *Journal of Sex Research, 21,* 56-67.

Bell, A. P., & Weinberg, M. S. (1978). *Homosexualities: A study of diversity among men and women.* New York: Simon & Schuster.

Bell, C., & Jenkins, E. (1991). Traumatic stress and children. *Journal of Health Care for the Poor and Underserved, 2,* 175-185.

Bell, C., & Mehta, H. (1979). The misdiagnosis of black patients with manic-depressive illness. *Journal of the National Medical Association, 72,* 141-145.

Bell, C. C., Thompson, J. P., Lewis, D., Redd, J., Shears, M., & Thompson, B. (1985). Misdiagnosis of alcohol-related organic brain syndromes: Implications for treatment. In F. L. Brisbane & M. Womble (Eds.), *Treatment of black alcoholics* (pp. 45-65). New York: Haworth.

Belle, D. (Ed.). (1982). *Lives in stress: Women and depression.* Beverly Hills, CA: Sage.

Benson, G. P., Haycraft, J. L., Steyaert, J. P., & Weigel, D. J. (1979). Mobility in sixth graders as related to achievement, adjustment, and socioeconomic status. *Psychology in the Schools, 16,* 444-447.

Berliner, L., & Ernest, E. (1984). Group work with pre-adolescent sexual assault victims. In I. R. Stuart & J. G. Greer (Eds.), *Victims of sexual aggressions: Treatment of children, women, and men* (pp. 105-126). New York: Van Nostrand Reinhold.

Berman, S., & Wandersman, A. (1990). Fear of cancer and knowledge of cancer: A review and proposed relevance to hazardous waste sites. *Social Science & Medicine, 31,* 81-90.

Billy, O. G., Tanfer, K., Grady, W. R., & Klepinger, D. H. (1993). The sexual behavior of men in the United States. *Family Planning Perspectives, 25*(2), 52-60.

Blake, W. M., & Darling, C. A. (1994). The dilemmas of the African American male. *Journal of Black Studies, 24*(4), 402-415.

Bloch, F. (1994). *Antidiscrimination law and minority employment.* Chicago: University of Chicago Press.

Block, C. R., Antigone, C., Jacob, A., & Przyblski, R. (1996). *Street gangs and crime: Patterns and trends in Chicago* (Research Bulletin). Chicago: Illinois Criminal Justice Information Authority.

Block, C. R., & Block, R. (1993). *Street gangs in Chicago.* Washington, DC: U.S. Department of Justice, National Institute of Justice.

Bloom, B., & Steinhart, D. (1993). *Why punish the children? A reappraisal of the children of incarcerated mothers in America.* San Francisco: National Council on Crime and Delinquency.

Bloomer, K. (1997, March 17). America's newest growth industry. *In These Times,* pp. 14-18.

Blum, D. (1990). Psychosocial support for the man with prostate cancer. *Primary Care & Cancer, 10,* 37-43.

Blumstein, A. (1993). Making rationality relevant—The American Society of Criminology 1992 Presidential Address. *Criminology, 31*(1), 1-16.

Bolton, F. G., Morris, L. A., & MacEachron, A. E. (1989). *Males at risk: The other side of child sexual abuse.* Newbury Park, CA: Sage.

Bonilla, L., & Porter, J. (1990). A comparison of Latino, black, and non-Hispanic whites' attitudes toward homosexuality. *Hispanic Journal of Behavioral Sciences, 12*(4), 437-452.

Booth, A., Johnson, D., White, L., & Edwards, J. (1986). Divorce and marital instability over the life course. *Journal of Family Issues, 7,* 421-442.

Borden, W. (1992). Narrative perspectives in psychosocial intervention following adverse life events. *Social Work, 37*(2), 135-141.

Botvin, G. J., Baker, E., Dusenbury, L., Tortu, S., & Botvin, E. M. (1990). Preventing adolescent drug abuse through a multi-modal cognitive-behavioral approach: Results of a three year study. *Journal of Consulting and Clinical Psychology, 58*(4), 437-446.

Bound, J., & Freeman, R. (1992). What went wrong? The erosion of gains in relative earnings among blacks. *Quarterly Journal of Economics, 107*(1), 201-232.

Bound, J., & Holzer, H. (1993). Industrial shifts, skill levels, and the labor market for whites and blacks. *Review of Economics and Statistics, 75*(3), 387-396.

Bowen, M. (1978). *Family therapy in clinical practice.* New York: Jason Aronson.

Bowman, P. J. (1989). Research perspectives on black men: Role strain and adaptation across the black adult male life cycle. In R. L. Jones (Ed.), *Black adult development and aging* (pp. 117-150). Berkeley, CA: Cobb and Henry.

Bowman, P. J. (1992). Coping with provider role strain: Adaptive cultural resources among Black husband-fathers. In A. K. H. Burlew, W. C. Banks, H. P. McAdoo, & D. A. Azibo (Eds.), *African American psychology: Theory, research, and practice* (pp. 135-151). Newbury Park, CA: Sage.

Bowman, P. J. (1993). The impact of economic marginality among African American husbands and fathers. In H. P. McAdoo (Ed.), *Family ethnicity: Strength in diversity* (pp. 120-137). Newbury Park, CA: Sage.

Boyd, H., & Allen, R. (Eds.). (1996). *Brotherman: The odyssey of black men in America—An anthology.* New York: One World.

Boyd-Franklin, N. (1989). *Black families in therapy: A multisystem approach.* New York: Guilford.

Boykin, A. W. (1983). The academic performance of Afro-American children. In J. T. Spence (Ed.), *Achievement and achievement motives: Psychological and sociological approaches* (pp. 321-371). San Francisco: W. H. Freeman.

Boykin, K. (1996). *One more river to cross: Black and gay in America.* New York: Doubleday.

Branch, T. (1988). *Parting of the waters: America in the King years, 1954-63.* New York: Simon & Schuster.

Brashears, F., & Roberts, M. (1996). The black church as resource for change. In S. L. Logan (Ed.), *The black family: Strengths, self-help, and positive change* (pp. 181-192). Boulder, CO: Westview.

Braus, P. (1996). Why does cancer cluster? *American Demographics, 18,* 36-41.

Brewer, D. A., Hawkins, J. D., Catalano, R. F., & Neckerman, H. J. (1995). Preventing serious, violent, and chronic offending: A review of selected strategies in childhood, adolescence, and the community. In J. C. Howell, B. Krisberg, J. D. Hawkins, & J. J. Wilson (Eds.), *A sourcebook: Serious, violent, and chronic juvenile delinquents* (pp. 61-141). Thousand Oaks, CA: Sage.

Brindis, C., Barth, R. P., & Loomis, A. B. (1987). Continuous counseling: Case management with teenage parents. *Social Casework: The Journal of Contemporary Social Work, 68,* 164-192.

Brindis, C. D. (1993, March). Keynote address at the Annual Conference of the Indiana Council on Adolescent Pregnancy, Indianapolis, IN.

Brockman, M. A., & Reeves, A. W. (1967). Relationship between transiency and test achievement. *Alberta Journal of Educational Research, 13,* 319-330.

Broman, C. L. (1987). Race differences in professional help seeking. *American Journal of Community Psychology, 15*(4), 473-489.

Brookins, C. C., & Robinson, T. L. (1995). Rites-of-passage as resistance to oppression. *Western Journal of Black Studies, 19,* 172-180.

Brophy, J., & Good, T. (1986). Teacher behavior and student achievement. In M. C. Wittrock (Ed.), *Handbook of research on teaching* (3rd ed., pp. 328-375). New York: Macmillan.

Brown, A. L., & Campione, J. C. (1994). Guided discovery in a community of learners. In K. McGilly (Ed.), *Classroom lessons: Integrating cognitive theory and classroom practice* (pp. 229-270). Cambridge: MIT Press.

Brown, C. (1965). *Manchild in the promised land.* New York: Signet.

Brown, S. (1990). *If the shoes fit: Final report and program implementation guide of the Maine Young Fathers Project.* Portland: Human Services Development Institute, University of Southern Maine.

Brown, W. K. (1978). Black gangs as family extensions. *International Journal of Offender Therapy and Comparative Criminology, 22*(1), 39-48.

Bursik, R., & Grasmick, H. (1993). *Neighborhoods and crime: The dimensions of effective community control.* New York: Lexington.

Bursik, R. J. (1988). Social disorganization and theories of crime and delinquency: Problems and prospect. *Criminology, 26,* 522.

Butts, J. B. (1989). Adolescent sexuality and teen pregnancy from a Black perspective. In N. Cervera & L. Videka-Sherman (Eds.), *Working with pregnant and parenting teenage clients* (pp. 146-157). Milwaukee, WI: Family Service America.

Butts, J. D. (1988). Sex therapy, intimacy, and the role of black population in the AIDS era. *Journal of the National Medical Association, 80,* 916-922.

Cairns, R. B., & Cairns, B. D. (1991). Social cognition and social networks: A developmental perspective. In D. J. Pepler & K. H. Rubin (Eds.), *The development and treatment of childhood aggression* (pp. 249-278). Hillsdale, NJ: Lawrence Erlbaum.

Campbell, B. M. (1986). *Successful women, angry men: Backlash in the two-career marriage.* New York: Random House.

Campbell, B. M. (1989). To be black, gifted, and alone. In N. Hare & J. Hare (Eds.), *Crisis in black sexual politics* (pp. 127-136). San Francisco: Black Think Tank.

Card, J. J., & Wise, L. L. (1978). Teenage mothers and teenage fathers: The impact of early childbearing on their personal and professional lives. *Family Planning Perspectives, 10,* 199-205.

Carnegie Council on Adolescent Development. (1993). *A matter of time: Risk and opportunity in nonschool hours.* New York: Author.

Carrera, M. A. (1992). Involving adolescent males in pregnancy and STD prevention programs. *Adolescent Medicine: State of the Art Reviews, 3,* 1-13.

Cass, V. C. (1979). Homosexual identity formation: A theoretical model. *Journal of Homosexuality, 4*(3), 219-235.

Cazenave, N. (1981). Black men in America: The quest for manhood. In H. P. McAdoo (Ed.), *Black families.* Beverly Hills, CA: Sage.

Chadiha, L. (1992). Black husbands' economic problems and resiliency during the transition to marriage. *Families in Society, 73,* 542-552.

Chatters, L. (1991) Physical health. In J. S. Jackson (Ed.), *Life in black America* (pp. 199-220). Newbury Park, CA: Sage.

Cheatham, H. E. (1990a). Africentricity and development of African-Americans. *Career Development Quarterly, 38,* 334-346.

Cheatham, H. E. (1990b). Empowering black families. In H. E. Cheatham & J. B. Stewart (Eds.), *Black families* (pp. 373-394). New Brunswick, NJ: Transaction Publishers.

Chestang, L. (1976). The black family and black culture: A study in copying. In M. Sotomayer (Ed.), *Cross-cultural perspectives in social work practice and education.* Houston, TX: University of Houston Graduate School of Social Work.

Children's Defense Fund. (1994). *The state of America's children: Yearbook, 1994.* Washington, DC: Author.

Christoffel, K. (1990). Violent death and injury in U.S. children and adolescents. *American Journal of Diseases of Childhood, 144,* 697-706.

Cimbolic, P. (1972). Counselor race and experience effects on black clients. *Journal of Counseling and Clinical Psychology, 39,* 328-332.

Clayton, L., & Byrd, W. (1993). The African-American cancer crisis, Part 1: The problem. *Journal of Health Care for the Poor and Underserved, 4,* 83-87.

Cloward, R., & Ohlin, L. E. (1960). *Delinquency and opportunity: A theory of delinquent gangs.* Glencoe, IL: Free Press.

Cochran, S. D., & Mays, V. M. (1994). Depressive distress among homosexually active African American men and women. *American Journal of Psychiatry, 151*(4), 524-529.

Cohen, E. C., Rachel, A., & Lotean, C. (1994). Producing equal-status interaction in the heterogeneous classroom. *American Educational Research Journal, 32,* 99-121.

Cohen, P., Johnson, J., Struening, E. L., & Brook, J. S. (1989). Family mobility as a risk for childhood psychopathology. In B. Cooper & T. Helgason (Eds.), *Epidemiology and the prevention of mental disorders.* New York: Routledge.

Coie, J. D., Underwood, M., & Lochman, J. E. (1991). Programmatic intervention with aggressive children in the school setting. In D. J. Pepler & K. H. Rubin (Eds.), *The development and treatment of childhood aggression* (pp. 389-410). Hillsdale, NJ: Lawrence Erlbaum.

Colarusso, C. A., & Nemiroff, R. A. (1987). Clinical implications of adult developmental theory. *American Journal of Psychiatry, 144,* 1263-1270.

Cole, M. (1996). *Cultural psychology: A once and future discipline.* Cambridge, MA: Belknap.

Coleman, D., & Baker, F. M. (1994). Misdiagnosis of schizophrenia among older, black veterans. *Journal of Nervous and Mental Disease, 182*(9), 527-528.

Collins, R. L. (1993). Responding to cultural diversity in schools. In L. A. Castenell, Jr., & W. F. Pinar (Eds.), *Understanding curriculum as racial text: Representations of identity and difference in education* (pp. 195-208). Albany: SUNY Press.

Comer, J. (1988, November). Educating poor minority children. *Scientific American, 259*(5), 42-48.

Comer, J. P. (1980). *School power: Implications of an intervention.* New York: Free Press.

Compton, B., & Galaway, B. (1994). *Social work processes.* Pacific Grove, CA: Brooks/Cole.

Connor, M. J. (1995). *What is cool: Understanding black manhood in America.* New York: Crown.

Constantino, G., Malgady, R. G., & Rogler, L. H. (1990). Culturally sensitive psychotherapy for Puerto Rican children and adolescents: A program of treatment outcome research. *Journal of Consulting and Clinical Psychology, 58*(6), 704-712.

Coppock Warfield, N. (1990). *Afrocentric theory and applications: Vol. 1. Adolescent rites of passage.* Washington, DC: Baobab Associates.

Coppock Warfield, N. (1992). The rites of passage movement: A resurgence of African-centered practices for socializing African American youth. *Journal of Negro Education, 61*(4), 471-482.

Cose, E. (1993). *The rage of a privileged class: Why are middle-class blacks angry? Why should America care?* New York: HarperCollins.

Courtwright, D. (1996). What human nature and the California Gold Rush tell us about crime in the inner city: Violence in America. *American Heritage,* pp. 38-51.

Covey, H., Menard, S., & Franzere, R. J. (1992). *Juvenile gangs.* Springfield, IL: Charles C Thomas.

Crawley, B. H. (1996). Effective programs and services for African American families and children: An African-centered perspective. In S. L. Logan (Ed.), *The black family: Strengths, self-help, and positive change* (pp. 112-130). Boulder, CO: Westview.

Crawley, B., & Freeman, E. (1993). Themes in the life views of older and younger African American males. *Journal of African American Studies, 1*(1), 15-29.

Cross, W. E. (1971). The Negro-to-black conversion experience. *Black World, 20,* 12-27.

Cross, W. E. (1991). *Shades of black diversity in African American identity.* Philadelphia: Temple University Press.

Cross, W. E. (1995). The psychology of Nigrescence: Revising the Cross model. In J. G. Ponterotto, J. M. Casas, L. A. Suzuki, & C. M. Alexander (Eds.), *Handbook of multicultural counseling* (pp. 93-122). Thousand Oaks, CA: Sage.

Cross, W. E., Parham, T. A., & Helms, J. E. (1991). The stages of black identity development: Nigresence models. In R. I. Jones (Ed.), *Black psychology* (3rd ed., pp. 319-338). Berkeley, CA: Cobb & Henry.

Cummings, J. (1986). Empowering minority students: A framework for intervention. *Harvard Educational Review, 56,* 18-36.

Curry, G. D., Ball, R., & Fox, R. J. (1994). *Gang crime and law enforcement record-keeping* (Research in brief). Washington, DC: National Institute of Justice.

Curry, G. D., & Spergel, I. (1988). Gang homicide, delinquency, and community. *Criminology, 26,* 381-405.

Curry, G. D., & Spergel, I. A. (1992). Gang involvement and delinquency among Hispanic and African-American adolescent males. *Journal of Research on Crime and Delinquency, 29*(3), 273-291.

Curtis, L. (1975). *Violence, race, and culture.* Lexington, MA: D. C. Heath.

Daly, A., Jennings, J., Beckett, J., & Leashore, B. (1995). Effective coping strategies of African Americans. *Social Work, 40,* 240-248.

D'Andrea, M., & Daniels, J. (1992). A career development program for inner-city youth. *Career Development Quarterly, 40,* 272-280.

Danziger, S., & Gottschalk, P. (1995). *America unequal.* New York: Russell Sage Foundation.

Darder, A. (1995). Bicultural identity and the development of voice: Twin issues in the struggle for cultural and linguistic democracy. In J. Frederickson (Ed.), *Reclaiming our voices* (pp. 35-52). Ontario: California Association for Bilingual Education.

D'Augelli, A. R. (1994). Identity development and sexual orientation: Toward a model of lesbian, gay, and bisexual development. In E. J. Trickett, R. J. Watts, & D. Birman (Eds.), *Human diversity: Perspectives on people in context* (pp. 312-333). San Francisco: Jossey-Bass.

Davis, J. (1994). College in black and white: Campus environment and academic achievement of African American males. *Journal of Negro Education, 63*(4), 620-633.

Davis, J. E., & Jordan, W. J. (1994). The effects of school context, structure, and experiences on African American males in middle and high school. *Journal of Negro Education, 63,* 570-587.

Davis, L. (1993). *Black and single.* Chicago: Noble Press.

Davis, L., & Proctor, E. (1989). *Race, gender, and class: Guidelines for practice with individuals, families, and groups.* Englewood Cliffs, NJ: Prentice Hall.

Davis, L. E. (1984). Essential components of group work with Black Americans. *Social Work With Groups, 7*(3), 97-109.

Davis, L. E. (1985). Groupwork with ethnic minorities of color. In M. Sandel, P. Glassen, R. Sarri, & R. Vinter (Eds.), *Individual change through small groups* (2nd ed., pp. 324-343). New York: Free Press.

Dawsey, D. (1996). *Living to tell about it: Young black men in America speak their piece.* New York: Anchor Books.

Decker, S. H. (1996). Gang violence as collective behavior. *Justice Quarterly, 13,* 243-264.

Decker, S. H., & Lauritsen, J. L. (1996). Leaving the gang: Breaking the bonds of membership. In C. R. Huff (Ed.), *Gangs in America* (2nd ed.). Thousand Oaks, CA: Sage.

Decker, S. H., & Pennell, S. (1996). *Understanding the illegal firearms market* (Research in brief). Washington, DC: National Institute of Justice.

Decker, S. H., & Van Winkle, B. (1994). "Slinging dope": The role of gangs and gang members in drug sales. *Justice Quarterly, 11,* 583-604.

Decker, S. H., & Van Winkle, B. (1996). *Life in the gang: Family, friends, and violence.* New York: Cambridge University Press.

Delpit, L. (1995). *Other people's children: Cultural conflict in the classroom.* New York: New Press.

Delpit, L. D. (1988). The silenced dialogue: Power and pedagogy in educating other people's children. *Harvard Educational Review, 58,* 280-298.

DeMarco, J. (1983). Gay racism. In M. J. Smith (Ed.), *Black men/white men: A gay anthology* (pp. 109-118). San Francisco: Gay Sunshine Press.

Demark-Wahnefrid, W., Strigo, T., Catoe, K., Conaway, M., Brunetti, M., Rimer, B., & Robertson, C. (1995). Knowledge, beliefs, and prior screening behavior among blacks and whites reporting for prostate cancer screening. *Journal of Urology, 46,* 346-351.

Devore, W., & Schlesinger, E.G. (1991). *Ethnic-sensitive social work practice* (3rd ed.). New York: Macmillan.

Diabetes Control and Complications Trial Research Group. (1993). The effect of intensive treatment of diabetes on the development and progression of long-term complications in insulin-dependent diabetes mellitus. *New England Journal of Medicine, 329,* 977-986.

Diabetes in the elderly. (1994). In V. Peragallo-Dittko, K. Godley, & J. Meyer (Eds.), *A core curriculum for diabetes educators* (2nd ed., pp. 477-496). Chicago: American Association of Diabetes Educators.

Dillard, J. M. (1980). Some unique career behavior characteristics of blacks: Career theories, counseling practice, and research. *Journal of Employment Counseling, 17,* 288-298.

Dodge, K. A. (1991). The structure and function of reactive and proactive aggression. In D. J. Pepler & K. H. Rubin (Eds.), *The development and treatment of childhood aggression* (pp. 201-218). Hillsdale, NJ: Lawrence Erlbaum.

Dohrenwend, B. P. (1966). Social status and psychological disorder: An issue of substance and an issue of method. *American Sociological Review, 31,* 14-34.

Dohrn, B. (1995, December). Undemonizing our children. *Education Digest, 61,* 4-6.

Douglass, F. (1874, June 25). *New National Era.*

Dowd, S. (1995). Therapeutic challenges in counseling African American gay men with HIV/AIDS. In W. Odets & M. Shernoff (Eds.), *The second decade of AIDS: A mental health practice handbook.* New York: Hatherleigh.

Dryfoos, J. (1990). *Adolescents at risk: Prevalence and prevention.* New York: Edna McConnell Clark Foundation.

Du Bois, W. E. B. (1968). *Black reconstruction.* Cleveland: Meridian Books. (Original work published 1935)

Du Bois, W. E. B. (1970). *The souls of black folk.* Greenwich, CT: Fawcett. (Original work published 1903)

Duncan, G. (1993). Racism as a developmental mediator. *Educational Forum, 57*(4), 360-370.

Duncan, G. (1997, November). *Black adolescent voices: Moral considerations in an informational age.* Paper presented at Voices of Care and Justice: Enhancing the Dialogue among Theorists, Researchers, and Practicitioners, the 23rd Annual Conference of the Association for Moral Education, Emory University, Atlanta, GA.

Duneier, M. (1992). *Slim's table: Race, respectability, and masculinity.* Chicago: University of Chicago Press.

Dupper, D. R., & Halter, A. P. (1994). Barriers in educating children from homeless shelters: Perspectives of school and shelter staff. *Social Work in Education, 16,* 39-45.

Durkheum, E. (1951). *Suicide, a study in sociology* (J. A. Spaulding & G. Simpson, Eds.; G. Simpson, Trans.). Glencoe, IL: Free Press.

Eckenrode, J., Rowe, E., Laird, M., & Brathwaite, J. (1995). Mobility as a mediator of the effects of child maltreatment on academic performance. *Child Development, 66,* 1130-1142.

344 ◪ WORKING WITH AFRICAN AMERICAN MALES

Edgar, T., Freimuth, V. S., & Hammond, S. L. (1988). Communicating the AIDS risk to college students: The problem of motivating change. *Health Education Research, 3*, 59-65.

The Education Trust. (1996). *Education watch: The 1996 Education Trust state and national data book.* Washington, DC: Author.

Edwards, K. (1997). *Individual development accounts: Creative savings for families and communities* (policy report). St. Louis: Center for Social Development, Washington University.

Einbender, A.,J. (1991). Treatment in the absence of maternal support. In W. N. Fredich (Eds.), *Casebook of sexual abuse treatment* (pp. 112-136). New York: Norton.

Elam, S. M., Rose, L. C., & Gallup, A. M. (1994, September). The 26th annual Phi Delta Kappa/Gallup poll of the public's attitudes toward the public schools. *Phi Delta Kappan, 76*, 41-56.

Eller, T. J., & Fraser, W. (1995). *Asset ownership of households: 1993* (Current Population Reports P70-47). Washington, DC: Government Printing Office.

Elliott, D., & Voss, H. (1974). *Delinquency and dropout.* Lexington, MA: D. C. Heath.

Elliott, D. S., Ageton, S. A., & Canter, R. J. (1980). Reconciling race and class differences in self-report and official estimates of delinquency. *American Sociological Review, 45*, 95-110.

Elliott, D. S., Huizinga, D., & Ageton, S. (1985). *Explaining delinquency and drug use.* Beverly Hills, CA: Sage.

Ellison, R. (1989). *Invisible man.* New York: Vintage. (Original work published 1947)

Engle, G. (1977). The need for a new medical model: A challenge for biomedicine. *Science, 196*, 129-136.

Engle, G. (1980). The clinical application of the biopsychosocial model. *American Journal of Psychiatry, 137*, 535-544.

Erickson, F. D. (1982). Taught cognitive learning in its immediate environments: A neglected topic in the anthropology of education. *Anthropology and Education Quarterly, 13*, 149-180.

Erickson, F. D. (1984). School literacy, reasoning and civility: An anthropologist's perspective. *Review of Educational Research, 54*, 525-546.

Erickson, F. D. (1987). Transformation and school success: The politics and culture of educational achievement. *Anthropology and Education Quarterly, 18*, 335-356.

Erickson, R. J., & Gecas, V. (1991). Social class and fatherhood. In F. W. Bozett & S. M. H. Hanson (Eds.), *Fatherhood and families in cultural context* (pp. 114-137). New York: Springer.

Erlanger, H. S. (1974). The empirical status of the subculture of violence thesis. *Social Problems, 22*, 280-292.

Ernst, F. A., Francis, R. A., Nevels, H., Collipp, B. S., & Lewis, A. (1991). Racial differences in affirmation of personal habit change to prevent HIV infection. *Preventive Medicine, 80*, 529-533.

Ernst, F. A., Francis, R. A., Nevels, H., & Lemeh, C. (1991). Condemnation of homosexuality in the black community: A gender-specific phenomenon? *Archives of Sexual Behavior, 20*(6), 579-585.

Ewalt, P. L., Freeman, E. M., Kirk, S. A., & Poole, D. L. (Eds.). (1996). *Multicultural issues in social work*. Washington, DC: NASW Press.

Faderman, L. (1984). The "new gay" lesbians. *Journal of Homosexuality, 10*(3/4), 85-95.

Faller, K. C. (1988). *Child sexual abuse: An interdisciplinary manual for diagnosis, case management, and treatment*. New York: Columbia University Press.

Farley, R. (1980). Homicide trends in United States. *Demography, 17,* 177-188.

Faubert, M., Locke, D. C., Sprinthall, N. A., & Howland, W. H. (1996). Promoting cognitive and ego development of African-American rural youth: A program of deliberate psychological education. *Journal of Adolescence, 19,* 533-543.

Federal Bureau of Investigation. (1995). *Uniform crime reports 1994*. Washington, DC: Government Printing Office.

Federal Bureau of Investigation. (1996). *Uniform crime reports 1995*. Washington, DC: Government Printing Office.

Felner, R. D., Primavera, J., & Cause, A. M. (1981). The impact of school transitions: A focus for preventive efforts. *American Journal of Community Psychology, 9,* 449-459.

Ferguson, R., & Filer, R. (1986). Do better jobs make better workers? Absenteeism from work among inner-city youth. In R. Freeman & H. Holzer (Eds.), *The black youth employment crisis*. Chicago: University of Chicago Press.

Ferguson, R. F. (1994). How professionals in community-based programs perceive and respond to the needs of Black male youth. In R. B. Mincy (Ed.), *Nurturing young black males* (pp. 59-98). Washington, DC: Urban Institute Press.

Fillenbaum, G. G., Heyman, A., Williams, K., Prosnit, B., & Burchett, B. (1990). Sensitivity and specificity of standardized screens for cognitive impairment and dementia among elderly black and white community residents. *Journal of Clinical Epidemiology, 43,* 651-660.

Finkelhor, D. (1986). *A source book on child sexual abuse*. Beverly Hills, CA: Sage.

Finney Hairston, C. (1991). Family ties during imprisonment: Important to who and for what? *Journal of Sociology and Social Welfare, 18*(1), 85-104.

Fishman, L. T. (1988). Prisoners and their wives: Marital and domestic effects of telephone contacts and home visits. *International Journal of Offender Therapy and Comparative Criminology, 32*(1), 55-65.

Fitzpatrick, K., & Boldizar, J. (1993). The prevalence and consequences of exposure to violence among African American youth. *Journal of the American Academy of Child and Adolescent Psychiatry, 32*(2), 424-431.

Fix, M., & Struyk, R. (1994). *Clear and convincing evidence*. Washington DC: Urban Institute Press.

Fleming, J. (1984). *Blacks in college: A comparative study of student success in black and white institutions*. San Francisco: Jossey-Bass.

Flores, B., Cousin, P., & Diaz, E. (1991). Transforming deficit myths about learning, language, and culture. *Language Arts, 68,* 369-379.

Folstein, M. F., Folstein, S. E., & McHugh, P. R. (1975). Mini-mental state: A practical method for grading the cognitive state of patients for the clinician. *Journal of Psychiatric Research, 12,* 189-198.

Fordham, S., & Ogbu, J. (1986). Black students' school success: Coping with the burden of "acting white." *Urban Review, 18,* 176-206.

Fox, J. A. (1995). *Trends in juvenile violence.* Washington, DC: Bureau of Justice Statistics, U.S. Department of Justice.

Frank, C. R. (1996, April). *Multiple positions and positionings in a bilingual homework center.* Paper presented at the annual meeting of the American Educational Research Association, New York City.

Franklin, A. J. (1989). Therapeutic interventions with urban black adolescents. In R. L. Jones (Ed.), *Black adolescents* (pp. 309-337). Berkeley, CA: Cobb & Henry.

Franklin, A. J. (1992). Therapy with African American men. *Families in Society, 73,* 350-355.

Franklin, A. J. (1993, July/August). The invisibility syndrome. *The Family Therapy Networker,* pp. 32-39.

Franklin, A. J. (1997, summer). Importance of friendship issues between African American men in a therapeutic support group. *Journal of African American Men, 3*(1), 29-43.

Franklin, C., II. (1992). Hey, home-yo, bro: Friendships among black men. In P. Nardi (Ed.), *Men's friendship* (pp. 201-214). Newbury Park, CA: Sage.

Franz, M. (Ed.). (1994). *Maximizing the role of nutrition in diabetes management.* Alexandria, VA: American Diabetes Association.

Frederich, W. (1995). *Psychotherapy with sexually abused boys.* Thousand Oaks, CA: Sage.

Freeman, E. M. (1990). Theoretical perspectives for practice with black families. In S. M. L. Logan, E. M. Freeman, & R. G. McRoy (Eds.), *Social work practice with black families: A culturally specific perspective* (pp. 38-52). New York: Longman.

Freeman, E. M., & O'Dell, K. (1993). Helping multicultural communities redefine self-sufficiency from the person-in-environment perspective. *Journal of Intergroup Relations, 40,* 38-53.

Freeman, H. (1990). Cancer in the socioeconomically disadvantaged. In *Cancer in the socioeconomically disadvantaged* (pp. 4-26). New York: American Cancer Society.

Freeman, R. (1992). Crime and the employment of disadvantaged youth. In G. Peterson & W. Vroman (Eds.), *Urban labor markets and job opportunities.* Washington, DC: Urban Institute Press.

Freeman, R. (1996, May/June). Labor market institutions and earnings inequality. *New England Economic Review,* pp. 157-168.

Freeman, R., & Holzer, H. (1986). *The black youth employment crisis.* Chicago: University of Chicago Press.

Freire, P. (1989). *Pedagogy of the oppressed.* New York: Continuum.

Freire, P. (1990). *Pedagogy of the oppressed.* New York: Continuum. (Original work published 1970)

Friedman, R., & Grossman, B. (Eds.). ([since] 1996). *Assets: An Quarterly Update for Innovators* [newsletter]. Washington, DC: Corporation for Enterprise Development.

Friedman, R., & Wilson, C. (1995). *State individual development accounts sourcebook.* Washington, DC: Corporation for Enterprise Development.

Furstenberg, F. F. (1976). *Unplanned parenthood: The social consequences of teenage childbearing.* New York: Free Press.

Furstenberg, F. F., Brooks-Gunn, J., & Morgan, S. P. (1987). *Adolescent mothers in later life.* New York: Cambridge University Press.

Gabriel, A., & McAnarney, E. R. (1983). Parenthood in two subcultures: White, middle-class couples and black, low-income adolescents in Rochester, New York. *Adolescence, 18,* 595-608.

Gambert, S. (1992). The crucial prostate exam. *Emergency Medicine, 21,* 25-40.

Gardner, H. (1991). *The unschooled mind: How children learn and how schools should teach.* New York: Basic Books.

Garibaldi, A. M. (1992). Educating and motivating African-American males to succeed. *Journal of Negro Education, 61,* 4-11.

Garland, J., Jones, H., & Kolodny, R. (1965). A model for stages of group development in social groups. In S. Bernstein (Ed.), *Explorations in group work.* Boston: Boston University Press.

Gary, L. (1985). Correlates of depressive symptoms among a select population of black males. *American Journal of Public Health, 75,* 1220-1222.

Gary, L. E., & Berry, G. L. (1985). Depressive symptomatology among black men. *Journal of Multicultural Counseling and Development, 13,* 121-129.

Gary, L. E., & Leashore, B. R. (1982). High risk status of black men. *Social Work, 27,* 54-58.

Gavin, J. R., III. (1996a). New program focuses on African Americans. *Diabetes Spectrum, 9*(2), 142.

Gavin, J. R., III. (1996b). Taming diabetes: The silent killer that prefers blacks. *Ebony, 51*(5), 118-122.

Gee, J. P. (1990). *Social linguistics and literacies: Ideology in discourse.* New York: Taylor & Francis.

George, J. C. (1993). *The black male crisis.* Cincinnati, OH: Zulema Enterprises.

Germain, C., & Gitterman, A. (1995). Ecological perspectives. In R. L. Edwards & J. G. Hopps (Eds.), *Encyclopedia of social work* (19th ed., pp. 816-824). Washington, DC: National Association of Social Workers Press.

Gibbs, J. T. (1980). The interpersonal orientation in mental health consultation: Toward a model of ethnic variations in consultation. *Journal of Community Psychology, 8,* 195-207.

Gibbs, J. T. (Ed.). (1988) *Young, black, and male in America: An endangered species.* Dover, MA: Auburn House.

Gil, E., & Johnson, T. C. (1993). *Sexualized children.* Rockville, MD: Launch Press.

Gilbert, G. (1974). The role of social work in black liberation. *Black Scholar, 6*(4), 16-23.

Giroux, H. (1985). Introduction. In P. Freire, *The politics of education: Culture, power, and liberation* (pp. iv-xxv) (D. Macedo, Trans.). New York: Bergin & Garvey.

Gittleman, M., & Howell, D. (1995). Changes in the structure and quality of jobs in the United States: Effects by race and gender, 1973-1990. *Industrial and Labor Relations Review, 48*(3), 420-439.

Gochros, J. S. (1966). Recognition and use of anger in Negro clients. *Social Work, 11,* 28-34.

Gold, M. (1970). *Delinquent behavior in America.* Belmont, CA: Brooks/Cole.

Goldstein, A. (1994). *The ecology of aggression.* New York: Plenum.

Gordon, J. U. (1993). A culturally specific approach to ethnic minority young adults. In E. M. Freeman (Ed.), *Substance abuse treatment: A family systems perspective* (pp. 71-99). Newbury Park, CA: Sage.

Gordon, R. (1976). Prevalence: The rare datum in delinquency measurement and its implications for the theory of delinquency. In M. W. Klein (Ed.), *The juvenile justice system.* Beverly Hills, CA: Sage.

Gottfredson, D. C. (1995). *Creating safe, disciplined, drug-free schools.* Paper prepared for the conference on implementing recent federal legislation, sponsored by the Office of Educational Research and Improvement, U.S. Department of Education, and the American Sociological Association, St. Petersburg, FL.

Gottfredson, G. D. (1985). *Victimization in schools.* New York: Plenum.

Gottlieb, G. K. (1996). Financial issues. In J. Sadavoy, L. F. Lazarus, L. F. Jarvik, & G. T. Grossberg (Eds.), *Comprehensive review of geriatric psychiatry* (Vol. 2, 2nd ed., pp. 1065-1085). Washington, DC: American Psychiatric Press.

Gray, D. (1991). *The plight of the African-American male: An executive summary of a legislative hearing.* Detroit, MI: Council President Pro Tem Gil, the Detroit City Council Youth Advisory Commission, and Wayne County Community College.

Gray-Little, B. (1982). Marital quality and power processes among black couples. *Journal of Marriage and the Family, 44,* 633-646.

Greaves, W. I. (1987). The black community. In H. Dalton & S. Burris (Eds.), *AIDS and the law* (pp. 281-289). New Haven, CT: Yale University Press.

Green, J. W. (1995). *Cultural awareness in the human services: A multi-ethnic approach.* Boston, MA: Allyn & Bacon.

Greenberg, D. (1988). *The construction of homosexuality.* Chicago: University of Chicago Press.

Greene, J. E., & Daugherty, S. L. (1961). Factors associated with school mobility. *Journal of Educational Sociology, 35,* 36-40.

Grier, W., & Cobbs, P. (1968). *Black rage.* New York: Basic Books.

Grier, W. H., & Cobbs, P. M. (1971). *Jesus bag.* New York: McGraw-Hill.

Griffith, E. E. H., & Baker, F. M. (1993). Psychiatric care of African Americans. In A. C. Gaw (Ed.), *Culture, ethnicity, and mental illness* (pp. 147-173). Washington, DC: American Psychiatric Press.

Griffith, E. E. H., & Bell, C. C. (1989). Recent trends in suicide and homicide among blacks. *Journal of the American Medical Association, 262,* 2265-2269.

Groce, J. T. (1988). Perceived factors in the early lives of black males that have influenced their later life development (Doctoral dissertation, Temple University). *Dissertation Abstracts International, 49,* 2155.

Grossman, B., & Friedman, R. E. (1997). *Building economic independence through individual development accounts* (Issues brief). Washington, DC: National Governors' Association.

Grossman, B., Sahay, P., & Friedman, R. E. (1996). *Designing your own individual development account demonstration: An information and resource handbook for community-based organizations* (rev. ed.). Washington, DC: Corporation for Enterprise Development.

Groves, P. A., & Ventura, L. A. (1983). The lesbian coming out process: Therapeutic considerations. *Personnel and Guidance Journal, 62*(3), 146-149.

Guerra, N. G., Tolan, P. H., & Hammond, W. R. (1994). Prevention and treatment of adolescent violence. In L. D. Eron, J. H. Gentry, & P. Schlegel (Eds.), *Reason to hope: A psychosocial perspective on violence and youth* (pp. 383-404). Washington, DC: American Psychological Association.

Gysbers, N. C., & Moore, E. J. (1987). *Career counseling: Skills and techniques for practitioners.* Englewood Cliffs, NJ: Prentice Hall.

Haberman, M. (1991, December). The pedagogy of poverty versus good teaching. *Phi Delta Kappan,* pp. 290-294.

Haberman, M. (1994, Spring). Gentle teaching in a violent society. *Educational Horizons,* pp. 131-135.

Hack, T. F., Osachuk, T. A. G., & Deluca, R. V. (1994). Group treatment for sexually abused preadolescent boys. *Families in Society, 15,* 217-228.

Hacker, A. (1992). *Two nations: Black and white, separate, hostile, unequal.* New York: Maxwell Macmillan.

Hagedorn, J. M. (1988). *People and folks: Gangs, crime, and the underclass in a rustbelt city.* Chicago: Lakeview Press.

Haley, A. (1992). *The autobiography of Malcolm X.* New York: Ballantine. (Original work published 1965)

Hammond, R., Kadis, P., & Yung, B. (1990, August 10-14). *Positive adolescents choices training (PACT): Preliminary findings of the effects of a school-based violence prevention program for African-American Adolescents.* Paper presented at the annual meeting of the American Psychological Association, Boston.

Hammond, R. W., & Yung, B. R. (1991). Preventing violence in at-risk African-American youth. *Journal of Health Care for the Poor and Underserved, 2,* 359-373.

Hammond, R. W., & Yung, B. (1993). Psychology's role in the public health response to assaultive violence among young African-American men. *American Psychologist, 48,* 142-154.

Hammond, R. W., & Yung, B. R. (1994). African Americans. In L. D. Eron, J. H. Gentry, & P. Schlegel (Eds.), *Reason to hope: A psychosocial perspective on violence and youth* (pp. 105-118). Washington, DC: American Psychological Association.

Haour-Knipe, M. (1989). International employment and children: Geographical mobility and mental health among children of professionals. *Social Science and Medicine, 28,* 197-205.

Hardy, J. B., & Zabin, L. S. (1991). *Adolescent pregnancy in an urban environment: Issues, programs, and evaluation.* Washington, DC: Urban Institute Press.

Hare, N., & Hare, J. (1984). *The endangered black family: Coping with the unisexualization and coming extinction of the black race.* San Francisco: Black Think Tank.

Hargrove, B., & Sedlacek, W. E. (1995). *Counseling interests among entering black university students over a ten-year period.* Counseling Center Report No. 6-95, University of Maryland at College Park.

Hargrow, A., & Hendricks, F. M. (in press). Career counseling African Americans in nontraditional fields. In B. Walsh, S. Osipow, R. Bingham, D. Brown, & C. Ward (Eds.), *Career counseling for African Americans.* Mahwah, NJ: Lawrence Erlbaum.

Harlow, C. (1989). *Injuries from crime* (Bureau of Justice Statistics, Special Report No. NCJ-116811). Washington, DC: U.S. Department of Justice.

Harper, M. S. (1992). Elderly issues in the African American community. In R. I. Braithwaite & S. E. Taylor (Eds.), *Health issues in the black community* (pp. 222-238). San Francisco: Jossey-Bass.

Harris, M. I. (1995). Summary. In *Diabetes in America* (2nd ed., pp. 1-14) (NIH Publication No. 95-1468). Bethesda, MD: National Institutes of Health.

Harry, J. (1990). A probability sample of gay males. *Journal of Homosexuality, 19*(1), 89-104.

Harvey, A. R. (1995). The issue of skin color in psychotherapy with African Americans. *Families in Society, 76*(1), 3-10.

Hatchett, S. J. (1991). Women and men. In J. S. Jackson (Ed.), *Life in black America* (pp. 84-104). Newbury Park, CA: Sage.

Hausman, J., Spivak, H., & Prothrow-Stith, D. (1994). Adolescents' knowledge and attitudes about and experience with violence. *Journal of Adolescent Health, 15,* 400-406.

Hayes, S. N., & Oziel, L. J. (1976). Homosexuality, behavior, and attitudes. *Archives of Sexual Behavior, 5,* 283-289.

Hays, R. B., Catania, J. A., McKusick, L., & Coates, T. J. (1990). Help-seeking for AIDS-related concerns: A comparison of gay men with various HIV diagnosis. *American Journal of Community Psychology, 18,* 743-754.

Hecht, M. L., Collier, M. J., & Ribeau, S. A. (1993). *African American communication: Ethnic identity and cultural interpretation.* Newbury Park, CA: Sage.

Heitgerd, J. L., & Bursik, R. J. (1987). Extracommunity dynamics and the ecology of delinquency. *American Journal of Sociology, 92,* 775-787.

Helms, J. E. (1990). *Black and white racial identity: Theory, research, and practice.* Westport, CT: Greenwood.

Helms, J. E. (1995). An update of Helms's white and people of color racial identity models. In J. G. Ponterotto, J. M. Casas, L. A. Suzuki, & C. M. Alexander (Eds.), *Handbook of multicultural counseling* (pp. 181-198). Thousand Oaks, CA: Sage.

Hendricks, F. M. (1994). Career counseling with African American college students. *Journal of Career Development, 21,* 117-126.

Hendricks, L. E. (1981). Black unwed adolescent fathers. In L. E. Gary (Ed.), *Black men* (pp. 131-138). Beverly Hills, CA: Sage.

Hendricks, L. E. (1988). Outreach with teenage fathers: A preliminary report on three ethnic groups. *Adolescence, 23*(91), 711-720.

Hendricks, L. E., & Hendricks, R. T. (1994). Efficacy of a day treatment program in management of diabetes for aging African Americans. *Activities, Adaptation, and Aging, 19*(2), 41-51.

Hendricks, L. E., Montgomery, T., & Fullilove, R. E. (1984). Educational achievement and locus of control among black adolescent fathers. *Journal of Negro Education, 53,* 182-188.

Hendricks, L. E., & Solomon, A. M. (1987). Reaching black adolescent parents through noneducational techniques. *Child and Youth Services, 9*(1), 111-124.

Hendricks, R. T., & Haas, L. B. (1991). Diabetes in minority populations. *Nurse Practitioner Forum, 2,* 199-202.

Heppner, M., O'Brien, K., Hinkelman, J., & Humphrey, C. (1994). Shifting the paradigm: The use of creativity in career counseling. *Journal of Career Development, 21,* 77-86.

Herek, G. M., & Capitanio, J. P. (1995). Black heterosexuals' attitudes toward lesbians and gay men in the United States. *Journal of Sex Research, 32*(2), 95-105.

Herrnstein, R., & Murray, C. (1994). *The bell curve: Intelligence and class structure in American life.* New York: Free Press.

Hill, P., Jr. (1992). *Coming of age: African American male rites-of-passage.* Chicago: African American Images.

Hill, R. (1972). *The strengths of black families.* New York: Emerson Hall.

Hilliard, A. (1976). *Alternatives to IQ testing: An approach to the identification of gifted minority children* (Final report to the California State Department of Education). Sacramento: Department of Education.

Hilliard, A. G. (1985). A framework for focused counseling on the African American man. *Journal of Non-White Concerns in Personnel and Guidance, 13,* 72-78.

Hindelang, M., Hirschi, T., & Weis, J. (1981). *Measuring delinquency.* Beverly Hills, CA: Sage.

Hirschi, T. (1969). *Causes of delinquency.* Berkeley: University of California Press.

Hirschi, T., & Hindelang, M. (1977). Intelligence and delinquency: A revisionist review. *American Sociological Review, 42,* 572-87.

Holland, J. L. (1970). *Self-directed search.* Palo Alto, CA: Consulting Psychologists Press.

Holzer, H. (1991). The spatial mismatch hypothesis: What does the evidence show? *Urban Studies, 28*(1), 105-122.

Holzer, H. (1996). *What employers want: Job prospects for less-educated workers.* New York: Russell Sage Foundation.

Holzer, H., & Ihlanfeldt, K. (1996, May/June). Spatial factors and the employment of blacks at the firm level. *New England Economic Review,* pp. 65-82.

hooks, b. (1994). *Killing rage: Ending racism.* New York: Owl Books.

hooks, b., & West, C. (1990). *Breaking bread: Insurgent black intellectual life.* Boston: South End Press.

Hotz, V. J., & Tienda, M. (1995). *Education and employment in a diverse society: Generating inequality through the school-to-work transition.* Unpublished manuscript, University of Chicago.

Houston, L. N. (1990). *Psychological principles and the black experience.* Lanham, MD: University Press of America.

Howard-Hamilton, M. (1995). Multicultural counseling trends and issues: Implications and imperatives for the next millenium. In W. M. Parker (Ed.), *Consciousness raising: A primer for multicultural counseling* (pp. 257-276). Springfield, IL: Charles C Thomas.

Huff, C. R. (1991). Denial, overreaction, and misidentification: A postscript on public policy. In C. R. Huff (Ed.), *Gangs in America.* Newbury Park, CA: Sage.

Hughes, M., & Sternberg, J. (1992). *The new metropolitan reality: Where the rubber meets the road in antipoverty policy.* Washington, DC: Urban Institute Press.

Huizinga, D., & Elliott, D. (1987). Juvenile delinquency: Prevalence, offender incidence, and arrest rates by race. *Crime and Delinquency, 33,* 206-223.

Hunter, J. (1990). Violence against lesbian and gay male youths. *Journal of Interpersonal Violence, 5*(3), 295-300.

Hunter, M. (1990). *The sexual abused male: Applications of treatment strategies* (Vol. 2). Lexington, MA: Lexington Books.

Hutson, R., Anglin, D., Kyriacou, D., Hart, J., & Spears, K. (1995). The epidemic of gang-related homicides in Los Angeles County from 1979 through 1994. *Journal of the American Medical Association, 274,* 1031-1036.

Icard, L. D. (1986). Black gay men and conflicting social identities: Sexual orientation versus racial identity. In J. Gripton & M. Valentich (Eds.), *Social work practice in sexual problems* (pp. 83-93). New York: Haworth.

Icard, L. D. (1996). Assessing the psychosocial well-being of African American gays: A multidimensional perspective. In J. F. Longres (Ed.), *Men of color: A context for service to homosexually active men* (pp. 25-49). Binghamton, NY: Harrington Park Press.

Icard, L. D., Longres, J. F., & Williams, J. H. (1996). An applied research agenda for homosexually active men of color. In J. F. Longres (Ed.), *Men of color: A context for service to homosexually active men* (pp. 139-164). Binghamton, NY: Harrington Park Press.

Icard, L. D., Schilling, R. F., El-Bassel, N., & Young, D. (1992). Preventing AIDS among black gay men and black gay and heterosexual male intravenous drug users. *Social Work, 37*(5), 440-445.

Icard, L. D., & Traunstein, D. M. (1987). Black, gay, alcoholic men: Their character and treatment. *Social Casework, 68,* 267-272.

Ingersoll, G. M., Seamman, J. R., & Eckerling, W. D. (1989). Geographic mobility and student achievement in an urban setting. *Educational Evaluation and Policy Analysis, 11,* 143-149.

Irwin, J., & Austin, J. (1994). *It's about time: America's imprisonment binge*. Belmont, CA: Wadsworth.

Issacs, M. (1992). *Violence: The impact of community violence on African-American children and families: Collaborative approaches to prevention and intervention*. Arlington, VA: National Center for Education in Maternal and Child Health.

Jackson, R. K., & McBride, W. D. (1986). *Understanding street gangs*. Placerville, CA: Copperhouse.

Jaroff, L. (1996, April 1). The man's cancer. *Time, 147*, 56-65.

Jason, L. A., Weine, A. M., Johnson, J. H., Warren-Sohlberg, L., Filippelli, L. A., Turner, E. Y., & Lardon, C. (1992). *Helping transfer students: Strategies for educational and social readjustment*. San Francisco: Jossey-Bass.

Jaynes, G., & Williams, R. (Eds.). (1989). *A common destiny: Blacks and American society*. Washington, DC: National Academy Press.

Jensen, A. R. (1969). How much can we boost IQ and scholastic achievement? *Harvard Educational Review, 39*, 1-23.

Jerome, N. W. (1988). Dietary intake and nutritional status of older U.S. blacks: An overview. In J. S. Jackson (Ed.), *The black American elderly: Research and physical and psychosocial health* (pp. 129-149). New York: Springer.

Johnson, C. M., Miranda, L., Sherman, A., & Weil, J. D. (1992). *Child poverty in America*. Washington, DC: Children's Defense Fund.

Johnson, G. J. (1989). Underemployment, underpayment, and psychosocial stress among working black men. *Western Journal of Black Studies, 13*, 57-65.

Johnson, J. (1982). Influence of assimilation on the psychosocial adjustment of black homosexual men. *Dissertation Abstracts International, 42*(11-B), 4620.

Johnson, R. A., & Lindblad, A. H. (1991). Effect of mobility on academic performance of sixth grade students. *Perceptual and Motor Skills, 72*, 547-552.

Johnston, L. D., O'Malley, P. M., & Bachman, J. G. (1995). *National survey results on drug use from the Monitoring the Future study, 1975-1994* (Vol. 1). Washington, DC: National Institute on Drug Abuse.

Jones, B., & Gay, B. (1982). Survey of psychotherapy with black males. *Journal of the American Psychiatric Association, 139*, 1174-1177.

Jones, B., & Gay, B. (1983). Black males and psychotherapy. *American Journal of Psychotherapy, 37*, 77-85.

Jones, B. E., Gray, B. A., & Jospitre, J. (1982). Survey of psychotherapy with black men. *American Journal of Psychiatry, 139*, 1174-1177.

Jones, B. E., Gray, B. A., & Parson, E. B. (1981). Manic-depressive illness among poor urban blacks. *American Journal of Psychiatry, 185*, 654-657.

Jones, D. L. (1979). African American clients: Clinical practice issues. *Social Work, 24*, 112-118.

Jones, E. E. (1985). Psychotherapy and counseling with black clients. In P. B. Pedersen (Ed.), *Handbook of cross-cultural counseling and therapy* (pp. 173-187). Westport, CT: Greenwood.

Jones, J. M. (1997). *Prejudice and racism* (2nd ed.). New York: McGraw-Hill.

Jones, R. (Ed.). (1989). *Black adolescents.* Berkeley, CA: Cobb & Henry.

Jorgensen, J. D., Hernandez, S. H., & Warren, R. C. (1986). Addressing the social needs of families of prisoners: A tool for inmate rehabilitation. *Federal Probation, 50*(4), 47-52.

Joseph, J. (1995). *Black youths, delinquency, and juvenile justice.* Westport, CT: Greenwood.

Juhn, C. (1992). Decline of male labor force participation: The role of declining market opportunities. *Quarterly Journal of Economics, 107*(1), 79-122.

Kachur, P., Stennies, G., Powell, K., Modzeleski, W., Stephens, R., Murphy, R., Kresnow, M., Sleet, D., & Lowry, R. (1996). School-associated violent deaths in the United States, 1992 to 1994. *Journal of the American Medical Association, 275,* 1729-1733.

Kain, J. (1992). The spatial mismatch hypothesis three decades later. *Housing Policy Debate, 3*(2), 371-462.

Kane, T. (1994). *College entry by blacks since 1970: The role of college costs, family background, and the returns to education.* Working paper, John F. Kennedy School of Government, Harvard University.

Kantor, H., & Brenzel, B. (1992). Urban education and the truly disadvantaged: The historical roots of the contemporary crisis, 1945-1990. *Teacher's College Record, 94,* 278-314.

Kaplan, H. B., Martin, S. S., Johnston, R. J., & Robbins, C. A. (1986). Escalation of marijuana use: Application of a general theory of deviant behavior. *Journal of Health and Social Behavior, 27,* 44-61.

Karenga, M. (1977). *Kwanzaa: Origin, concepts, practice.* Los Angeles: Kawaida.

Kasarda, J. (1995). Industrial restructuring and the changing locations of jobs. In R. Farley (Ed.), *State of the union* (Vol. 1). New York: Russell Sage Foundation.

Katz, J. (1976). *Gay American history: Lesbians and gay men in the U.S.A.* New York: Thomas Y. Crowell.

Keating, D. P. (1990). Adolescent thinking. In S. S. Feldman & G. R. Elliott (Eds.), *At the threshold: The developing adolescent* (pp. 54-89). Cambridge, MA: Harvard University Press.

Keeley, K., & Weiss, C. (1993). *Savings groups: A tool for community organizations.* Washington, DC: Corporation for Enterprise Development.

Kendall, P. C., Ronan, K. R., & Epps, J. (1991). Aggression in children/adolescents: Cognitive-behavioral treatment perspectives. In D. J. Pepler & K. H. Rubins (Eds.), *The development and treatment of childhood aggression.* Hillsdale, NJ: Lawrence Erlbaum.

King, A. E. O. (1993a). African American males in prison: Are they doing time or is the time doing them? *Journal of Sociology & Social Welfare, 20*(4), 9-27.

King, A. E. O. (1993b). Helping inmates cope with family separation and role strain: A group work approach. *Social Work With Groups, 16*(4), 43-55.

King, A. E. O. (1993c). The impact of incarceration on African American families: Implications for practice. *Families in Society, 74*(3), 145-153.

King, A. E. O. (1994). An Afrocentric cultural awareness program for incarcerated African American males. *Journal of Multicultural Social Work, 3*(4), 17-28.

King, J. (1991). Dysconscious racism: Ideology, identity, and the miseducation of teachers. *Journal of Negro Education, 60*(2), 133-146.

Kinsey, A. C., Pomeroy, W., & Martin, C. E. (1948). *Sexual behavior in the human male.* Philadelphia: W. B. Saunders.

Kirschenman, J. (1991). *Gender within race in the labor market.* Unpublished manuscript, University of Chicago.

Kirschenman, J., & Neckerman, K. (1991). We'd love to hire them but . . . In C. Jencks & P. Peterson (Eds.), *The urban underclass.* Washington DC: Brookings Institution.

Kiselica, M. S. (1995). *Multicultural counseling with teenage fathers: A practical guide.* Newbury Park, CA: Sage.

Kiselica, M. S. (1996). Parenting skills training with teenage fathers. In M. Andronico (Ed.), *Men in groups: Insights, interventions, and psychoeducational work* (pp. 283-300). Washington, DC: American Psychological Association.

Kiselica, M. S., & Murphy, D. K. (1994). Developmental career counseling with teenage parents. *Career Counseling Quarterly, 42,* 238-244.

Kiselica, M. S., & Pfaller, J. (1993). Helping teenage parents: The independent and collaborative roles of school counselors and counselor educators. *Journal of Counseling and Development, 72,* 42-48.

Kiselica, M. S., Rotzien, A., & Doms, J. (1994). Preparing teenage fathers for parenthood: A group psychoeducational approach. *Journal for Specialists in Group Work, 19,* 83-94.

Kitchur, M., & Bell, R. (1989). *International Journal of Group Psychotherapy, 39*(3), 285-310.

Klein, M. (1995). *The American street gang.* New York: Oxford University Press.

Klein, M., & Maxson, C. (1994). Gangs and crack cocaine trafficking. In D. MacKenzie & C. Uchida (Eds.), *Drugs and crime: Evaluating public policy initiatives* (pp. 42-58). Newbury Park, CA: Sage.

Klein, M., Maxson, C., & Cunningham, L. (1991). Crack, street gangs, and violence. *Criminology, 29,* 623-650.

Klinman, D. G., & Sander, J. H. (1985). *The teen parent collaboration: Reaching and serving the teenage father.* New York: Bank Street College of Education.

Kotlowitz, A. (1991). *There are no children here: The story of two boys growing up in the other America.* New York: Doubleday.

Kozol, J. (1991). *Savage inequalities: Children in America's schools.* New York: Harper Perennial.

Kunjufu, J. (1986). *Countering the conspiracy to destroy black boys* (2 vols.). Chicago: African American Images.

Landrine, H., & Klonoff, E. (1992). Culture and health-related schemas: Review and proposal for interdisciplinary integration. *Health Psychology, 11,* 267-276.

Lanier, C. S. (1991). Dimensions of father-child interaction in a New York State prison population. *Journal of Offender Rehabilitation, 16*(3/4), 27-42.

Larsen, K. S., Cate, R., & Reed, M. (1983). Anti-black attitudes, religious orthodoxy, permissiveness, and sexual information: A study of the attitudes of heterosexuals toward homosexuality. *Journal of Sex Research, 19,* 105-118.

Larsen, K. S., Reed, M., & Hoffman, S. (1980). Attitudes of heterosexuals toward homosexuality: A Likert-type scale and construct validity. *Journal of Sex Research, 16,* 245-257.

Larson, J. (1994). Violence prevention in the schools: A review of selected programs and procedures. *School Psychology Review, 23,* 151-164.

Lawson, A., & Rhode, D. L. (Eds.). (1993). *The politics of pregnancy: Adolescent sexuality and public policy.* New Haven, CT: Yale University Press.

Lawson, E., & Thompson, A. (1995). Black men make sense of marital stress and divorce. *Family Relations, 44,* 211-218.

Leake, D. O., & Leake, B. L. (1992). Islands of hope: Milwaukee's African-American immersion schools. *Journal of Negro Education, 61,* 24-29.

Leashore, B. (1991). Social policies, black males, and black families. In R. Staples (Ed.), *The black family: Essays and studies* (4th ed.). Belmont, CA: Wadsworth.

LeCompte, M., & Goebel, S. (1987). Can bad data produce good program planning? An analysis of record keeping on school dropouts. *Education and Urban Society, 19,* 250-268.

Lee, C. (1991). Big picture talkers/words walking without masters: The instructional implications of ethnic voices for an expanded literacy. *Journal of Negro Education, 60*(3), 291-304.

Lee, C. C. (1989). Counseling the black adolescent: Critical roles and functions for counseling professionals. In R. L. Jones (Ed.), *Black adolescents* (pp. 293-308). Berkeley, CA: Cobb & Henry.

Lee, C. C. (1990). Black male development: Counseling the "native son." In D. Moore & F. Leafgren (Eds.), *Problem solving strategies and interventions for men in conflict.* Alexandria, VA: AACD Press.

Lee, C. C., & Bailey, D. F. (1997). Counseling African American male youth and men. In C. C. Lee (Ed.), *Multicultural issues in counseling: New approaches to diversity* (2nd ed.). Alexandria, VA: American Counseling Association.

Lee, V. E., & Croninger R. G. (1995). *The social organization of safe high schools.* Paper presented at the Goals 2000, Reauthorization of the Elementary and Secondary Education Act, and the School-to-Work Opportunities Act conference, Palm Beach, FL.

Leigh, D. (1990). *Does training work for displaced workers?* Kalamazoo MI: W. E. Upjohn Institute for Employment Research.

Leonard, J. (1990). The impact of affirmative action regulation and equal opportunity law on black employment. *Journal of Economic Perspectives, 4*(4), 47-64.

Leonard, P. Y. (1985). Vocational theory and the vocational behavior of black males: An analysis. *Journal of Multicultural Counseling and Development, 13,* 91-105.

Leopold, N., Cooper, J., & Clancy, C. (1996). Sustained partnership in primary care. *Journal of Family Practice, 42*(2), 129-137.

Lerman, R. I., & Ooms, T. J. (Eds.). (1993). *Young unwed fathers: Changing roles and emerging policies.* Philadelphia: Temple University Press.

Levant, R. F., & Pollack, W. S. (Eds.). (1995). *A new psychology of men.* New York: Basic Books.

Levin, H., & Hopfenberg, W. (1991). Accelerated schools for at-risk students. *Education Digest, 56,* 47-50.

Levine, M. (1966). Residential change and school adjustment. *Community Mental Health Journal, 2,* 61-69.

Lewis, J. (1994). *How I survived prostate cancer and so can you: A guide for diagnosing and treating prostate cancer.* New York: Health Education Literary Publishers.

Lichtenstein, A. A., & Kroll, M. A. (1990). *The fortress economy: The economic role of the U.S. prison system.* Philadelphia: American Friends Service Committee.

Liebow, E. (1967). *Tally's corner.* Boston: Little, Brown.

Lipson, L. G., Kato-Palmer, S., Boggs, W. L., et al. (1988) Black Americans. *Diabetes Forecast, 4*(9), 34-37.

Lisella, L. C., & Serwatka, T. S. (1996). Extracurricular participation and academic achievement in minority students in urban schools. *The Urban Review, 28,* 63-80.

Littrup, P., Lee, F., & Mettlin, C. (1992). Prostate cancer screening: Current trends and future implications. *CA: A Cancer Journal for Clinicians, 42,* 198-211.

Lloyd, E. (1993). Prisoners' link with their children: Research on benefits for children and their parents. *Issues in Criminology and Legal Psychology, 20,* 27-31.

Locke, D. C. (1989). Fostering the self-esteem of African-American children. *Elementary School Guidance and Counseling, 23,* 254-259.

Locke, D. C. (1998). *Increasing multicultural understanding: A comprehensive model.* Thousand Oaks, CA: Sage.

Locke, D. C., & Covington, R. O. (1992). A peer mentor program for African American students. *Journal of the Southeastern Association of Educational Opportunity Program Personnel, 11*(2), 16-23.

Locke, D. C., & Faubert, M. (1993). Getting on the right track: A program for African American high school students. *The School Counselor, 41,* 129-133.

Locke, D. C., & Zimmerman, N. A. (1987). The effects of peer counseling training on the psychological maturity of African-American students. *Journal of College Student Personnel, 28,* 525-532.

Logan, S. L., & Joyce, J. (1996). Helping black families who are providing care for people with AIDS. In S. L. Logan (Ed.), *The black family: Strengths, self-help, and positive change* (pp. 53-66). Boulder, CO: Westview.

Loiacano, D. K. (1989). Gay identity issues among black Americans: Racism, homophobia, and the need for validation. *Journal of Counseling & Development, 68,* 21-25.

Loiacano, D. K. (1993). Gay identity issues among black Americans: Racism, homophobia, and the need for validation. In L. D. Garnets & D. C. Kimmel (Eds.), *Psychological perspectives on lesbian & gay male experiences* (pp. 364-375). New York: Columbia University Press.

Lubell, D., & Soong, W. (1982). Group theory with sexually abused adolescents. *Canadian Journal of Psychiatry, 27,* 311-315.

Lum, D. (1996). *Social work practice and people of color: A process-stage approach* (3rd ed.). Pacific Grove, CA: Brooks/Cole.

Madhubuti, H. (1990). *Black men: Obsolete, single, dangerous? The Afrikan American family in transition.* Chicago. Third World Press.

Majors, R. (1991). Nonverbal behaviors and communication styles among African Americans. In R. Jones (Ed.), *Black psychology* (3rd ed., pp. 269-294). Berkeley, CA: Cobb & Henry.

Majors, R., & Billson, J. M. (1992). *Cool pose: The dilemmas of black manhood in America.* New York: Lexington.

Majors, R., & Nikelly, A. (1983). Serving the black minority: A new direction for psychotherapy. *Journal of Non-White Concerns in Personnel and Guidance, 11,* 142-151.

Mandell, J. G., & Damon, L. (1989). *Group treatment for sexually abused children.* New York: Guilford.

Manns, W. (1981). Support systems of significant others in black families. In H. P. McAdoo (Ed.), *Black families* (pp. 238-251). Beverly Hills, CA: Sage.

Marable, M. (1983). *How capitalism underdeveloped black America.* Boston: South End Press.

Marchant, K. H., & Medway, F. J. (1987). Adjustment and achievement associated with mobility in military families. *Psychology in the Schools, 24,* 289-294.

Marsiglio, W. (1986). Teenage fatherhood: High school completion and educational attainment. In A. B. Elster & M. E. Lamb (Eds.), *Adolescent fatherhood* (pp. 67-88). Hillsdale, NJ: Lawrence Erlbaum.

Marsiglio, W. (1987), Adolescent fathers in the United States: Their initial living arrangements, marital experience, and educational outcomes. *Family Planning Perspectives, 19,* 240-251.

Maslow, A. H. (1970). *Motivation and personality.* New York: Harper.

Mauer, M. (1990). *Young black men and the criminal justice system: A growing national problem.* Washington, DC: The Sentencing Project.

Mauer, M. (1994). *Americans behind bars: The international use of incarceration, 1992-1993.* Washington, DC: The Sentencing Project.

Maxson, C. L., & Klein, M. W. (1990). Street gang violence: Twice as large or half as large? In C. R. Huff (Ed.), *Gangs in America.* Newbury Park, CA: Sage.

Maxson, C. L., Whitlock, M., & Klein, M. W. (1996, November 22). *Resistance to street gang membership.* Paper presented to the American Society of Criminology, Chicago.

Maxson, C. L., Woods, K., & Klein, M. W. (1996, February). Street gang migration: How big a threat? *National Institute of Juvenile Justice Journal, 230,* 26-31.

Mays, V. C., Cochran, S. D., Bellinger, G., Smith, R. G., Henley, N., Daniels, M., Tibbits, T., Victorriane, G. D., Osei, K. O., & Birt, D. K. (1992). The language of black gay men's sexual behavior: Implications for AIDS risk reduction. *Journal of Sex Research, 29*(3), 425-434.

Mays, V. M. (1989). AIDS prevention in black populations: Methods of a safer kind. In V. M. Mays, G. W. Albee, & S. F. Schneider (Eds.), *Primary prevention of AIDS: Psychological approaches* (pp. 264-279). Newbury Park, CA: Sage.

McAdoo, H. P. (1992). Upward mobility and parenting in middle-income black families. In A. Burlew, W. C. Banks, H. P. McAdoo, & D. A. Azibo (Eds.), *African American psychology: Theory, research, and practice* (pp. 63-86). Newbury Park, CA: Sage.

McAdoo, H. P. (1996). *Black families.* Thousand Oaks, CA: Sage.

McAdoo, J. L. (1993). The roles of African American fathers: An ecological perspective. *Families in Society, 74*(11), 28-35.

McBride, W. D., & Jackson, R. K. (1989, June). In L.A. County, a high-tech assist in the war on drugs. *The Police Chief,* pp. 28-29.

McCall, N. (1994). *Makes me wanna holler: A young black man in America.* New York: Vintage.

McCurdy, K., & Daro, D. (1993). *Current trends in child abuse reporting and fatalities: The results of the 1992 Annual Fifth State Survey.* Chicago: National Committee for Prevention of Child Abuse.

McDaniels, C., & Gysbers, N. C. (1992). *Counseling for career development: Theories, resources, and practice.* San Francisco: Jossey-Bass.

McDavis, R., & Parker, W. (1988). Counseling black people. In N. A. J. Vacc, J. Wittmer, & S. DeVaney (Eds.), *Experiencing and counseling multicultural and diverse populations* (pp. 127-150). Muncie, IN: Accelerated Development.

McDermott, R. P. (1987). The exploration of minority school failure, again. *Anthropology and Education Quarterly, 18,* 361-364.

McIntosh, P. (1989). White privilege: Unpacking the invisible knapsack. *Peace and Freedom, 2,* 10-12.

McLanahan, S., & Sandefur, G. (1994). *Growing up with a single parent: What hurts, what helps.* Cambridge, MA: Harvard University Press.

McLaren, P. (1989). *Life in schools: An introduction to critical pedagogy in the foundations of education.* New York: Longman.

Mehrabian, A. (1981). *Silent messages.* Belmont, CA: Wadsworth.

Meier, D. (1995). *The power of their ideas: Lessons for America from a small school in Harlem.* Boston: Beacon.

Mendel, M. D. (1995). *The male survivor: The impact of sexual abuse.* Newbury Park, CA: Sage.

Mercer, J. (1979). *The system of multicultural pluralistic assessment (S.O.M.P.A.).* New York: Psychological Corp.

Merton, R. K. (1957). *Social theory and social structure.* Glencoe, IL: Free Press.

Messner, S., & Rosenfeld, R. (1994). *Crime and the American dream.* Belmont, CA: Wadsworth.

Meth, R. L., & Passick, R. S. (Eds.). (1990). *Men in therapy: The challenge of change.* New York: Guilford.

Meyer, C. H. (1993). *Assessment in social work practice.* New York: Columbia University Press.

Mfusi, K. (1996). *No free ride: From the mean streets to the mainstream.* New York: Ballantine.

Mickelson, R. (1990). The attitude-achievement paradox among black adolescents. *Sociology of Education, 63,* 44-61.

Mieszkowski, P., & Mills, E. (1993). The causes of metropolitan suburbanization. *Journal of Economic Perspectives, 7*(3), 135-148.

Miller, C. H. (1974). Career development theory in perspective. In E. L. Herr (Ed.), *Vocational guidance and human development* (pp. 235-262). Boston: Houghton Mifflin.

Miller, R. H. (1991). *Reflections of a black cowboy.* Englewood Cliffs, NJ: Silver Burdett Press.

Mincy, R. B. (1994a). Introduction. In R. B. Mincy (Ed.), *Nurturing young black males* (pp. 7-29). Washington, DC: Urban Institute Press.

Mincy, R. (Ed.). (1994b). *Nurturing young black males.* Washington, DC: Urban Institute Press.

Minton, H. L., & McDonald, G. J. (1984). Homosexual identity formation as a developmental process. *Journal of Homosexuality, 9*(2/3), 91-104.

Monteiro, K. P., & Fuqua, V. (1993/1994). African American gay youth: One form of manhood. *The High School Journal, 77,* 20-38.

Moody, C., & Moody, C. (1989). Elements of effective black schools. In W. Smith & E. Chunn (Eds.), *Black education: A quest for equity and excellence* (pp. 176-186). New Brunswick, NJ: Transaction Publishers.

Moore, D., & Leafgren, F. (Eds.). (1990). *Problem-solving strategies and interventions for men in conflict.* Alexandria, VA: American Counseling Association.

Moore, K. A., & Burt, M. R. (1982). *Private crisis, public cost: Policy perspectives on teenage childbearing.* Washington DC: Urban Institute Press.

Moore, K. A., Simms, M. C., & Betsey, C. L. (1986). *Choice and circumstance: Racial differences in adolescent sexuality and fertility.* New Brunswick, NJ: Transaction Books.

Morin, S. F. (1993). AIDS: The challenge to psychology. In L. D. Garnets & D. C. Kimmel (Eds.), *Psychological perspectives on lesbian and gay male experiences* (pp. 557-566), New York: Columbia University Press.

Morrison, G. M., Furlong, M. J., & Morrison, R. L. (1994). School violence to school safety: Reframing the issue for school psychologists. *School Psychology Review, 23,* 236-256.

Moss, P., & Tilly, C. (1995). *Soft skills and race.* Working paper, Russell Sage Foundation.

Mundy, P., Robertson, J., Greenblatt, M., & Robertson, M. (1989). Residential instability in adolescent inpatients. *Journal of the American Academy of Child and Adolescent Psychiatry, 28,* 176-181.

Murray, C. (1984). *Losing ground: American social policy, 1950-1980*. New York: Basic Books.

Murrell, P. C. (1994). In search of responsive teaching for African American males: An investigation of students' experiences of middle school mathematics curriculum. *Journal of Negro Education, 63,* 556-569.

Myers, H. F., Anderson, N. B., & Strickland, T. L. (1989). A biobehavioral perspective on stress and hypertension in black adults. In R. L. Jones (Ed.), *Black adult development and aging*. Berkeley, CA: Cobb & Henry.

Myers, L. J. (1988). *Understanding an Afrocentric world view: Introduction to optimal psychology*. Dubuque, IA: Kendall/Hunt.

Nardi, P. (1992). Seamless souls: An introduction to men's friendships. In P. Nardi (Ed.), *Men's friendships* (pp. 1-14). Newbury Park, CA: Sage.

National Center for Health Statistics. (1991). *Health United States, 1990*. Hyattsville, MD: Author.

National Center for Health Statistics. (1992). Unpublished data tables from the NCHS Mortaliiy Tapes, FBI-SHR. Atlanta, GA: Centers for Disease Control.

National Center on Addiction and Substance Abuse (CASA). (1994). *Cigarettes, alcohol, marijuana: Gateways to illicit drug use*. New York: Author.

National Center on Addiction and Substance Abuse (CASA). (1996). *The National Survey of American Attitudes on Substance Abuse II: Teens and their parents*. New York: Author.

National Center on the Educational Quality of the Workforce. (1995). *First findings from the EQW National Employer Survey*. Unpublished report, University of Pennsylvania.

National Diabetes Information Clearinghouse. (1989). *Diabetes dateline* (Vol. 10, No. 1, pp. 1-2). Bethesda, MD: Author.

National Diabetes Information Clearinghouse. (1990). *Diabetes dateline* (Vol. 11, No. 1, pp. 1-3). Bethesda, MD: Author.

National Diabetes Information Clearinghouse. (1992). *Diabetes in Black Americans* (NIH Publication No. 93-3266). Bethesda, MD: Author.

National Education Goals Panel. (1995). *The National Education Goals Report: Vol. 1, National data; Vol. 2, State data*. Washington DC: Government Printing Office.

National Institute of Education & U.S. Department of Health, Education, and Welfare. (1978). *Violent schools—safe schools* (The safe school study report to Congress, No. 1). Washington, DC: Government Printing Office.

National Institute of Justice. (1995, November). *Drug use forecasting: 1994 annual report on adult and juvenile arrests*. Washington, DC: Government Printing Office.

National Research Council. (1996). *Understanding violence against women*. Washington, DC: National Academy Press.

Neighbors, H. W. (1985). Seeking professional help for personal problems: Black Americans' use of health and mental health services. *Community Mental Health Journal, 21*(3), 156-166.

Newman, B. S., & Muzzonigro, P. G. (1993). The effects of traditional family values on the coming out process of gay male adolescents. *Adolescence, 28,* 213-225.

Nobles, W. W. (1988). *Hawk project profile: A federation of manhood training and development programs.* Oakland, CA: Institute for the Advanced Study of Black Family Life & Culture, Inc.

Nobles, W. W. (1991). African philosophy: Foundations for black psychology. In R. L. Jones (Ed.), *Black psychology* (3rd ed., pp. 47-64). Berkeley, CA: Cobb & Henry.

Nobles, W. W., Goddard, L. L., & Cavil, W. (1985). *Black teenage parenting and early childhood education: Basic curriculum plan.* Oakland, CA: Black Family Institute.

Noddings, N. (1992). *The challenge to care in schools.* New York: Teachers College Press.

Noddings, N. (1995). Teaching themes of care. *Phi Delta Kappan, 76,* 675-679.

Noguera, P. A. (1995). Preventing and producing violence: A critical analysis of responses to school violence. *Harvard Educational Review, 65,* 189-212.

Noldon, D. F., & Sedlacek, W. E. (1995). *Trends in attitudes, skills, and behavior of black university students over a ten-year period.* Counseling Center Report, No. 5-95, University of Maryland at College Park.

Oakes, J. (1982). The reproduction of inequity: The content of secondary school tracking. *Urban Review, 14,* 107-120.

Oakes, J. (1992). Can tracking research inform practice? Technical, normative, and political considerations. *Educational Researcher, 21,* 12-21.

Oetting, E. R., & Beauvais, F. (1987). Peer cluster theory, socialization characteristics, and adolescent drug use: A path analysis. *Journal of Counseling Psychology, 34,* 205-213.

Ogbu, J. U. (1978). *Minority education and caste: The American system in cross-cultural perspective.* New York: Academic Press.

Ogbu, J. U. (1982). Cultural discontinuities and schooling. *Anthropology and Education Quarterly, 13,* 290-307.

Ogbu, J. U. (1983). Minority status and schooling in plural societies. *Comparative Education Review, 27,* 168-190.

Ogbu, J. U. (1987). Variability in minority school performance: A problem in search of an explanation. *Anthropology and Education Quarterly, 18,* 312-334.

Ogbu, J. U. (1991). Minority status and literacy in comparative perspective. In S. R. Graubard (Ed.), *Literacy: An overview by 14 experts* (pp. 141-168). New York: Noonday.

Okocha, A. G. (1994). Preparing racial ethnic minorities for the workforce 2000. *Journal of Multicultural Counseling and Development, 22,* 106-114.

Oliver, M. L. (1997). Building wealth: Another way to fight poverty. *The Ford Foundation Report,* Winter, pp. 8-9.

Oliver, M. L., & Shapiro, T. M. (1995). *Black wealth/white wealth: A new perspective on racial inequality.* New York: Routledge.

Oliver, W. (1984). Black males and the tough guy image: A dysfunctional compensatory adaptation. *Western Journal of Black Studies, 8,* 201-202.

Oliver, W. (1989). Black males and social problems: Prevention through Afrocentric socialization. *Journal of Black Studies, 20*(1), 15-39.

Olweus, D. (1991). Bully/victim problems among school children: Basic facts and effects of a school-based intervention program. In D. J. Pepler & K. H. Rubin (Eds.), *The development and treatment of childhood aggression* (pp. 411-448). Hillsdale, NJ: Lawrence Erlbaum.

Oubre, C. F. (1978). *Forty acres and a mule: The Freedmen's Bureau and black land ownership.* Baton Rouge: Louisiana State University Press.

Oyserman, D., Gant, L., & Ager, J. (1995). A socially contextualized model of African American identity: Possible selves and school persistence. *Journal of Personality & Social Psychology, 69,* 1216-1232.

Ozawa, M. (1986). Non-whites and the demographic imperative in social welfare spending. *Social Work, 3,* 440-446.

Pace, D. (1993). *Community relations concepts.* Placerville, CA: Copperhouse.

Page-Adams, D., & Sherraden, M. (1996). *What we know about effects of asset accumulation.* Working Paper 96-1, Center for Social Development, Washington University, St. Louis.

Parham, T. A., & Austin, N. L. (1994). Career development and African Americans: A contextual reappraisal using the nigrescence construct. *Journal of Vocational Behavior, 44,* 139-154.

Parker, S., Tong, T., Bolden, S., & Wingo, P. (1997, January/February). Cancer statistics, 1997. *CA: A Cancer Journal for Clinicians,* pp. 5-27.

Pearson, D. (1994). The black man: Health issues and implications for clinical practice. *Journal of Black Studies, 25*(1), 81-98.

Pedersen, F. A., & Sullivan, E. J. (1964). Relationships among geographic mobility and emotional disturbances in children. *American Journal of Orthopsychiatry, 34,* 575-580.

Pepler, D. J., King, G., & Byrd, W. (1991). A social-cognitively based social skills training program for aggressive children. In D. J. Pepler & K. H. Rubin (Eds.), *The development and treatment of childhood aggression* (pp. 361-379). Hillsdale, NJ: Lawrence Erlbaum.

Perkins, U. E. (1986). *Harvesting new generations: The positive development of black youth.* Chicago: Third World Press.

Perkins, U. E. (1987). *Explosion of Chicago's black street gangs.* Chicago: Third World Press.

Perry, J. L., & Locke, D. C. (1985). Career development of black men: Implications for school guidance services. *Journal of Multicultural Counseling and Development, 13,* 106-111.

Peters, S., Wyatt, G., & Finkelhor, D. (1986). Prevalence. In D. Finkelhor et al. (Eds.), *A source book on child sexual abuse.* Beverly Hills, CA: Sage.

Peterson, J. L. (1992). Black men and their same-sex desires and behaviors. In G. Herdt (Ed.), *Gay culture in America: Essays from the field* (pp. 147-164). Boston: Beacon.

Peterson, J. L., Coates, T. J., Catania, J. A., Middleton, L., Hilliard, B., & Hearst, N. (1992). High-risk sexual behavior and condom use among gay and bisexual African American men. *American Journal of Public Health, 82*(11), 1490-1494.

364   🕮   WORKING WITH AFRICAN AMERICAN MALES

Peterson, J. L., Coates, T. J., Catania, J. A., Hilliard, B., Middleton, L., & Hearst, N. (1995). Help-seeking for AIDS high-risk sexual behavior among gay and bisexual African American men. *AIDS Education and Prevention, 7*(1), 1-9.

Peterson, J. L., & Marin, G. (1988). Issues in the prevention of AIDS among black and Hispanic men. *American Psychologist, 34,* 871-877.

Pfeiffer, E. (1975). A short portable mental status questionnaire for the assessment of organic brain deficits in elderly patients. *Journal of the American Geriatrics Society, 23,* 433-441.

Pfeiffer, E. (1979). A short psychiatric evaluation schedule. In Bayer Symposium VII, *Brain function in old age* (pp. 228-236). Berlin: Springer-Verlag.

Phillips, F. B. (1990). NTU psychotherapy: An Afrocentric approach. *Journal of Black Psychology, 17,* 55-74.

Pierce, L., & Pierce, R. (1984). Race as a factor in the sexual abuse of children. *Social Work Research and Abstracts, 20*(2), 9-14.

Pierce, R., & Pierce, L. H. (1985). The sexually abused child: A comparison of male and female victims. *Child Abuse & Neglect, 54,* 910-811.

Pi-Sunyer, F. X. (1990). Obesity and diabetes in blacks. *Diabetes Care, 13*(11), 1144-1149.

Pleck, J. H. (1995). The gender role strain paradigm: An update. In R. F. Levant & W. S. Pollack (Eds.), *A new psychology of men* (pp. 11-32). New York: Basic Books.

Poitier, V. L., Niliwaambieni, M., & Lamar Rowe, C. (1997). A rite of passage approach designed to preserve the families of substance-abusing African American women. *Child Welfare, 76*(1), 173-195.

Polite, V. C. (1994). The method in the madness: African American males, avoidance schooling, and chaos theory. *Journal of Negro Education, 63*(4), 588-601.

Porter, E. (1986). *Treating the young male victims of sexual assault: Issues and intervention strategies.* Syracuse, NY: Safer Society Press.

Porter, F. A., Block, L. C., & Sgroi, S. N. (1982). Treatment of the sexually abused child. In S. G. Sgroi (Ed.), *Handbook of clinical intervention in child sexual abuse* (pp. 109-145). Lexington, MA: Lexington Books.

Powell, C. (1995). *My American journey.* New York: Ballantine.

Prentiss, T. M. (1996, April). *The relationship of learning process and social context: A cross-case analysis of the social construction of homework centers.* Paper presented at the annual meeting of the American Educational Research Association, New York City.

Price, J., Colvin, T., & Smith, D. (1993). Prostate cancer: Perceptions of African-American males. *Journal of the National Medical Association, 85,* 941-947.

Prothrow-Stith, D. (1991). *Deadly consequences: How violence is destroying our teenage population and a plan to begin solving the problem.* New York: Harper Collins.

Prothrow-Stith, D., & Weissman, M. (1991). *Deadly consequences.* New York: Harper Collins.

Rabin, S. (1994). How to sell across cultures. *American Demographics, 16,* 56-57.

Radloff, L. S. (1977). The CES-D scale: A self-report depression scale for research in the general population. *Applied Psychological Measures, 3,* 385-401.

Rainey Ranson, E. (1994). Doing time together: An exploratory study of incarcerated fathers and their kids. *Dissertation Abstracts International, 54*(10-A), 3884.

Raskin, P. (Ed.). *Medical management of non-insulin-dependent (Type II) diabetes* (3rd ed.). Alexandria, VA: American Diabetes Association.

Ratzki, A., & Fisher, A. (1989/1990). Life in a restructured school. *Educational Leadership, 47,* 46-51.

Raymond, N. R., & D'Eramo-Melkus, G. (1993). Insulin-dependent diabetes and obesity in the black and Hispanic population: Culturally sensitive management. *The Diabetes Educator, 19,* 313-317.

Redd, M. L. (1989). Alcoholism and drug addiction among black adults. In R. L. Jones (Ed.), *Black adult development and aging.* Berkeley, CA: Cobb & Henry.

Rees, A. (1966). Information networks in labor markets. *American Economic Review, 56*(2), 559-566.

Reiss, A. (1988). Co-offending and criminal careers. In M. Tonry & N. Morris (Eds.), *Crime and delinquency* (Vol. 10). Chicago: University of Chicago Press.

Remnick, D. (1996, April 29 and May 6). Dr. Wilson's neighborhood. *The New Yorker,* pp. 96-107.

Reno calls for crime prevention programs. (1993, July 11). *Star Tribune,* p. 1A.

Resnick, G., Burt, M. R., Newmark, L., & Reilly, L. (1992). *Youth at risk: Definitions, prevalence, and approaches to service delivery.* Washington, DC: Urban Institute Press.

Reynolds, R. (1993, July). Kids who kill. *Black Enterprise,* p. 47.

Rich, J. A., & Stone, D. A. (1996). The experience of violent injury for young African American men: The meaning of being a sucker. *Journal of General Internal Medicine, 11,* 77-82.

Ridley, C. R. (1984). Clinical treatment of the nondisclosing black client: A therapeutic paradox. *American Psychologist, 39*(11), 1234-1244.

Rivara, F. P., Sweeney, P. J., & Henderson, B. F. (1986). Black teenage fathers: What happens when the child is born? *Pediatrics, 78,* 151-158.

Rivera, D., Jackson, J., & Jackson, J. (1993). Our current concerns. *National Rainbow Coalition Newsletter, 1*(12).

Robins, L. N., & Przybeck, T. R. (1985). Age of onset of drug use as a factor in drug and other disorders. *National Institute of Drug Abuse Research Series, 56,* 178-192.

Robinson, B. E. (1988). *Teenage fathers.* Lexington, MA: Lexington Books.

Rogers, C. M., & Terry, T. (1984). Clinical interventions with boy victims of sexual abuse. In I. Stewart & J. Greer (Eds.), *Victims of sexual aggression* (pp. 91-104). New York: Van Nostrand Reinhold.

Rogoff, B. (1994). Developing understanding of the idea of communities of learners. *Mind, Culture, and Activity, 1,* 209-229.

Rose, H. (1990). *Race place and risk: Black homicide in urban America.* Albany: State University of New York Press.

Ross, S., & Jackson, J. (1991). Teachers' expectations for black males' and black females' academic achievement. *Personality and Social Psychology Bulletin, 17*(1), 78-82.

Rosseau, R. (1996). Project Kofi. In E. Wattenberg & Y. Pearson (Eds.), *Defining excellence for school-linked services: A summary of the proceedings of the conference held September 14, 1995, at the University of Minnesota* (pp. 21-22). Minneapolis: Center for Urban and Regional Affairs.

Rotheram, M. J., & Phinney, J. S. (1987). Definitions and perspectives in the study of children's ethnic socialization. In J. S. Phinney & M. J. Rotheram (Eds.), *Children's ethnic socialization: Pluralism and development* (pp. 10-28). Newbury Park, CA: Sage.

Rotheram-Borus, M. J. (1993). Multicultural issues in the delivery of group interventions. *Special Services in the Schools, 8,* 179-188.

Rotheram-Borus, M. J., Bahlburg, H. F. L., Rosario, M., Koopman, C., Haignere, C. S., Exner, T. M., Matthieu, M., Henderson, R., & Gruen, R. S. (1992). Lifetime sexual behaviors among predominantly minority male runaways and gay/bisexual adolescents in New York City. *AIDS Education and Prevention,* Supplement, 34-42.

Rotheram-Borus, M. J., & Koopman, C. (1991). Sexual risk behavior, AIDS knowledge, and beliefs about AIDS among predominantly minority gay and bisexual male adolescents. *AIDS Education and Prevention, 3*(4), 305-312.

Rowan, B. (1990). Commitment and control: Alternative strategies for the organizational design of schools. In C. B. Cazden (Ed.), *Review of research in education* (pp. 353-389). Washington DC: American Educational Research Association.

Ruhm, C. (1995). *Is high school employment consumption or investment?* Working paper, National Bureau of Economic Research.

Russell, D. E. H. (1983). The incidence and prevalence of intra-familiar and extra-familiar sexual abuse of female children. *Child Abuse & Neglect, 7*(33), 133-146.

Ryan, R., Longres, J. F., & Roffman, R. A. (1996). Sexual identity, social support, and social networks among African-, Latino-, and European American men in an HIV prevention program. In J. F. Longres (Ed.), *Men of color: A context for service to homosexually active men* (pp. 1-24). Binghamton, NY: Harrington Park Press.

Sack, W. H. (1977). Children of imprisoned fathers. *Psychiatry, 40,* 163-174.

Salguero, C. (1984). The role of ethnic factors in adolescent pregnancy and motherhood. In M. Sugar (Ed.), *Adolescent parenthood* (pp. 75-98). New York: SP Medical and Scientific Books.

Salter, A. C. (1988). Victim identification and behavior of sexually abused children. In *Treating child sex offenders and victims: A practical guide* (pp. 223-245). Newbury Park, CA: Sage.

Sampson, R. (1991). Black male genocide: A final solution to the race problem in America. In B. P. Bowser (Ed.), *Black adolescents: Parenting and education in the community context.* Lanham, MD: University Press.

Samuel, M., & Winkelstein, W., Jr. (1987). Prevalence of human immunodeficiency virus infection in ethnic minority homosexual/bisexual men. *Journal of American Medical Association, 257*(14), 1901-1902.

Sanchez-Jankowski, M. (1991). *Islands in the street: Gangs and American urban society.* Berkeley: University of California Press.

Sander, J. H., & Rosen, J. L. (1987). Teenage fathers: Working with the neglected partner in adolescent childbearing. *Family Planning Perspectives, 19,* 107-110.

Sanders, W. (1995). *Gang-bangs and drive-bys: Grounded culture and juvenile gang violence.* New York: Aldine.

Santiago, J. V. (Ed.). (1994). *Medical management of insulin-dependent (Type I) diabetes* (2nd ed.). Alexandria, VA: American Diabetes Association.

Sautter, C. (1995). Standing up to violence. *Phi Delta Kappan, 76,* K1-K12.

Savin-Williams, R. C. (1990). *Gay and lesbian youth: Expressions of identity.* New York: Hemisphere Publishing.

Scanlon, E., & Emerson, S. (1997). *Home mortgage lending in St. Louis: An analysis of 1992 and 1994 Home Mortgage Disclosure Act data.* Working paper, Center for Social Development, Washington University, St. Louis.

Schacht, A., Kerlinshy, D., & Carlson, C. (1990). Group therapy with sexually abused boys: Leadership projective identification and counter-transference issues. *International Journal of Group Psychotherapy, 40,* 401-417.

Scher, M., Stevens, M., Good, G., & Eichenfield, G. A. (1987). *Handbook of counseling and psychotherapy with men.* Newbury Park, CA: Sage.

Schiele, J. H. (1996). Afrocentricity: An emerging paradigm in social welfare practice. *Social Work, 41*(3), 284-294.

Schilit, J. (1989). Study four: Homeless families and children in South Florida. In D. S. Fike (Ed.), *The South Florida homelessness studies of 1989: A summary of key findings* (Vol. 3). Miami: Barry College.

Schinke, S. P., Botvin, G. J., & Orlandi, M. A. (1991). *Substance abuse in children and adolescents: Evaluation and intervention.* Newbury Park, CA: Sage.

Schneider, D., Greenberg, M., & Choi, D. (1993). Black leaders' perceptions of the Year 2000 public health goals for black Americans. *American Journal of Public Health, 83*(8), 1171-1173.

Schneller, D. P. (1976). *The prisoner's family: A study of the effects of imprisonment on the families of prisoners.* San Francisco: R & E Research Associates.

Schorr, L. (1988). *Within our reach: Breaking the cycle of disadvantage.* New York: Doubleday.

Scott-Jones, D., Roland, E. J., & White, A. B. (1989). Antecedents and outcomes of pregnancy in black adolescents. In R. L. Jones (Ed.), *Black adolescents* (pp. 341-371). Berkeley, CA: Cobb & Henry.

Sebold, J. (1987). Indicators of child sexual abuse in males: Social casework. *Journal of Contemporary Social Work, 68,* 75-80.

Sedlacek, W. E., & Brooks, G. C., Jr. (1976). *Racism in American education: A model for change.* Chicago: Nelson-Hall.

Seidler, V. (1992). Rejection, vulnerability, and friendship. In P. Nardi (Ed.), *Men's friendships* (pp. 15-34). Newbury Park, CA: Sage.

Shakoor, B., & Chalmers, D. (1991). Co-victimization of African-American children who witness violence: Effects on cognitive, emotional, and behavioral development. *Journal of the National Medical Association, 83,* 233-238.

Shakur, S. (1993). *Monster.* New York: Atlantic Monthly Press.

Shakur, S. (1994). *Monster: The autobiography of an L.A. gang member.* New York: Penguin.

Shannon, L. (1982). *Assessing the relationship of adult criminal careers to juvenile careers: A summary.* Washington, DC: Government Printing Office.

Shapiro, C. (1993). *When part of the self is lost: Helping clients heal after sexual and reproductive losses.* San Francisco: Jossey-Bass.

Shaw, C., & McKay, H. (1942). *Juvenile delinquency and urban areas.* Chicago: University of Chicago Press.

Shaw, R. (1987). *Children of imprisoned fathers.* London: Hodder & Stoughton.

Sherraden, M. (1988). Rethinking social welfare: Toward assets. *Social Policy, 18*(3), 37-43.

Sherraden, M. (1989). Individual development accounts. *Entrepreneurial Economy Review, 8*(5), 1-22.

Sherraden, M. (1990). *Stakeholding: A new direction in social policy* (Report No. 2). Washington, DC: Progressive Policy Institute.

Sherraden, M. (1991). *Assets and the poor: A new American welfare policy.* New York: M. E. Sharpe.

Sherraden, M., & Adamek, M. (1984). Explosive imagery and misguided policy. *Social Service Review, 58*(4), 539-555.

Sherraden, M. S., & Ninacs, W. (Eds.). (1998). Community economic development [Special issue]. *Journal of Community Practice.*

Shilkoff, D. (1983). The use of male-female co-leadership in an early adolescent girls' activity group. *Social Work With Groups, 6*(2), 67-80.

Short, J. F., Jr., & Strodtbeck, F. L. (1965). *Group process and gang delinquency.* Chicago: University of Chicago Press.

Siegel, K., Bauman, L. J., Christ, G. H., & Krown, S. (1988). Patterns of change in sexual behavior among gay men in New York City. *Archives of Sexual Behavior, 17*(6), 481-497.

Silverberg, J. (1989). Sexual problems in people with diabetes. *Diabetes Dialogue, 36*(2), 15-17.

Simmons, R. (1991a). Some thoughts on the challenges facing black gay intellectuals. In E. Hemphill (Ed.), *Brother to brother: New writings by black gay men* (pp. 211-228). Boston: Alyson.

Simmons, R. (1991b). Tongues untied: An interview with Marlon Riggs. In E. Hemphill (Ed.), *Brother to brother: New writings by black gay men* (pp. 189-199). Boston: Alyson.

Slaby, R. G., Barham, J., Eron, L. D., & Wilcox, B. L. (1994). Policy recommendations: Prevention and treatment of youth violence. In L. D. Eron, J. H. Gentry, & P. Schlegel (Eds.), *Reason to hope: A psychosocial perspective on violence and youth* (pp. 447-456). Washington, DC: American Psychological Association.

Slaughter-Defoe, D., & Richards, H. (1995). Literacy for empowerment: The case of black males. In V. L. Godsen & D. A. Wagner (Eds.), *Literacy among African*

American youth: Issues in learning, teaching, and schooling (pp. 125-147). Cresskill, NJ: Hampton.

Slavin, R. E., Madden, N. A., Dolan, L. J., Wasch, B. A., Ross, S. M., & Smith, L. J. (1994, April). Whenever and wherever we choose: The replication of success for all. *Phi Delta Kappan, 75,* 639-647.

Smith, E. J. (1981). Cultural and historical perspectives in counseling blacks. In D. W. Sue (Ed.), *Counseling the culturally different: Theory and practice* (pp. 141-185). New York: John Wiley.

Smith, L. A. (1988). Black adolescent fathers: Issues for service provision. *Social Work, 33*(3), 269-271.

Smith, L. A. (1989). *Windows on opportunities: An exploration in program development for black adolescent fathers.* Unpublished doctoral dissertation, City University of New York.

Smitherman, G. (1977). *Talkin' and testifyin': The language of black America.* Boston: Houghton Mifflin.

Solomon, A. (1992). Clinical diagnosis among diverse populations: A multicultural perspective. *Families and Society: The Journal of Contemporary Human Services, 73*(6), 371-377.

Spergel, I. (1995). *The youth gang problem: A community approach.* New York: Oxford University Press.

Spergel, I., & Curry, G. D. (1993). The National Youth Gang Survey: A research and development process. In A. Goldstein & C. R. Huff (Eds.), *The gang intervention handbook.* Champaign, IL: Research Press.

Sprinthall, N. A., & Scott, J. R. (1989). Promoting psychological development, math achievement, and success attribution of female students through deliberate psychological education. *Journal of Counseling Psychology, 36,* 440-446.

Spurlock, J. (1982). Black Americans. In A. Gaw (Ed.), *Cross-cultural psychiatry* (pp. 163-178). Littleton, MA: John Wright-PSG Publishing.

Staples, B. (1994). *Parallel time: Growing up in black and white.* New York: Avon.

Staples, R. (1978). Masculinity and race: The dual dilemma of black men. *Journal of Social Issues, 34,* 169-183.

Staples, R. (1982). *Black masculinity: The black male's role in American society.* San Francisco: Black Scholar Press.

Staples, R. (1985). Changes in black family structure: The conflict between family ideology and structural conditions. *Journal of Marriage and the Family, 53,* 221-230.

Staples, R. (1991). *The black family: Essays and studies* (4th ed.). Belmont, CA: Wadsworth.

Staples, R., & Bowlin-Johnson, L. (1993). *Black families at the crossroads: Challenges and prospects.* San Francisco: Jossey-Bass.

Stark, E. (1993). The myth of black violence. *Social Work, 38*(4), 485-491.

State of Missouri, House of Representatives. (1997). *Family Development Accounts,* H.R. 302. Jefferson City: House of Representatives.

Staub, E. (1996). Cultural-societal roots of violence: The examples of the genocidal violence and contemporary youth violence in the United States. *The American Psychologist, 51*(2), 117-133.

Stewart, C. (1991). Black, gay (and invisible)—double jeopardy. *New Republic, 205*(23), 13-15.

Stewart, M. (1992). The educational status of black males in America: The agony and the ecstasy. *Negro Educational Review, 43*(1-2), 28-30.

Stolar, M. (1995, August 24-26). *Diabetes educators: Making a difference.* Paper presented at the American Association of Diabetes Educators annual meeting, Boston.

Stoy, D., Curtis, R., & Dameworth, K. (1995). The successful recruitment of elderly black subjects in a clinical trial: The Crisp program. *Journal of the National Medical Association, 87,* 280-287.

Strasburger, V. C. (1995). *Adolescents and the media: Medical and psychological impact.* Thousand Oaks, CA: Sage.

Stricker, G., & Gold, J. (Eds.). (1993). *Comprehensive handbook of psychotherapy integration.* New York: Plenum.

Strickland, W. (1989, November). The future of black men. *Essence,* pp. 50-52, 112.

Strike, K. A., & Soltis, J. F. (1985). *The ethics of teaching.* New York: Teachers College Press.

Strong, E. K., Hansen, J., & Campbell, D. P. (1994). *Strong interest inventory.* Palo Alto: CA: Consulting Psychologists Press.

Sturkie, K. (1983). Structured group treatment for sexually abused children. *Health and Social Work, 8,* 299-308.

Sue, D. W., & Sue, D. (1990). *Counseling the culturally different: Theory and practice* (2nd ed.). New York: Wiley Interscience.

Sue, S., McKinney, H., Allen, D., & Hall, J. (1974). Delivery of community mental health services to black and white clients. *Journal of Consulting and Clinical Psychology, 42,* 794-801.

Sullivan, M. L. (1985). *Teen fathers in the inner city: An exploratory ethnographic study* (Report No. UD 024 536). New York: Vera Institute of Justice. (ERIC Document Reproduction Service No. ED 264 316)

Sussman, L. (1996). Sociocultural concerns of diabetes care. In D. Haire-Joshu (Ed.), *Management of diabetes mellitus: Perspectives of care across the life span* (pp. 473-512). St. Louis, MO: C. V. Mosby.

Sutton, A. (1996). African American men in group therapy. In M. Andronico (Ed.), *Men in groups: Insights, interventions, psychoeducational work.* Washington, DC: American Psychological Association.

Sutton, S. (1996). *Weaving a tapestry of resistance: The places, power and poetry of a sustainable society.* Westport, CT: Bergen Garvey.

Swan, A. L. (1981). *Families of black prisoners.* Boston: G. K. Hall

Szapocznik, J., & Kurtines, W. (1980). Acculturation, biculturalism, and adjustment among Cuban Americans. In A. M. Padilla (Ed.), *Acculturation: Theory, models, and some new findings.* Boulder, CO: American Association for the Advancement of Science.

Tanfer, K. (1993). National Survey of Men: Design and execution. *Family Planning Perspectives, 25*(2), 83-86.

Targonski, P., Guinan, P., & Phillips, C. (1991). Prostate cancer: The stage disadvantage in the black male. *Journal of the National Medical Association, 83,* 1094-1096.

Taylor, C. S. (1993). *Girls, gangs, women, and drugs.* East Lansing: Michigan State University Press.

Taylor, R., Leashore, B., & Tolliver, S. (1988). An assessment of the provider role as perceived by black males. *Family Relations, 37,* 426-431.

Taylor, R. J. (1988). Structural determinants of religious participation among black Americans. *Review of Religious Research, 30,* 114-125.

Taylor, R. J., & Chatters, L. M. (1986a). Church-based informal support among elderly blacks. *Gerontology, 26,* 637-642.

Taylor, R. J., & Chatters, L. M. (1986b). Patterns of informal support to elderly black adults: The role of family and church members. *Social Work, 31,* 432-438.

Taylor, R. J., & Chatters, L. M. (1989). Family, friend, and church support networks of black Americans. In R. L. Jones (Ed.), *Black adult development and aging.* Berkeley, CA: Cobb & Henry.

Taylor, R. J., Neighbors, H. W., & Broman, C. L. (1989). Evaluation by black Americans of the social service encounter during a serious personal problem. *Social Work, 34,* 205-211.

Taylor, R. J., Thornton, M. C., & Chatters, L. M. (1987). Black Americans' perceptions of sociohistorical role of the church. *Journal of Black Studies, 18*(2), 123-138.

Thomas, C. (1993). *Black and blue: Profiles of blacks in IBM.* Atlanta, GA: Aaron Press.

Thrasher, F. (1927). *The gang.* Chicago: University of Chicago Press.

Timberlake, E. M., & Sabatino, C. A. (1994). Homeless children: Impact of school attendance on self-esteem and loneliness. *Social Work in Education, 12,* 9-20.

Tinney, J. S. (1986). Why a black gay church? In J. Beam (Ed.), *In the life: A black gay anthology* (pp. 70-86). Boston: Alyson.

Tobias, R. (1989). Educating black urban adolescents. In R. Jones (Ed.), *Black adolescents* (pp. 207-228). Berkeley, CA: Cobb & Henry.

Trent, W., & McPartland, J. (1981). *Race comparisons of student course enrollment and extracurricular membership in segregated and desegregated high schools.* Paper presented at the American Educational Research Association annual meeting, Los Angeles.

Troiden, R. R. (1979). Becoming homosexual: A model of gay identity acquisition. *Psychiatry, 24,* 362-373.

Trotter, A. (1991). Rites of passage. *Executive Express, 13,* 48-49.

Tucker, C., Chennault, S., Brody, G., Fraser, K., Gaskin, V., Dunn, C., & Frisby, C. (1995). A parent, community public schools, and university involved partnership education program to examine and boost academic achievement and adaptive functioning skills of African-American students. *Journal of Research & Development in Education, 28,* 175-185.

Tucker, M., & Mitchell-Kernan, C. (Eds.). (1995). *The decline in marriage among African Americans.* New York: Russell Sage Foundation.

Tull, E. S., & Roseman, W. H. (1995). Diabetes in African Americans. In National Institutes of Health (Ed.), *Diabetes in America* (2nd ed., pp. 613-630). Bethesda, MD: Editor.

Turner, S., Norman, E., & Zunz, S. (1995). Enhancing resiliency in girls and boys: A case for gender specific adolescent prevention programming. *Journal of Primary Prevention, 16*(8), 25-38.

Urquiza, A. J., & Capra, M. (1990). The impact of sexual abuse: Initial and long-term effects. In M. Hunter (Ed.), *The sexual abused male: Vol. 1. Prevalence, impact, and treatment* (pp. 105-136). Lexington, MA: Lexington.

U.S. Bureau of the Census. (1991a). *Marital status and living arrangements: May 1990* (Current Population Reports, Series P-20, No. 450). Washington, DC: Government Printing Office.

U.S. Bureau of the Census. (1991b). *Money, income, and poverty status of families and persons in the United States* (Current Population Reports, Series P-60, No. 181). Washington, DC: Government Printing Office.

U.S. Bureau of the Census. (1992). *Poverty in the United States, 1991* (Current Population Reports, Series P-60, No. 181). Washington, DC: Government Printing Office.

U.S. Bureau of the Census. (1993). *Statistical abstract of the United States: 1993.* Washington DC: Government Printing Office.

U.S. Bureau of the Census. (1995a). *Asset ownership of households* (Current Population Reports, Series P-70, No. 47). Washington, DC: Government Printing Office.

U.S. Bureau of the Census. (1995b). *Statistical abstract of the United States: 1995* (115th ed.). Washington, DC: Government Printing Office.

U.S. Bureau of the Census. (1996a). *Household and family characteristics, March, 1996* (Current Population Reports. Series P-20, No. 495). Washington, DC: Government Printing Office.

U.S. Bureau of the Census. (1996b). *Statistical abstract of the United States: 1996* (116th ed.). Washington, DC: Government Printing Office.

U.S. Bureau of the Census. (1997). *Selected characteristics of the population by race, March 1997.* Washington, DC: Government Printing Office.

U.S. Bureau of the Census. (1998). *Educational attainment in the United States: March 1997.* (Current Population Reports). Washington, DC: Government Printing Office.

U.S. Congress. (1996). *The Personal Responsibility and Work Opportunity Act,* PL 104-193. Washington: U.S. Government Printing Office.

U.S. Department of Health and Human Services. (1986). Chemical dependency and diabetes. In *Report of the Secretary's Task Force on Black and Minority Health* (Vol. 7, pp. 189-374). Washington, DC: Author.

U.S. Department of Health and Human Services. (1989). *Report of the Secretary's Task Force on Black and Minority Health: Vol. 1. Executive summary* (DHHS Publication No. 241-80-841/05306). Washington, DC: Government Printing Office.

U.S. Department of Health and Human Services. (1990). *Health status of minorities and low income groups.* Washington, DC: Government Printing Office.

U.S. Department of Justice, Federal Bureau of Investigation. (1995a). *Crime in the United States, 1994.* Washington, DC: Government Printing Office.

U.S. Department of Justice. (1995b). *Prisoners in 1994* (NCJ-151654). Washington, DC: Government Printing Office.

U.S. Department of Justice. (1995c). *Sourcebook of criminal justice statistics—1994* (NCJ-154591). Washington, DC: Government Printing Office.

U.S. Department of Justice. (1996). *HIV in prisons, 1994* (NCJ-158-020). Washington, DC: Government Printing Office.

U.S. Department of Labor. (1994). *Occupational outlook handbook.* Washington, DC: Government Printing Office.

U.S. General Accounting Office. (1990). *Drug education: School-based programs seen as useful but impact unknown* (GAO/HRD 91-27; Report to the Chairman, Committee on Governmental Affairs, U.S. Senate). Washington, DC: Government Printing Office.

U.S. Senate. (1995). *The Assets for Independence Act,* S. 1212, 104th Congress. Washington: Government Printing Office.

Van Sertima, I. (1976). *They came before Columbus.* New York: Random House.

Vaz, R., Smolen, P., & Miller, C. (1983). Adolescent pregnancy: Involvement of the male partner. *Journal of Adolescent Health Care, 4,* 246-250.

Violato, C., & Genius, M. (1993). Problems of research in male child sexual abuse: A review. *Journal of Child Sexual Abuse, 2,* 33-54.

Voight, L., Thornton, W., Barrile, L., & Seaman, J. M. (1994). *Criminology and justice.* New York: McGraw-Hill.

Vontress, C. E. (1995). The breakdown of authority: Implications for counseling young African American males. In J. G. Ponterotto, J. M. Casas, L. A. Suzuki, & C. M. Alexander (Eds.), *Handbook of multicultural counseling* (pp. 457-472). Thousand Oaks, CA: Sage.

Vosler, N., & Robertson, J. (1998). Nonmarital co-parenting: Knowledge-building for practice. *Families in Society: The Journal of Contemporary Human Service, 79*(2), 149-159.

Walker, S., Spohn, C., & Delone, M. (1996). *The color of justice: Race, ethnicity, and crime in America.* Belmont, CA: Wadsworth.

Walling, D. R. (1990). *Meeting the needs of transient students.* Bloomington, IN: Phi Delta Kappa.

Warnath, C. E. (1975). Vocational theories: Direction to nowhere. *Personnel and Guidance Journal, 53,* 422-428.

Washington, B. T. (1909). *The story of the Negro* (2 vols.). New York: Doubleday, Page.

Washington, C. S. (1987). Counseling black men. In M. Scher, M. Stevens, G. Good, & G. A. Eichenfield (Eds.), *Handbook of counseling and psychotherapy with men* (pp. 192-202). Newbury Park, CA: Sage.

Washington, V., & Newman, J. (1991). Setting our own agenda: Exploring the meaning of gender disparities among blacks in higher education. *Journal of Negro Education, 60,* 19-35.

Watts, N. B., Spanheimer, R. G., Di Girolamo, M., et al. (1990). Prediction of glucose responses to weight loss in patients with non-insulin-dependent diabetes mellitus. *Archives of Internal Medicine, 150,* 803-806.

Weine, A. M., Kuraski, K. S., Jason, L. A., Danner, K. E., & Johnson, J. H. (1993). An evaluation of preventive tutoring programs for transfer students. *Child Study Journal, 23,* 135-152.

Wells-Barnett, I. B. (1969). *On lynchings.* New York: Arno. (Original work published 1892)

Wetzel, J. (1989). American youth: A statistical snapshot. In *Youth and America's future: The William T. Grant commission on work, family, and citizenship.* Washington, DC: William T. Grant Commission.

Whetstone, M. (1996, March). What happens when the woman makes more than the man? *Ebony,* pp. 30-34.

White, J. L. (1984). *The psychology of blacks: An Afro-American perspective.* Englewood Cliffs, NJ: Wadsworth.

William, J., & Gold, M. (1972). From delinquent behavior to official delinquency. *Social Problems, 20,* 209-229.

Williams, C. W. (1991). *Black teenage mothers: Pregnancy and child rearing from their perspective.* Lexington, MA: Lexington Books.

Williams, J. H., Stiffman, A. R., & O'Neal, J. L. (1998) Violence among African American youths: An analysis of environmental and behavioral risk factors. *Social Work Research, 22*(1), 3-13.

Williams, M. W. (1990). Polygamy and the declining male to female ratio in black communities: A social inquiry. In H. E. Cheatham & J. B. Stewart (Eds.), *Black families: Interdisciplinary perspectives* (pp. 171-193). New Brunswick, NJ: Transaction Publishers.

Williams, O. J. (1995, September 25). Treatment for African American men who batter. *CURA Reporter,* pp. 6-10.

Williams, O. J. (1998). Healing and confronting the African American man who batters. In R. Carrillo & J. Tello (Eds.), *Family violence and men of color: Healing the wounded male spirit.* New York: Springer.

Williams, O. J., & Becker, L. R. (1994) Domestic partner abuse treatment programs and cultural competence: The results of a national study. *Violence and Victims, 8*(3), 287-296.

Williams, W. S. (1972). Black economic and cultural development: A prerequisite to vocational choice. In R. Jones (Ed.), *Black psychology* (pp. 233-245). New York: Harper & Row.

Wilson, A. (1990). *Black-on-black violence: The psychodynamics of black self-annihilation in service of white domination.* New York: Afrikan World InfoSystems.

Wilson, A. N. (1991) *Understanding black adolescent male violence: Its remediation and prevention.* New York: Afrikan World InfoSystems.

Wilson, J. & Herrnstein, R. (1985). *Crime and human nature.* New York: Simon & Schuster.

Wilson, W. J. (1987). *The truly disadvantaged.* Chicago: University of Chicago Press.

Wilson, W. J. (1996). *When work disappears.* New York: Knopf.

Wing, R. R., Koeske, R., Epstein, L. H., et al. (1987). Long-term effects of modest weight loss in Type II diabetic patients. *Archives of Internal Medicine, 147,* 1749-1753.

Wingert, P. (1990, January 29). Fewer blacks on campus. *Newsweek,* p. 75.

Wolfe, D. M., & Kolb, D. A. (1980). Career development, personal growth, and experimental learning. In J. W. Springer (Ed.), *Issues in career and human resource development.* Madison, WI: American Society for Training and Development.

Wolff, E. N. (1995). *Top heavy: A study of the increased inequality of wealth in America.* New York: Twentieth Century Fund.

Wolfgang, M., & Ferracuti, F. (1967). *The subculture of violence: Toward an integrated theory in criminology.* London: Tavistock.

Wright, J. W. (1993). African American male sexual behavior and the risk for HIV infection. *Human Organization, 52*(4), 421-431.

Wright, R. (1945). *Black boy: A record of childhood and youth.* New York: Harper.

Wright, W. J. (1991-1992). The endangered black male child. *Educational Leadership, 49,* 14-16.

Wyatt, G. E. (1982). Identifying stereotypes of Afro-American sexuality and their impact upon sexual behavior. In B. A. Bass, G. E. Wyatt, & G. J. Powell (Eds.), *The Afro-American family: Assessment, treatment, and research issues* (pp. 333-346). New York: Grune & Stratton.

Wyatt, G. (1985). The sexual abuse of Afro American and White American women in childhood. *Child Abuse & Neglect, 9,* 231-240.

Wynn, M. (1992). *Empowering African-American males to succeed: A ten-step approach for parents and teachers.* South Pasadena, CA: Rising Sun Publishing.

Yalom, I. (1995). *The theory and practice of group psychotherapy* (4th ed.). New York: Basic Books.

Zatz, M. S. (1987). The changing forms of racial/ethnic biases in sentencing. *Journal of Research in Crime and Delinquency, 24*(1), 69-92.

Zeldin, S., & Price, L. A. (1995). Creating supportive communities for adolescent development: Challenges to scholars. *Journal of Adolescent Research, 10,* 6-14.

Ziesemer, C., Marcoux, L., & Marwell, B. E. (1994). Homeless children: Are they different from other low-income children? *Social Work, 39,* 658-668.

Index

About the Editor

Larry E. Davis is Professor of Social Work and Psychology in the George Warren Brown School of Social Work at Washington University in St. Louis, Missouri, where he is chairholder of the E. Desmond Lee Professorship to encourage scholarship on and understanding of racial and ethnic diversity. His areas of interest include race, gender, and class dynamics on clinical practice and organizational behavior. Currently, he is conducting research on African American high school students' decisions to stay in school. Prior publications include *Race, Gender, and Class: Guidelines for Practice With Individuals, Families, and Groups; Ethnic Issues in Adolescent Mental Health;* and *Black and Single: Finding and Choosing a Partner Who Is Right for You.*

About the Contributors

Paula Allen-Meares is currently Dean of and Professor in the University of Michigan School of Social Work. Research interests include the tasks and functions of social workers employed in educational settings and the organizational variables that influence service delivery; repeat births among adolescents and young adults, health care utilization, and social integration factors which influence sexual behavior and parenthood; and maternal psychiatric disorders and their direct and indirect effects on parenting skills and developmental outcomes of offspring. In addition, she has published on such topics as conceptual frameworks for social work, research methodologies, and racial/ethnic minority youths. Published books include *Intervention With Children and Adolescents* and *Social Work Services in Schools.* She is Principal Investigator of a Kellogg Foundation Grant on Global Program for Youth and Co-Principal Investigator of the NIMH Center on Poverty, Risk, and Mental Illness. She is currently Editor-in-Chief of the *Journal of Social Work Education.*

Elizabeth Allison is affiliated with the University of Tennessee College of Social Work.

Ron Avi Astor, MSW, PhD, is Assistant Professor of Social Work and Education at the University of Michigan. His research focuses on school violence and children's moral reasoning about violence. His projects have been funded by the Fulbright Foundation, the National Academy of Education/Spencer Foundation, the National Institute of Mental Health, the H. F. Guggenheim Foundation, and the Israeli government. Currently, he is researching how children think about issues of poverty and violence and how culture influences children's understanding of violence.

F. M. Baker, MD, MPH, is Associate Professor of Psychiatry at Maryland School of Medicine in Baltimore. She has written extensively on the clinical treatment of the African American elderly.

Gilbert Botvin, PhD, has been a member of the full-time faculty of Cornell University Medical College since 1980 and currently is Professor in both the Department of Public Health and the Department of Psychiatry. He also is Director of Cornell's Institute for Prevention Research and an Attending Psychologist at New York Hospital–Cornell Medical Center. He is author or coauthor of 147 scientific journal articles and book chapters, and his groundbreaking work has received national and international attention. He was the first prevention researcher to receive the prestigious MERIT award from the National Institute on Drug Abuse and also is the recipient of the Society of Prevention Research's Disque Dean Presidential Award for Prevention Excellence. The SPR has appointed him to be the inaugural editor of its new journal, *Prevention Science.*

Kristin Cole, MS, is Associate Research Scholar at Columbia University School of Social Work and currently involved in a National Cancer Institute study to reduce cancer risks among economically disadvantaged youths in greater New York City. She has contributed papers on services to families of high-risk youths, prevention services to high-risk youths, and methodological issues in conducting prevention research in ethnic-racial communities.

G. David Curry is Associate Professor of Criminology and Criminal Justice at the University of Missouri–St. Louis. He is coauthor with Scott H. Decker of *Confronting Gangs: Crime and Community* as well as other publications. He has been a member of gang advisory boards for the City of Chicago, the Boys and Girls Clubs of America, and the Juvenile Detention and Correctional Association. He has served as a consultant to the St. Louis Police Department, the Safer Foundation, the National Youth Gang Center, the Southern Poverty Law Center, the NAACP, and Legal Services Corporation.

Timothy Davey is Assistant Professor at the University of Tennessee College of Social Work in Nashville. He has served as an evaluator of the HERO Homeless Education program since 1995. His current research focuses on the mental health of homeless families and on evaluations of interventions designed to reduce stress and isolation of homeless children and youths.

Scott H. Decker is Professor of Criminology and Criminal Justice at the University of Missouri–St. Louis. He earned his PhD in criminology from Florida State University in 1976. His primary research areas include the offenders perspective, criminal justice policy, and gangs. His book *Life in the Gang: Family, Friends, and Violence* (1996) won the Academy of Criminal Justice Sciences Award for Outstanding Book in 1998. He is currently engaged in the evaluation of the Safe Futures project in the city of St. Louis.

Garrett Albert Duncan is Assistant Professor of African and Afro-American Studies and Education at Washington University. Formerly a teacher educator in Southern California, he received his PhD in education from Claremont Graduate School in 1994 after an 8-year career as a public school science teacher. He received numerous awards for his teaching and scholarship, including Teacher of the Year from the students of Pomona High School, a Distinguished Alumni Award from Cal Poly Pomona, the Christa McAuliffe Fellowship from the U.S. Department of Education, a National Science Teacher Fellowship from the National Science Foundation, and a Minority Postdoctoral Fellowship in African and Afro-American Studies and Education.

Anderson J. Franklin, PhD, is Professor in the Clinical Psychology and Social Personality Psychology doctoral programs at City University of New York. He is a Fellow in the American Psychological Association's Society for the Study of Ethnic and Minority Issues (Division 45) where he also serves as Associate Editor of their journal *Cultural Diversity and Ethnic Minority Psychology.* He is a psychotherapist in private practice working with African American males in individual, group, marital, and family therapy and for many years has run therapeutic support groups for black males.

Edith M. Freeman is Professor at the University of Kansas School of Social Welfare, where she is also Director of the PhD Program. She teaches at both the MSW and PhD levels. Her research focus is on children and families, substance abuse, and cultural diversity issues especially related to the black family. She has published many books and articles on those topics, including *Substance Abuse Treatment: A Family Systems Approach,* "Empowering

African American Males and Their Non-Parenting Peers," "The Use of Storytelling Techniques With African-American Males: Implications for Substance Abuse Prevention," and *The Black Family: A Culturally Specific Approach.*

Fredericka Hendricks is Assistant Professor of Psychology at Austin Peay State University in Clarksville, Tennessee. Her primary focus is career development.

Leo E. Hendricks, PhD, LICSW, CDE, is Director of LHCA's Diabetes Self-Management Skills Training Center located in Wheaton, Maryland. The Center is recognized by the American Diabetes Association for quality patient education and provides diabetes self-management skills training for persons with Type I, Type II, and gestational diabetes. It is dedicated to helping people accept greater responsibility for their health. As an epidemiolgist, licensed independent clinical social worker, and a certified diabetes educator, he has focused on the areas of diabetes management, treatment, and support groups since 1994. He is an active member of the American Diabetes Association and the American Association of Diabetes Educators.

Harry J. Holzer is Professor of Economics at Michigan State University. He received his PhD from Harvard in 1983. He is also a National Fellow in the Harvard program on poverty and social inequality and an affiliate of the Institute for Research on Poverty at the University of Wisconsin. He has worked extensively on the labor market problems of minority youths and other disadvantaged workers. His books include *The Black Youth Employment Crisis* (with Richard B. Freeman, 1986) and *What Employers Want: Job Prospects for Less-Educated Workers* (1996).

Janice Joseph, PhD, is Professor of the Criminal Justice Program at Richard Stockton College of New Jersey. She received her MA and PhD degrees from York University, Toronto, Canada. Her research interests include violence against women, women and criminal justice, youth violence, juvenile delinquency, gangs, and minorities and criminal justice. Significant publications include a book, *Black Youths, Delinquency, and Juvenile Justice,* several journal articles on delinquency, gangs, and elderly abuse, and chapters on domestic violence.

Anthony E. O. King, PhD, is Assistant Dean for Liberal Arts at Cuyahoga Community College. In addition to his research on social work practice with incarcerated African American males and their families, he has published and presented nationally on violence among African American males and the impact of incarceration on African American males, their families, and their communities. He has extensive experience working with incarcerated men and women and has served as a consultant for numerous state, federal and private nonprofit social service programs and agencies. His present research focuses on African Americans' attitudes toward marriage, male/female relationships, and the impact of rites-of-passage training on adults.

Mark S. Kiselica, PhD, NCC, is Associate Professor in and Chair of the Department of Counseling and Personnel Services at the College of New Jersey. He is a licensed psychologist, a national certified counselor, and president of the Society for the Psychological Study of Men and Masculinity (Division 51 of the American Psychological Association). He is the founder of the American School Counselor Association National Professional Interest Network on Teen Parents, a member of the Teen Pregnancy Task Force of Bucks County, Pennsylvania, and a former member of the board of directors of the Indiana Council on Adolescent Pregnancy. He also serves as a consulting scholar to the Federal Fatherhood Initiative.

Paula Kleinman, PhD, is a research scientist at Columbia University's Joseph L. Mailman School of Public Health. Her research interests focus on substance abuse, research methods, and race/ethnic studies, and she has published more than 30 papers on these subjects.

Courtland C. Lee, PhD, is Professor of Counselor Education at the University of Virginia. He has authored two books on counseling African American males, edited or coedited four books on multicultural counseling, and published numerous articles and book chapters on counseling across cultures. He is past president of the *Association for Multicultural Counseling and Development* and former editor of the *Journal of Multicultural Counseling and Development* and the *Journal of African American Men.*

Don C. Locke is Director of the North Carolina State University doctoral program in adult and community college education at the Asheville Graduate Center. Immediately prior to assuming his present position in July 1993, he was Professor and Head of the Department of Counselor Education at North Carolina State University in Raleigh. He is the recipient of the Professional Development Award from the American Counseling Association (1996), and the Professional Recognition Award from the American Counseling Association

Foundation (1998). He is author or coauthor of more than 60 publications, with a current focus on multicultural issues. His 1992 book, *Increasing Multicultural Understanding*, was a Sage Publications best-seller, and the second edition was released in 1998. The second edition of *Psychological Techniques for Teachers* was published in 1995. His coauthored book, *Culture and Diversity Issues in Counseling*, was published in 1996.

Sadye M. L. Logan, PhD, is Associate Professor of Social Welfare at the University of Kansas. She teaches graduate-level courses on family practice and clinical practice. She has authored and coauthored numerous articles and two books, *The Black Family: Strengths, Self-Help, and Positive Change* and *Social Work Practice With Black Families*.

Ruth G. McRoy, PhD, is Ruby Lee Piester Centennial Professor of Services to Children and Families at the University of Texas at Austin. She holds a joint appointment in African American Studies and is Director of the Center for Social Work Research. She teaches graduate and undergraduate courses on African American families and social work practice with groups. She has numerous publications on such topics as racial identity development, transracial adoptions, and cultural diversity. She is coeditor, with Edith Freeman and Sadye Logan, of *Social Work Practice With Black Families*.

Heather Ann Meyer, EdM, is a doctoral candidate in the combined education and psychology program at the University of Michigan. Her research focuses on how children understand the context of the school as it relates to school violence. Her most recent work explores the ways teachers think about issues of gender and school violence.

Mary Nakashian is Vice President and Director of Program Demonstration at the National Center on Addiction and Substance Abuse (CASA) at Columbia University. Before coming to CASA in 1994, she was Executive Deputy Commissioner of the City of New York Human Resources Administration. She also previously worked for the Connecticut State Department of Income Maintenance. She received her undergraduate degree in international relations and a graduate degree in organizational psychology. She is an adjunct faculty member at the New York University Wagner School of Public Affairs.

William R. Penuel is Research Social Scientist at SRI International. He is author of numerous presentations and articles on the evaluation of education programs for homeless children and youths and in the past served as the

Homeless Education Coordinator for the Metropolitan Nashville Public Schools. His current research focuses on the assessment and evaluation of technology-based projects designed to support teachers, principals, and district administrators in implementing collaborative school reform initiatives targeted to at-risk students.

Robert Pierce, PhD, is Associate Professor of Social Work at George Warren Brown School of Social Work at Washington University in St. Louis, Missouri. His writing and research focuses on African American children in the child welfare system (child protective services); cross-cultural policy and practice issues in child welfare; health issues in African Americans (organ transplants and cancer); and help seeking and functioning among African American males diagnosed with prostate cancer.

Ronald Pitner, MSW, is a doctoral candidate in the joint social psychology and social work PhD program at the University of Michigan. His research focuses on the process of stereotyping and violence. He has also conducted research on the role of culture and interpersonal practice.

Shirley Salmon-Davis is a licensed clinical social worker in private practice in St. Louis, Missouri. A native of Jamaica, she received her MSW degree from Howard University. She specializes in child and family therapy. She is also a certified criminal justice specialist and works with criminal offenders.

Steven Schinke, PhD, is Professor in the School of Social Work at Columbia University, where he teaches research methods to doctoral students. Prior to joining Columbia in 1986, he served on the faculty of the University of Washington School of Social Work in Seattle. His research interests center on prevention training, with a special focus on substance abuse and minority culture adolescents. He has published over 170 articles on preventive interventions and skills training for adolescents and currently is Principal Investigator of research studies to develop and test preventive interventions among high-risk youths. He presently serves as a consulting editor for *Addictive Behaviors, Behavioral Medicine Abstracts, Children and Youth Services Review, Journal of Adolescent Research, Journal of Family Violence, Journal of Social Service Research,* and *Research on Social Work Practice.*

Michael Sherraden is Benjamin E. Youngdahl Professor of Social Development and Director of the Center for Social Development at Washington University in St. Louis. He is author of *Assets and the Poor: A New American*

Welfare Policy (1991), which proposes individual development accounts (IDAs) and matched savings accounts for the poor. He currently directs the evaluation of a 6-year (1997-2003) IDA demonstration at 13 sites around the country, supported by a consortium of 10 foundations. He is coeditor of *Alternatives to Social Security: An International Inquiry* (1997), where he points out that a major challenge in asset-based social security systems is to make them inclusive and progressive.

Bertha Sherrill is a school social worker for the Metropolitan Nashville Public Schools. She helped start the HERO Homeless Education Program in Nashville in 1992, a tutoring and enrichment program for school-age children and youths living in area shelters and has served as the program's social worker since that time.

Christopher Williams, PhD, is Assistant Professor of Psychology at the Institute for Prevention Research at Cornell University Medical College in New York City. His research focuses on the etiology and prevention of substance use among inner-city youths, and he has published articles and book chapters on the socioemotional development and aggression-related behavior of children and adolescents. He has made numerous scientific presentations at national conferences and holds memberships in several professional organizations including the Society for Research and Child Development and the American Psychological Association. He earned his PhD from Northwestern University and completed his postdoctoral training in child and adolescent psychiatry at Columbia University.

James Herbert Williams, PhD, is Assistant Professor of Social Work at George Warren Brown School of Social Work at Washington University in St. Louis. In addition to teaching, he is involved in research and community work. His current areas of research examine African American family structure, risk and protective factors for childhood and adolescent antisocial behaviors, co-morbidity of mental illness and violence in African American adolescents, predictors of transitions in adolescent from nonviolent to violent offending, and barriers and challenges to service utilization in high crime communities. He is on the editorial board of *Journal of Applied Social Sciences.*

Oliver J. Williams, Executive Director of the Institute on Domestic Violence in the African American Community, is Associate Professor in the Graduate School of Social Work at the University of Minnesota in Minneapolis. He is a practitioner as well as an academician. As a practitioner, he has worked in the field of domestic violence for more than 20 years and has provided individual, couples, and family counseling. He has been a child welfare and delinquency worker, worked in battered women's shelters, and developed and conducted counseling on partner abuse treatment programs. As an academician, his research and publications have centered on creating effective service delivery strategies that will reduce violent behavior among African Americans. Additionally, he writes about ethnically sensitive practice as well as aging and elder maltreatment. He has conducted training nationally on research and service delivery issues in the areas of child abuse, partner abuse, and elder maltreatment. He also serves on several national advisory boards focused on the issue of domestic violence.